医学教学图谱

人体局部解剖

Atlas of
Human Regional Anatomy 图谱

主编

陈金宝　刘　强

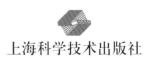

上海科学技术出版社

图书在版编目（CIP）数据

人体局部解剖图谱 / 陈金宝，刘强主编 . —上海：上海科学技术出版社，2016.4
（医学教学图谱）
ISBN 978-7-5478-2745-1

Ⅰ. ①人…　Ⅱ. ①陈…　②刘…　Ⅲ. ①局部解剖学 – 图谱

Ⅳ. ① R323-64

中国版本图书馆 CIP 数据核字（2015）第 170075 号

人体局部解剖图谱

主编　陈金宝　刘　强

上海世纪出版股份有限公司
上海科学技术出版社　　出版
（上海钦州南路 71 号　邮政编码 200235）
上海世纪出版股份有限公司发行中心发行
200001　上海福建中路 193 号　www.ewen.co
浙江新华印刷技术有限公司印刷
开本 787×1092　1/16　印张 17.25
字数：400 千字
2016 年 4 月第 1 版　2016 年 4 月第 1 次印刷
ISBN 978-7-5478-2745-1/R · 962
定价：88.00 元

内容提要

　　本书是为了适应我国高等医学教育改革和发展的需要，根据我国 5 年制和 7 年制高等医学院校学生的培养目标和临床需求而编写的教学图谱。全书采用汉英对照的形式，根据解剖学教学的要求，按照普通高等教育国家级规划教材《局部解剖学》的内容顺序编排，从头部、颈部、胸部、腹部、盆部、背部、上肢和下肢 8 个方面对人体结构进行了逐层解剖，充分显示了浅组织、筋膜、肌肉、骨骼、血管、神经的相互位置关系，同时还采用了断面解剖和临床的一些影像，从不同侧面展示结构关系。

　　本书采取人工绘制和标本拍摄相结合的方式，人工绘制的图像色泽艳丽、结构清晰、边界明确、形态典型；标本拍摄的图像更直观、更真实、更实用。两者结合使用相互补充、相互对照，可为医学生、临床医生及解剖工作者更好地了解和掌握正常人体结构提供参考与指导。

编委名单

主　编
陈金宝　刘　强

副主编
段坤昌　齐亚力　周艳芬
季雪芳　陆　宇

编　委
（按姓氏笔画排序）
刘　强　齐亚力　李　亮　杨　雄　陈金宝
季雪芳　周艳芬　段坤昌　傅　强

主编简介

陈金宝

1944 年生，山东单县人，1963 年考入中国医科大学医疗系学习，1969 年毕业。1994 年晋升为教授，2000 年获得国务院特殊津贴。一直在中国医科大学从事医学图像制作和医学图像处理的研究及资源库建设等工作。

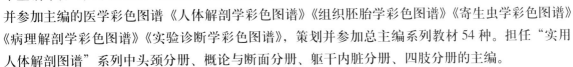

发表论文及出版

在国家级杂志发表的论文、编写出版的教材及专著共 140 余篇（部）。其中主编专著《医学摄影》，副主编《断面解剖与 MRI CT ECT 对照图谱》，策划并参加主编的医学彩色图谱《人体解剖学彩色图谱》《组织胚胎学彩色图谱》《寄生虫学彩色图谱》《病理解剖学彩色图谱》《实验诊断学彩色图谱》，策划并参加总主编系列教材 54 种。担任"实用人体解剖图谱"系列中头颈分册、概论与断面分册、躯干内脏分册、四肢分册的主编。

承担课题

国家"九五"重点攻关课题"人体解剖学课件""组织胚胎学课件"2 项，国家新世纪网络建设工程课题"人体解剖学网络课程""组织胚胎学网络课程"2 项，教育部重大研究课题子课题 1 项，"药理学"国家级优秀网络课程 1 项，辽宁省科委课题 1 项，辽宁省教育厅课题 1 项。

获得奖励

卫生部奖 6 项，教育部奖 1 项，美国医学电教学会（HESCA）奖 1 项。

辽宁省科技进步一等奖"现代医学教育资源库"1 项，辽宁省优秀教学成果一等奖 1 项，辽宁省优秀教学成果二等奖 2 项，辽宁省优秀教学成果三等奖 1 项，辽宁省优秀课件一等奖 1 项，沈阳市科技进步三等奖 1 项。

曾任职务

中国医科大学教育技术中心主任，网络教育学院常务副院长。卫生部继续医学教育和乡村医生教育的视听教育专家，中华医学会教育技术分会委员、常务委员、副主任委员、主任委员、名誉主任委员，教育部高等医药院校现代教育技术与计算机教学指导委员会委员，中国电化教育协会理事、医学委员会主任委员，辽宁省高等院校电化教育研究会副理事长等职。

主编简介

刘　强

1975 年生，辽宁省丹东市人，1994 年考入中国医科大学日语临床医学专业学习，2000 年毕业，硕士学位。一直从事医学教育管理、教育技术研究、教学资源库建设等工作。

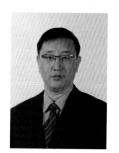

担任职务

中国医科大学网络教育学院院长，教育技术中心主任；中华医学会教育技术分会第七届委员会委员，虚拟仿真应用研究专业学组副组长；辽宁省医学会医学教育学分会第五届委员会教育技术与应用学组委员。

获得奖励

制作的《药理学》《护理学基础》课程获得国家级精品资源共享课程（网络教育），制作的《生活方式与健康》课程获得国家级精品视频公开课程，制作十余门辽宁省精品视频公开课和精品资源共享课等。

编写教材及专著

参与编写"成人高等教育基础医学教材""成人高等教育护理学专用教材""成人高等教育药学专用教材"，由上海科学技术出版社出版。担任"实用人体解剖图谱"系列中头颈分册、概论与断面分册、躯干内脏分册、四肢分册的副主编。

承担课题

2008 年教育部课题：继续教育改革和发展战略与政策研究行业继续教育子课题"乡村医生继续教育现状改革和发展研究"；2011 年辽宁省课题：中国医科大学临床医学本科综合改革试点专业建设立项子课题"优质教学资源建设与共享项目"。

前　言

　　局部解剖学是在系统解剖学研究人体器官、系统和功能的基础上，按照人体的部位（头部、颈部、胸部、腹部、盆部、背部、上肢和下肢），由浅入深对各部结构的形态、位置及相互关系等进行描述的学科。

　　局部解剖学是一门形态学科，虽然国内已经出版了一些局部解剖学教材和参考书，但由于插图多为黑白色，且数量不够，不能完全满足学习者的需求。本书是为了适应我国高等医学教育改革和发展的需要，根据我国5年制和7年制高等医学院校学生的培养目标和临床需求而编写的。全书分头部、颈部、胸部、腹部、盆部与会阴、脊柱区、上肢和下肢共8章。在内容方面除了借鉴国内外同类图谱的优点外，力求做到科学性、先进性和适用性的统一。本图谱注重局部解剖学的科学性、临床科学的实用性，把局部解剖学和临床应用相结合。

　　本图谱按照内容的需要，进行逐层解剖，充分显示浅组织、筋膜、肌肉、骨骼、血管、神经的相互位置关系。此外，还采用了断面解剖和临床的一些影像，从不同侧面展示结构关系。在表现形式上，我们采取人工绘制和标本拍摄相结合的方法。人工绘制的图像色泽艳丽、结构清晰、边界明确、形态典型。标本拍摄的图像更直观、更真实、更实用。两者结合使用相互补充、相互对照，为医学生掌握正常人体结构提供方便。

　　在图谱的编绘过程中，参阅了大量国内外出版的解剖学图谱和专著。在此，对出版社和其他编者表示衷心的感谢。

　　由于作者的水平限制，本图谱难免存在不当或错误，敬请学界专家和读者给予批评指正。

陈金宝

2015 年 12 月

目　录

第五章
盆部与会阴

第八章 下肢

第一节

表面解剖

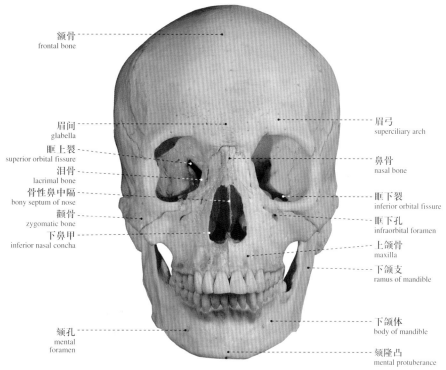

图 1　颅（前面观）
Skull (anterior aspect)

額骨
frontal bone

眉间
glabella

眶上裂
superior orbital fissure

泪骨
lacrimal bone

骨性鼻中隔
bony septum of nose

颧骨
zygomatic bone

下鼻甲
inferior nasal concha

颏孔
mental foramen

眉弓
superciliary arch

鼻骨
nasal bone

眶下裂
inferior orbital fissure

眶下孔
infraorbital foramen

上颌骨
maxilla

下颌支
ramus of mandible

下颌体
body of mandible

颏隆凸
mental protuberance

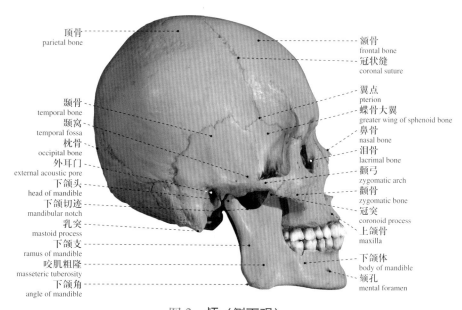

图 2　颅（侧面观）
Skull (lateral aspect)

顶骨
parietal bone

颞骨
temporal bone

颞窝
temporal fossa

枕骨
occipital bone

外耳门
external acoustic pore

下颌头
head of mandible

下颌切迹
mandibular notch

乳突
mastoid process

下颌支
ramus of mandible

咬肌粗隆
masseteric tuberosity

下颌角
angle of mandible

额骨
frontal bone

冠状缝
coronal suture

翼点
pterion

蝶骨大翼
greater wing of sphenoid bone

鼻骨
nasal bone

泪骨
lacrimal bone

颧弓
zygomatic arch

颧骨
zygomatic bone

冠突
coronoid process

上颌骨
maxilla

下颌体
body of mandible

颏孔
mental foramen

面 部

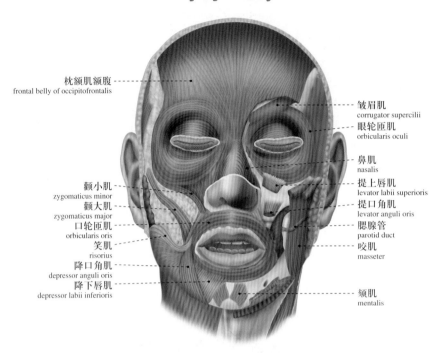

枕额肌额腹
frontal belly of occipitofrontalis

皱眉肌
corrugator supercilii

眼轮匝肌
orbicularis oculi

鼻肌
nasalis

提上唇肌
levator labii superioris

提口角肌
levator anguli oris

腮腺管
parotid duct

咬肌
masseter

颏肌
mentalis

颧小肌
zygomaticus minor

颧大肌
zygomaticus major

口轮匝肌
orbicularis oris

笑肌
risorius

降口角肌
depressor anguli oris

降下唇肌
depressor labii inferioris

图 3　面部肌肉（前面观）
Facial muscles（anterior aspect）

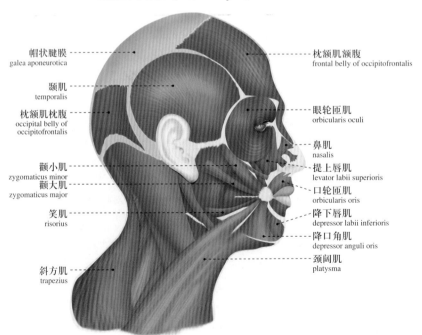

帽状腱膜
galea aponeurotica

颞肌
temporalis

枕额肌枕腹
occipital belly of occipitofrontalis

颧小肌
zygomaticus minor

颧大肌
zygomaticus major

笑肌
risorius

斜方肌
trapezius

枕额肌额腹
frontal belly of occipitofrontalis

眼轮匝肌
orbicularis oculi

鼻肌
nasalis

提上唇肌
levator labii superioris

口轮匝肌
orbicularis oris

降下唇肌
depressor labii inferioris

降口角肌
depressor anguli oris

颈阔肌
platysma

图 4　面部肌肉（侧面观）
Facial muscles（lateral aspect）

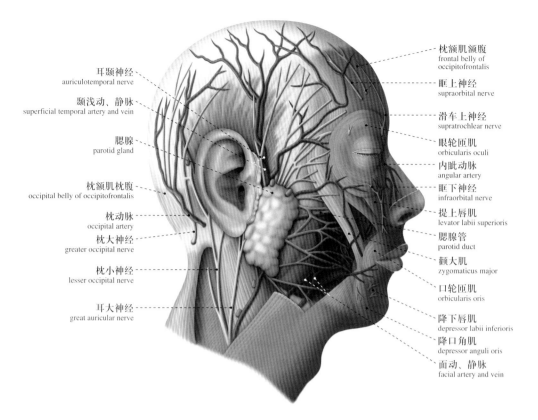

耳颞神经
auriculotemporal nerve

颞浅动、静脉
superficial temporal artery and vein

腮腺
parotid gland

枕额肌枕腹
occipital belly of occipitofrontalis

枕动脉
occipital artery

枕大神经
greater occipital nerve

枕小神经
lesser occipital nerve

耳大神经
great auricular nerve

枕额肌额腹
frontal belly of occipitofrontalis

眶上神经
supraorbital nerve

滑车上神经
supratrochlear nerve

眼轮匝肌
orbicularis oculi

内眦动脉
angular artery

眶下神经
infraorbital nerve

提上唇肌
levator labii superioris

腮腺管
parotid duct

颧大肌
zygomaticus major

口轮匝肌
orbicularis oris

降下唇肌
depressor labii inferioris

降口角肌
depressor anguli oris

面动、静脉
facial artery and vein

图 5　面部浅层结构
Facial superficial structure

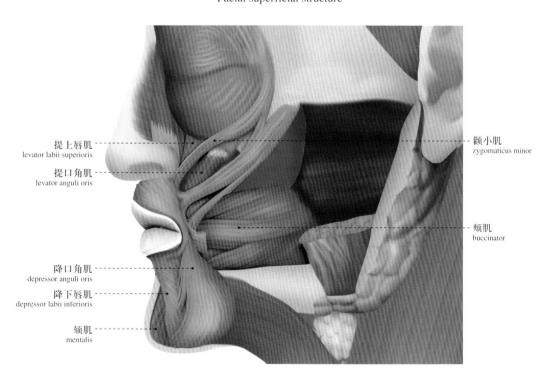

提上唇肌
levator labii superioris

提口角肌
levator anguli oris

降口角肌
depressor anguli oris

降下唇肌
depressor labii inferioris

颏肌
mentalis

颧小肌
zygomaticus minor

颊肌
buccinator

图 6　口部肌肉浅层（侧面观）
Superficial layer of the mouth muscles (lateral aspect)

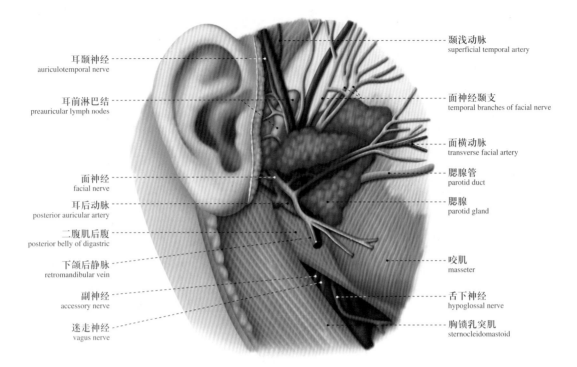

颞浅动脉
superficial temporal artery

耳颞神经
auriculotemporal nerve

面神经颞支
temporal branches of facial nerve

耳前淋巴结
preauricular lymph nodes

面横动脉
transverse facial artery

腮腺管
parotid duct

面神经
facial nerve

腮腺
parotid gland

耳后动脉
posterior auricular artery

二腹肌后腹
posterior belly of digastric

下颌后静脉
retromandibular vein

咬肌
masseter

副神经
accessory nerve

舌下神经
hypoglossal nerve

迷走神经
vagus nerve

胸锁乳突肌
sternocleidomastoid

图 7　腮腺及穿经腮腺的结构

Parotid gland and structure passes through the parotid gland

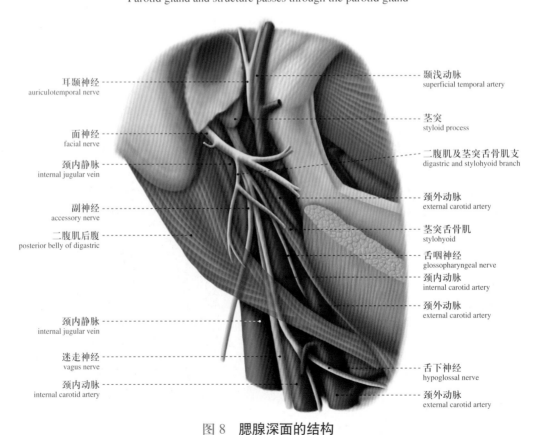

耳颞神经
auriculotemporal nerve

颞浅动脉
superficial temporal artery

茎突
styloid process

面神经
facial nerve

二腹肌及茎突舌骨肌支
digastric and stylohyoid branch

颈内静脉
internal jugular vein

颈外动脉
external carotid artery

副神经
accessory nerve

茎突舌骨肌
stylohyoid

二腹肌后腹
posterior belly of digastric

舌咽神经
glossopharyngeal nerve

颈内动脉
internal carotid artery

颈内静脉
internal jugular vein

颈外动脉
external carotid artery

迷走神经
vagus nerve

舌下神经
hypoglossal nerve

颈内动脉
internal carotid artery

颈外动脉
external carotid artery

图 8　腮腺深面的结构

Structure of the deep surface of the parotid gland

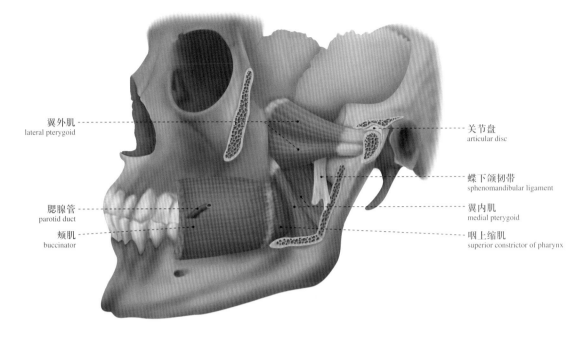

翼外肌
lateral pterygoid

腮腺管
parotid duct

颊肌
buccinator

关节盘
articular disc

蝶下颌韧带
sphenomandibular ligament

翼内肌
medial pterygoid

咽上缩肌
superior constrictor of pharynx

图 9　咀嚼肌
Masticatory muscles

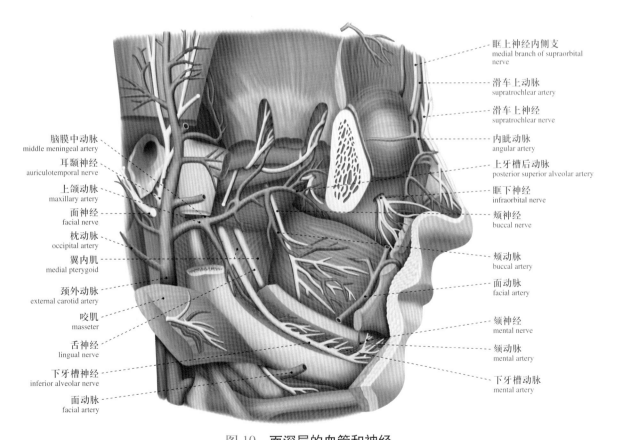

脑膜中动脉
middle meningeal artery

耳颞神经
auriculotemporal nerve

上颌动脉
maxillary artery

面神经
facial nerve

枕动脉
occipital artery

翼内肌
medial pterygoid

颈外动脉
external carotid artery

咬肌
masseter

舌神经
lingual nerve

下牙槽神经
inferior alveolar nerve

面动脉
facial artery

眶上神经内侧支
medial branch of supraorbital nerve

滑车上动脉
supratrochlear artery

滑车上神经
supratrochlear nerve

内眦动脉
angular artery

上牙槽后动脉
posterior superior alveolar artery

眶下神经
infraorbital nerve

颊神经
buccal nerve

颊动脉
buccal artery

面动脉
facial artery

颏神经
mental nerve

颏动脉
mental artery

下牙槽动脉
mental artery

图 10　面深层的血管和神经
Blood vessels and nerves of the deep layer

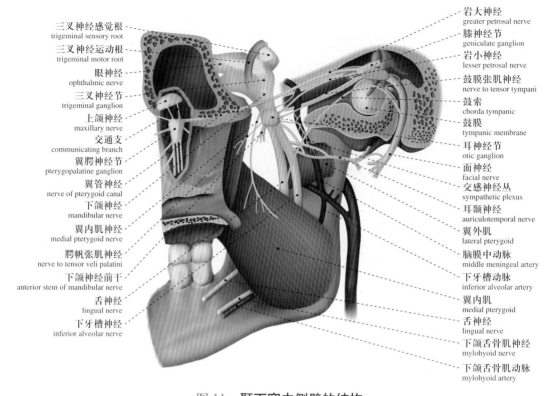

三叉神经感觉根
trigeminal sensory root

三叉神经运动根
trigeminal motor root

眼神经
ophthalmic nerve

三叉神经节
trigeminal ganglion

上颌神经
maxillary nerve

交通支
communicating branch

翼腭神经节
pterygopalatine ganglion

翼管神经
nerve of pterygoid canal

下颌神经
mandibular nerve

翼内肌神经
medial pterygoid nerve

腭帆张肌神经
nerve to tensor veli palatini

下颌神经前干
anterior stem of mandibular nerve

舌神经
lingual nerve

下牙槽神经
inferior alveolar nerve

岩大神经
greater petrosal nerve

膝神经节
geniculate ganglion

岩小神经
lesser petrosal nerve

鼓膜张肌神经
nerve to tensor tympani

鼓索
chorda tympanic

鼓膜
tympanic membrane

耳神经节
otic ganglion

面神经
facial nerve

交感神经丛
sympathetic plexus

耳颞神经
auriculotemporal nerve

翼外肌
lateral pterygoid

脑膜中动脉
middle meningeal artery

下牙槽动脉
inferior alveolar artery

翼内肌
medial pterygoid

舌神经
lingual nerve

下颌舌骨肌神经
mylohyoid nerve

下颌舌骨肌动脉
mylohyoid artery

图 11　颞下窝内侧壁的结构
Structure of the medial wall of the infratemporal fossa

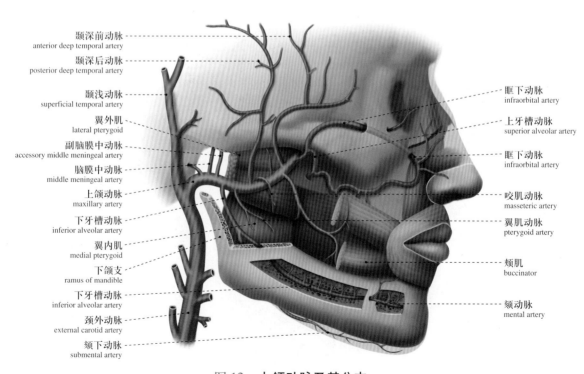

颞深前动脉
anterior deep temporal artery

颞深后动脉
posterior deep temporal artery

颞浅动脉
superficial temporal artery

翼外肌
lateral pterygoid

副脑膜中动脉
accessory middle meningeal artery

脑膜中动脉
middle meningeal artery

上颌动脉
maxillary artery

下牙槽动脉
inferior alveolar artery

翼内肌
medial pterygoid

下颌支
ramus of mandible

下牙槽动脉
inferior alveolar artery

颈外动脉
external carotid artery

颏下动脉
submental artery

眶下动脉
infraorbital artery

上牙槽动脉
superior alveolar artery

眶下动脉
infraorbital artery

咬肌动脉
masseteric artery

翼肌动脉
pterygoid artery

颊肌
buccinator

颏动脉
mental artery

图 12　上颌动脉及其分支
Maxillary artery and its branches

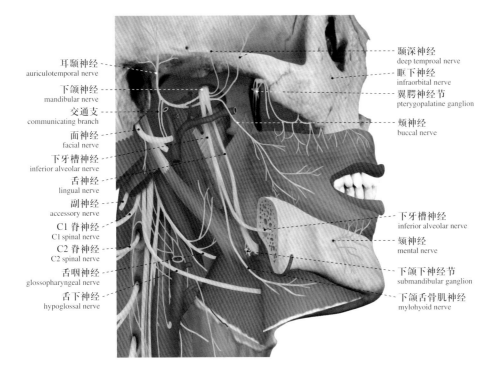

耳颞神经
auriculotemporal nerve

下颌神经
mandibular nerve

交通支
communicating branch

面神经
facial nerve

下牙槽神经
inferior alveolar nerve

舌神经
lingual nerve

副神经
accessory nerve

C1 脊神经
C1 spinal nerve

C2 脊神经
C2 spinal nerve

舌咽神经
glossopharyngeal nerve

舌下神经
hypoglossal nerve

颞深神经
deep temproal nerve

眶下神经
infraorbital nerve

翼腭神经节
pterygopalatine ganglion

颊神经
buccal nerve

下牙槽神经
inferior alveolar nerve

颏神经
mental nerve

下颌下神经节
submandibular ganglion

下颌舌骨肌神经
mylohyoid nerve

图 13　头颈部运动神经支配
Motor innervation of the head and neck

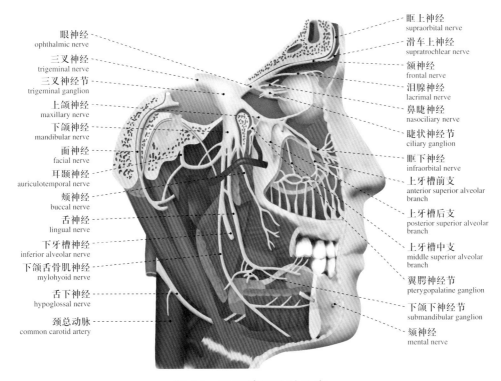

眼神经
ophthalmic nerve

三叉神经
trigeminal nerve

三叉神经节
trigeminal ganglion

上颌神经
maxillary nerve

下颌神经
mandibular nerve

面神经
facial nerve

耳颞神经
auriculotemporal nerve

颊神经
buccal nerve

舌神经
lingual nerve

下牙槽神经
inferior alveolar nerve

下颌舌骨肌神经
mylohyoid nerve

舌下神经
hypoglossal nerve

颈总动脉
common carotid artery

眶上神经
supraorbital nerve

滑车上神经
supratrochlear nerve

额神经
frontal nerve

泪腺神经
lacrimal nerve

鼻睫神经
nasociliary nerve

睫状神经节
ciliary ganglion

眶下神经
infraorbital nerve

上牙槽前支
anterior superior alveolar branch

上牙槽后支
posterior superior alveolar branch

上牙槽中支
middle superior alveolar branch

翼腭神经节
pterygopalatine ganglion

下颌下神经节
submandibular ganglion

颏神经
mental nerve

图 14　三叉神经及其分支
Trigeminal nerve and its branches

颅 部

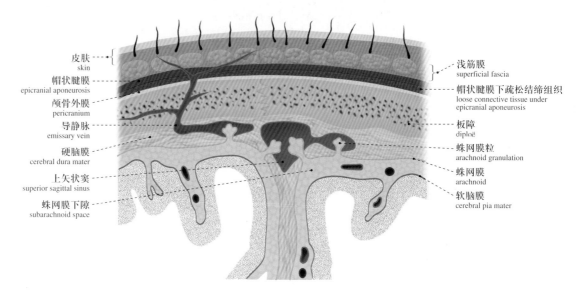

皮肤
skin

帽状腱膜
epicranial aponeurosis

颅骨外膜
pericranium

导静脉
emissary vein

硬脑膜
cerebral dura mater

上矢状窦
superior sagittal sinus

蛛网膜下隙
subarachnoid space

浅筋膜
superficial fascia

帽状腱膜下疏松结缔组织
loose connective tissue under
epicranial aponeurosis

板障
diploë

蛛网膜粒
arachnoid granulation

蛛网膜
arachnoid

软脑膜
cerebral pia mater

图 15　颅顶结构（冠状面观）
Parietal structure (coronal aspect)

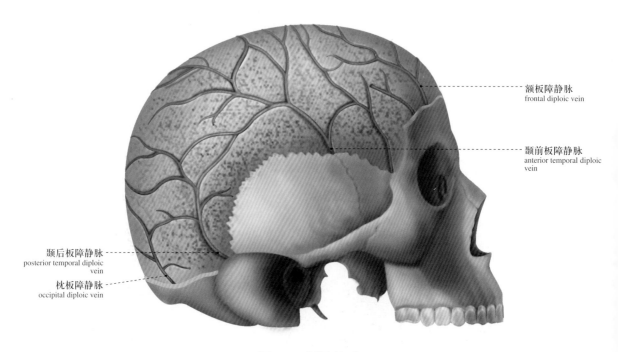

额板障静脉
frontal diploic vein

颞前板障静脉
anterior temporal diploic
vein

颞后板障静脉
posterior temporal diploic
vein

枕板障静脉
occipital diploic vein

图 16　板障静脉
Diploic veins

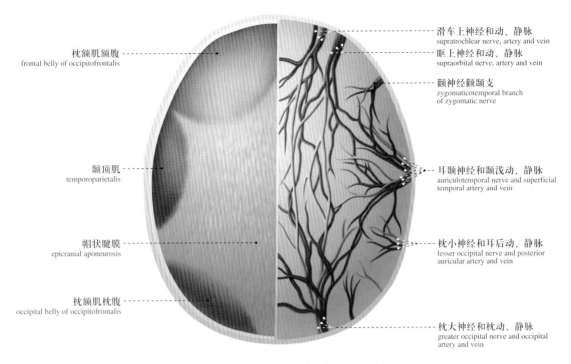

滑车上神经和动、静脉
supratrochlear nerve, artery and vein

眶上神经和动、静脉
supraorbital nerve, artery and vein

颧神经颧颞支
zygomaticotemporal branch
of zygomatic nerve

耳颞神经和颞浅动、静脉
auriculotemporal nerve and superficial
temporal artery and vein

枕小神经和耳后动、静脉
lesser occipital nerve and posterior
auricular artery and vein

枕大神经和枕动、静脉
greater occipital nerve and occipital
artery and vein

枕额肌额腹
frontal belly of occipitofrontalis

颞顶肌
temporoparietalis

帽状腱膜
epicranial aponeurosis

枕额肌枕腹
occipital belly of occipitofrontalis

图 17　枕额肌及颅顶部的血管和神经
Occipitofrontalis and parietal blood vessels and nerves

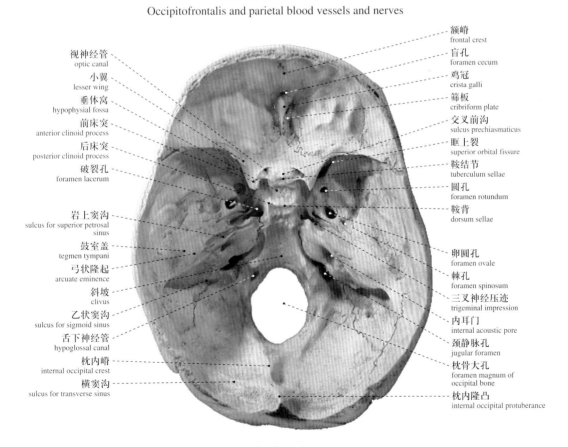

视神经管
optic canal

小翼
lesser wing

垂体窝
hypophysial fossa

前床突
anterior clinoid process

后床突
posterior clinoid process

破裂孔
foramen lacerum

岩上窦沟
sulcus for superior petrosal
sinus

鼓室盖
tegmen tympani

弓状隆起
arcuate eminence

斜坡
clivus

乙状窦沟
sulcus for sigmoid sinus

舌下神经管
hypoglossal canal

枕内嵴
internal occipital crest

横窦沟
sulcus for transverse sinus

额嵴
frontal crest

盲孔
foramen cecum

鸡冠
crista galli

筛板
cribriform plate

交叉前沟
sulcus prechiasmaticus

眶上裂
superior orbital fissure

鞍结节
tuberculum sellae

圆孔
foramen rotundum

鞍背
dorsum sellae

卵圆孔
foramen ovale

棘孔
foramen spinosum

三叉神经压迹
trigeminal impression

内耳门
internal acoustic pore

颈静脉孔
jugular foramen

枕骨大孔
foramen magnum of
occipital bone

枕内隆凸
internal occipital protuberance

图 18　颅底（内面观）
Base of the skull (internal aspect)

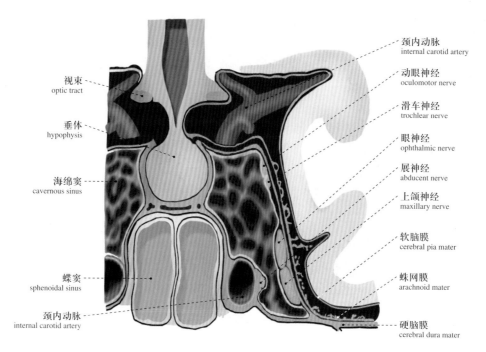

视束
optic tract

垂体
hypophysis

海绵窦
cavernous sinus

蝶窦
sphenoidal sinus

颈内动脉
internal carotid artery

颈内动脉
internal carotid artery

动眼神经
oculomotor nerve

滑车神经
trochlear nerve

眼神经
ophthalmic nerve

展神经
abducent nerve

上颌神经
maxillary nerve

软脑膜
cerebral pia mater

蛛网膜
arachnoid mater

硬脑膜
cerebral dura mater

图 19　海绵窦
Cavernous sinus

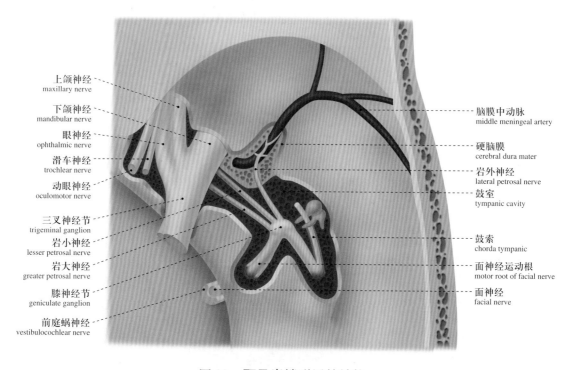

上颌神经
maxillary nerve

下颌神经
mandibular nerve

眼神经
ophthalmic nerve

滑车神经
trochlear nerve

动眼神经
oculomotor nerve

三叉神经节
trigeminal ganglion

岩小神经
lesser petrosal nerve

岩大神经
greater petrosal nerve

膝神经节
geniculate ganglion

前庭蜗神经
vestibulocochlear nerve

脑膜中动脉
middle meningeal artery

硬脑膜
cerebral dura mater

岩外神经
lateral petrosal nerve

鼓室
tympanic cavity

鼓索
chorda tympanic

面神经运动根
motor root of facial nerve

面神经
facial nerve

图 20　颞骨岩嵴附近的结构
Structure near the petrous crest

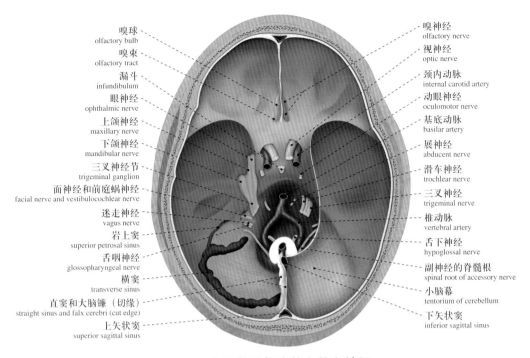

图 21　小脑幕及颅底的血管和神经
Tentorium of cerebellum and blood vessels and nerves of skull base

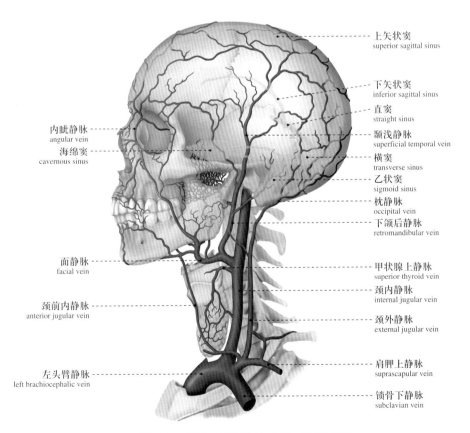

图 22　颅内外静脉的交通（侧面观）
Intracranial and extracranial venous traffic (lateral aspect)

第四节

头部断层解剖

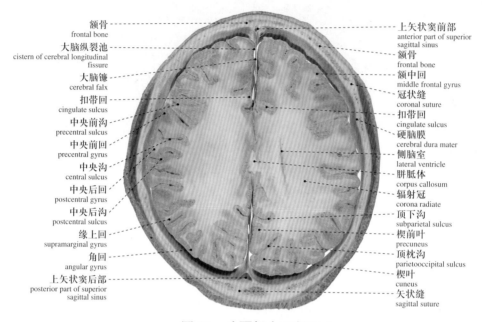

额骨
frontal bone

大脑纵裂池
cistern of cerebral longitudinal fissure

大脑镰
cerebral falx

扣带回
cingulate sulcus

中央前沟
precentral sulcus

中央前回
precentral gyrus

中央沟
central sulcus

中央后回
postcentral gyrus

中央后沟
postcentral sulcus

缘上回
supramarginal gyrus

角回
angular gyrus

上矢状窦后部
posterior part of superior sagittal sinus

上矢状窦前部
anterior part of superior sagittal sinus

额骨
frontal bone

额中回
middle frontal gyrus

冠状缝
coronal suture

扣带回
cingulate sulcus

硬脑膜
cerebral dura mater

侧脑室
lateral ventricle

胼胝体
corpus callosum

辐射冠
corona radiate

顶下沟
subparietal sulcus

楔前叶
precuneus

顶枕沟
parietooccipital sulcus

楔叶
cuneus

矢状缝
sagittal suture

图 23　头颈部水平断面 1
Horizontal section of the head and neck 1

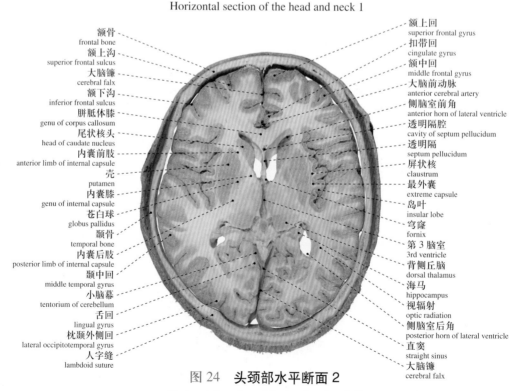

额骨
frontal bone

额上沟
superior frontal sulcus

大脑镰
cerebral falx

额下沟
inferior frontal sulcus

胼胝体膝
genu of corpus callosum

尾状核头
head of caudate nucleus

内囊前肢
anterior limb of internal capsule

壳
putamen

内囊膝
genu of internal capsule

苍白球
globus pallidus

颞骨
temporal bone

内囊后肢
posterior limb of internal capsule

颞中回
middle temporal gyrus

小脑幕
tentorium of cerebellum

舌回
lingual gyrus

枕颞外侧回
lateral occipitotemporal gyrus

人字缝
lambdoid suture

额上回
superior frontal gyrus

扣带回
cingulate gyrus

额中回
middle frontal gyrus

大脑前动脉
anterior cerebral artery

侧脑室前角
anterior horn of lateral ventricle

透明隔腔
cavity of septum pellucidum

透明隔
septum pellucidum

屏状核
claustrum

最外囊
extreme capsule

岛叶
insular lobe

穹窿
fornix

第 3 脑室
3rd ventricle

背侧丘脑
dorsal thalamus

海马
hippocampus

视辐射
optic radiation

侧脑室后角
posterior horn of lateral ventricle

直窦
straight sinus

大脑镰
cerebral falx

图 24　头颈部水平断面 2
Horizontal section of the head and neck 2

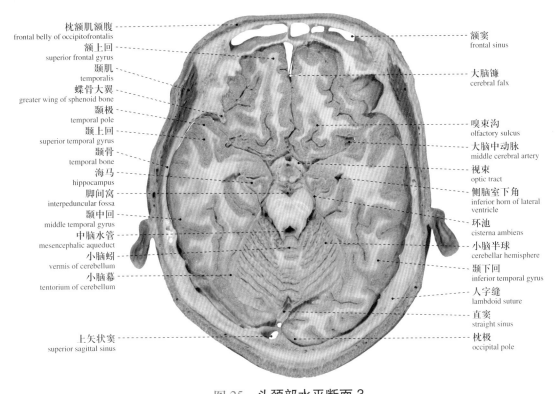

枕额肌额腹
frontal belly of occipitofrontalis

额上回
superior frontal gyrus

颞肌
temporalis

蝶骨大翼
greater wing of sphenoid bone

颞极
temporal pole

颞上回
superior temporal gyrus

颞骨
temporal bone

海马
hippocampus

脚间窝
interpeduncular fossa

颞中回
middle temporal gyrus

中脑水管
mesencephalic aqueduct

小脑蚓
vermis of cerebellum

小脑幕
tentorium of cerebellum

上矢状窦
superior sagittal sinus

额窦
frontal sinus

大脑镰
cerebral falx

嗅束沟
olfactory sulcus

大脑中动脉
middle cerebral artery

视束
optic tract

侧脑室下角
inferior horn of lateral ventricle

环池
cisterna ambiens

小脑半球
cerebellar hemisphere

颞下回
inferior temporal gyrus

人字缝
lambdoid suture

直窦
straight sinus

枕极
occipital pole

图 25 头颈部水平断面 3
Horizontal section of the head and neck 3

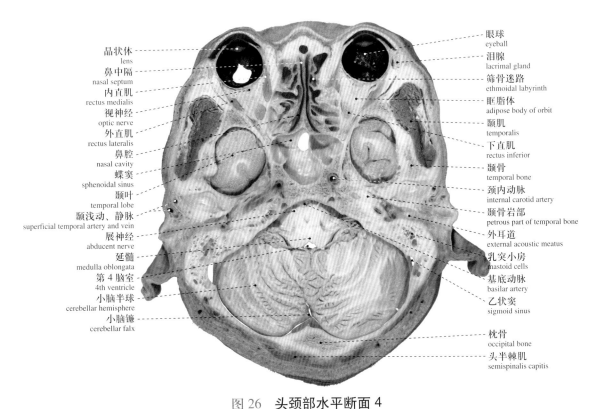

晶状体
lens

鼻中隔
nasal septum

内直肌
rectus medialis

视神经
optic nerve

外直肌
rectus lateralis

鼻腔
nasal cavity

蝶窦
sphenoidal sinus

颞叶
temporal lobe

颞浅动、静脉
superficial temporal artery and vein

展神经
abducent nerve

延髓
medulla oblongata

第 4 脑室
4th ventricle

小脑半球
cerebellar hemisphere

小脑镰
cerebellar falx

眼球
eyeball

泪腺
lacrimal gland

筛骨迷路
ethmoidal labyrinth

眶脂体
adipose body of orbit

颞肌
temporalis

下直肌
rectus inferior

颞骨
temporal bone

颈内动脉
internal carotid artery

颞骨岩部
petrous part of temporal bone

外耳道
external acoustic meatus

乳突小房
mastoid cells

基底动脉
basilar artery

乙状窦
sigmoid sinus

枕骨
occipital bone

头半棘肌
semispinalis capitis

图 26 头颈部水平断面 4
Horizontal section of the head and neck 4

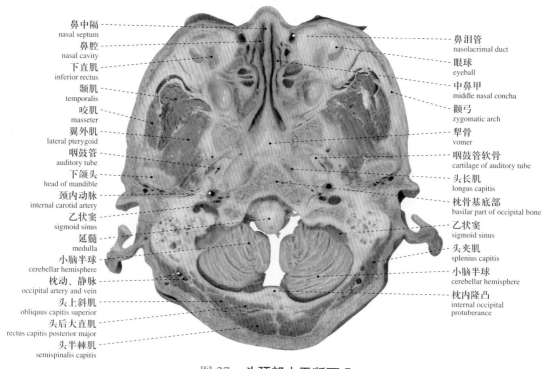

鼻中隔
nasal septum

鼻腔
nasal cavity

下直肌
inferior rectus

颞肌
temporalis

咬肌
masseter

翼外肌
lateral pterygoid

咽鼓管
auditory tube

下颌头
head of mandible

颈内动脉
internal carotid artery

乙状窦
sigmoid sinus

延髓
medulla

小脑半球
cerebellar hemisphere

枕动、静脉
occipital artery and vein

头上斜肌
obliquus capitis superior

头后大直肌
rectus capitis posterior major

头半棘肌
semispinalis capitis

鼻泪管
nasolacrimal duct

眼球
eyeball

中鼻甲
middle nasal concha

颧弓
zygomatic arch

犁骨
vomer

咽鼓管软骨
cartilage of auditory tube

头长肌
longus capitis

枕骨基底部
basilar part of occipital bone

乙状窦
sigmoid sinus

头夹肌
splenius capitis

小脑半球
cerebellar hemisphere

枕内隆凸
internal occipital protuberance

图 27　头颈部水平断面 5

Horizontal section of the head and neck 5

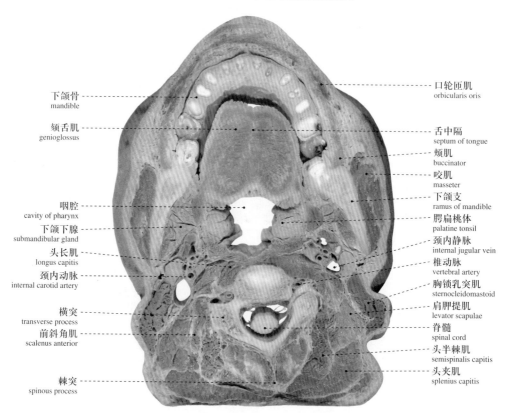

下颌骨
mandible

颏舌肌
genioglossus

咽腔
cavity of pharynx

下颌下腺
submandibular gland

头长肌
longus capitis

颈内动脉
internal carotid artery

横突
transverse process

前斜角肌
scalenus anterior

棘突
spinous process

口轮匝肌
orbicularis oris

舌中隔
septum of tongue

颊肌
buccinator

咬肌
masseter

下颌支
ramus of mandible

腭扁桃体
palatine tonsil

颈内静脉
internal jugular vein

椎动脉
vertebral artery

胸锁乳突肌
sternocleidomastoid

肩胛提肌
levator scapulae

脊髓
spinal cord

头半棘肌
semispinalis capitis

头夹肌
splenius capitis

图 28　头颈部水平断面 6

Horizontal section of the head and neck 6

第一节

颈部分区与体表投影

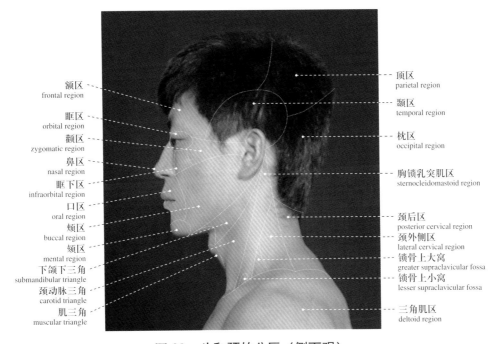

额区
frontal region

眶区
orbital region

颧区
zygomatic region

鼻区
nasal region

眶下区
infraorbital region

口区
oral region

颊区
buccal region

颏区
mental region

下颌下三角
submandibular triangle

颈动脉三角
carotid triangle

肌三角
muscular triangle

顶区
parietal region

颞区
temporal region

枕区
occipital region

胸锁乳突肌区
sternocleidomastoid region

颈后区
posterior cervical region

颈外侧区
lateral cervical region

锁骨上大窝
greater supraclavicular fossa

锁骨上小窝
lesser supraclavicular fossa

三角肌区
deltoid region

图 29　头和颈的分区（侧面观）
Regions of the head and neck (lateral aspect)

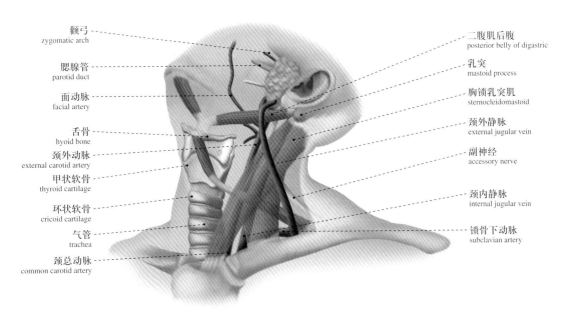

颧弓
zygomatic arch

腮腺管
parotid duct

面动脉
facial artery

舌骨
hyoid bone

颈外动脉
external carotid artery

甲状软骨
thyroid cartilage

环状软骨
cricoid cartilage

气管
trachea

颈总动脉
common carotid artery

二腹肌后腹
posterior belly of digastric

乳突
mastoid process

胸锁乳突肌
sternocleidomastoid

颈外静脉
external jugular vein

副神经
accessory nerve

颈内静脉
internal jugular vein

锁骨下动脉
subclavian artery

图 30　颈部有关器官的体表投影
Surface projection of the relevant organs of the neck

第二节

颈部层次结构

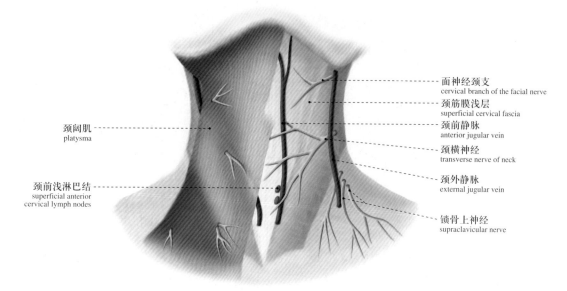

颈阔肌
platysma

颈前浅淋巴结
superficial anterior
cervical lymph nodes

面神经颈支
cervical branch of the facial nerve

颈筋膜浅层
superficial cervical fascia

颈前静脉
anterior jugular vein

颈横神经
transverse nerve of neck

颈外静脉
external jugular vein

锁骨上神经
supraclavicular nerve

图 31　颈阔肌及颈部浅层结构
Platysma and superficial structure of the neck

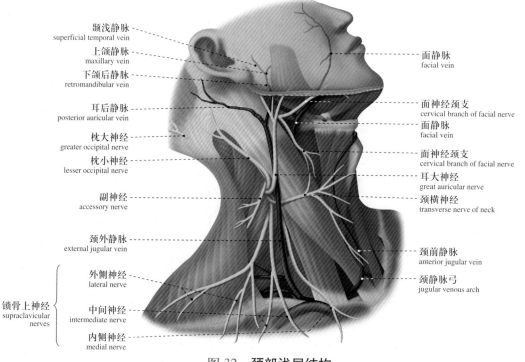

颞浅静脉
superficial temporal vein

上颌静脉
maxillary vein

下颌后静脉
retromandibular vein

耳后静脉
posterior auricular vein

枕大神经
greater occipital nerve

枕小神经
lesser occipital nerve

副神经
accessory nerve

颈外静脉
external jugular vein

锁骨上神经
supraclavicular
nerves

外侧神经
lateral nerve

中间神经
intermediate nerve

内侧神经
medial nerve

面静脉
facial vein

面神经颈支
cervical branch of facial nerve

面静脉
facial vein

面神经颈支
cervical branch of facial nerve

耳大神经
great auricular nerve

颈横神经
transverse nerve of neck

颈前静脉
anterior jugular vein

颈静脉弓
jugular venous arch

图 32　颈部浅层结构
Superficial structure of the neck

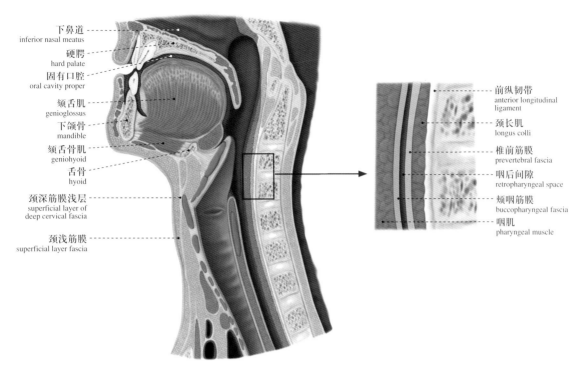

下鼻道
inferior nasal meatus

硬腭
hard palate

固有口腔
oral cavity proper

颏舌肌
genioglossus

下颌骨
mandible

颏舌骨肌
geniohyoid

舌骨
hyoid

颈深筋膜浅层
superficial layer of
deep cervical fascia

颈浅筋膜
superficial layer fascia

前纵韧带
anterior longitudinal
ligament

颈长肌
longus colli

椎前筋膜
prevertebral fascia

咽后间隙
retropharyngeal space

颊咽筋膜
buccopharyngeal fascia

咽肌
pharyngeal muscle

图 33　颈筋膜（正中矢状面）
Cervical fascia (median sagittal section)

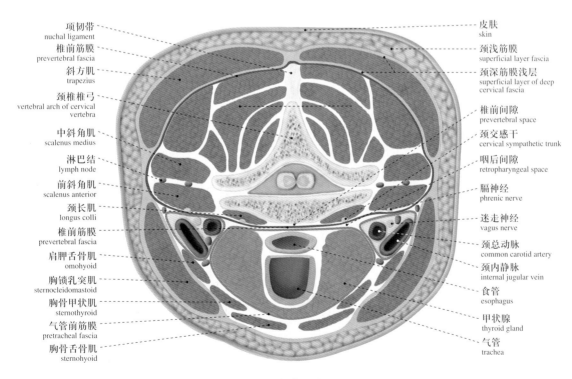

项韧带
nuchal ligament

椎前筋膜
prevertebral fascia

斜方肌
trapezius

颈椎椎弓
vertebral arch of cervical
vertebra

中斜角肌
scalenus medius

淋巴结
lymph node

前斜角肌
scalenus anterior

颈长肌
longus colli

椎前筋膜
prevertebral fascia

肩胛舌骨肌
omohyoid

胸锁乳突肌
sternocleidomastoid

胸骨甲状肌
sternothyroid

气管前筋膜
pretracheal fascia

胸骨舌骨肌
sternohyoid

皮肤
skin

颈浅筋膜
superficial layer fascia

颈深筋膜浅层
superficial layer of deep
cervical fascia

椎前间隙
prevertebral space

颈交感干
cervical sympathetic trunk

咽后间隙
retropharyngeal space

膈神经
phrenic nerve

迷走神经
vagus nerve

颈总动脉
common carotid artery

颈内静脉
internal jugular vein

食管
esophagus

甲状腺
thyroid gland

气管
trachea

图 34　颈筋膜（水平断面）
Cervical fascia (horizontal section)

第三节

颈前区

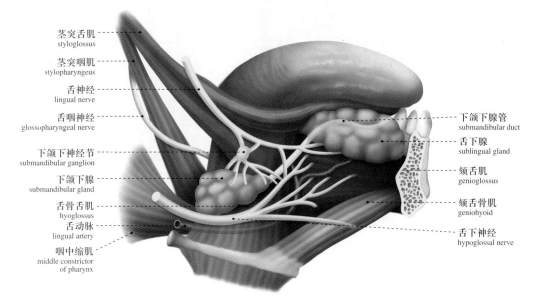

荃突舌肌
styloglossus

荃突咽肌
stylopharyngeus

舌神经
lingual nerve

舌咽神经
glossopharyngeal nerve

下颌下神经节
submandibular ganglion

下颌下腺
submandibular gland

舌骨舌肌
hyoglossus

舌动脉
lingual artery

咽中缩肌
middle constrictor
of pharynx

下颌下腺管
submandibular duct

舌下腺
sublingual gland

颏舌肌
genioglossus

颏舌骨肌
geniohyoid

舌下神经
hypoglossal nerve

图 35　下颌下三角内结构
Submandibular triangle structure

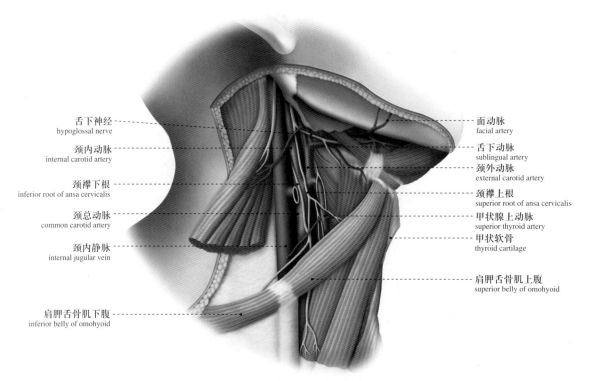

舌下神经
hypoglossal nerve

颈内动脉
internal carotid artery

颈襻下根
inferior root of ansa cervicalis

颈总动脉
common carotid artery

颈内静脉
internal jugular vein

肩胛舌骨肌下腹
inferior belly of omohyoid

面动脉
facial artery

舌下动脉
sublingual artery

颈外动脉
external carotid artery

颈襻上根
superior root of ansa cervicalis

甲状腺上动脉
superior thyroid artery

甲状软骨
thyroid cartilage

肩胛舌骨肌上腹
superior belly of omohyoid

图 36　颈动脉三角内结构
Carotid triangle structure

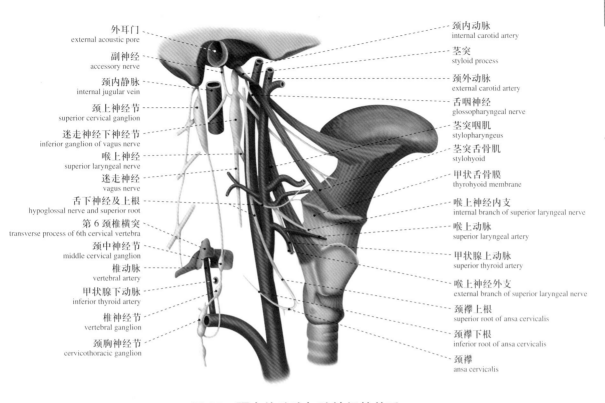

外耳门
external acoustic pore

副神经
accessory nerve

颈内静脉
internal jugular vein

颈上神经节
superior cervical ganglion

迷走神经下神经节
inferior ganglion of vagus nerve

喉上神经
superior laryngeal nerve

迷走神经
vagus nerve

舌下神经及上根
hypoglossal nerve and superior root

第 6 颈椎横突
transverse process of 6th cervical vertebra

颈中神经节
middle cervical ganglion

椎动脉
vertebral artery

甲状腺下动脉
inferior thyroid artery

椎神经节
vertebral ganglion

颈胸神经节
cervicothoracic ganglion

颈内动脉
internal carotid artery

茎突
styloid process

颈外动脉
external carotid artery

舌咽神经
glossopharyngeal nerve

茎突咽肌
stylopharyngeus

茎突舌骨肌
stylohyoid

甲状舌骨膜
thyrohyoid membrane

喉上神经内支
internal branch of superior laryngeal nerve

喉上动脉
superior laryngeal artery

甲状腺上动脉
superior thyroid artery

喉上神经外支
external branch of superior laryngeal nerve

颈襻上根
superior root of ansa cervicalis

颈襻下根
inferior root of ansa cervicalis

颈襻
ansa cervicalis

图 37　颈内外动脉与脑神经的关系

Relationship between carotid internal artery and cranial nerve

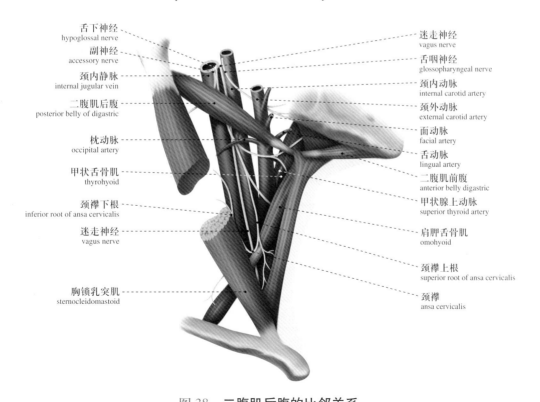

舌下神经
hypoglossal nerve

副神经
accessory nerve

颈内静脉
internal jugular vein

二腹肌后腹
posterior belly of digastric

枕动脉
occipital artery

甲状舌骨肌
thyrohyoid

颈襻下根
inferior root of ansa cervicalis

迷走神经
vagus nerve

胸锁乳突肌
sternocleidomastoid

迷走神经
vagus nerve

舌咽神经
glossopharyngeal nerve

颈内动脉
internal carotid artery

颈外动脉
external carotid artery

面动脉
facial artery

舌动脉
lingual artery

二腹肌前腹
anterior belly digastric

甲状腺上动脉
superior thyroid artery

肩胛舌骨肌
omohyoid

颈襻上根
superior root of ansa cervicalis

颈襻
ansa cervicalis

图 38　二腹肌后腹的比邻关系

Adjacent to the posterior belly of digastric relationship

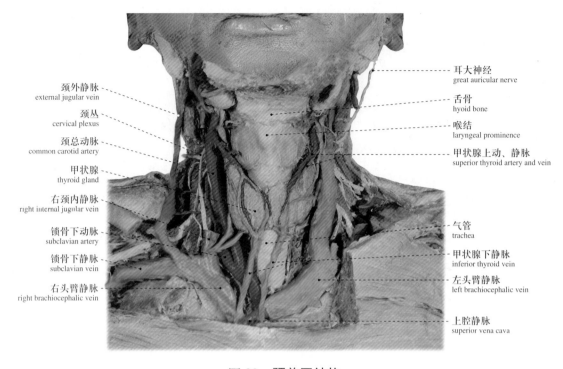

颈外静脉
external jugular vein

颈丛
cervical plexus

颈总动脉
common carotid artery

甲状腺
thyroid gland

右颈内静脉
right internal jugular vein

锁骨下动脉
subclavian artery

锁骨下静脉
subclavian vein

右头臂静脉
right brachiocephalic vein

耳大神经
great auricular nerve

舌骨
hyoid bone

喉结
laryngeal prominence

甲状腺上动、静脉
superior thyroid artery and vein

气管
trachea

甲状腺下静脉
inferior thyroid vein

左头臂静脉
left brachiocephalic vein

上腔静脉
superior vena cava

图 39　颈前区结构
Structure of anterior region of the neck

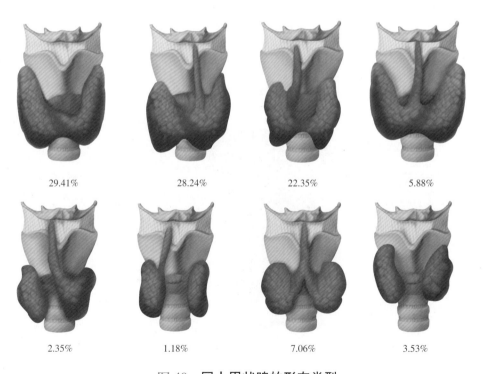

29.41%　　28.24%　　22.35%　　5.88%

2.35%　　1.18%　　7.06%　　3.53%

图 40　国人甲状腺的形态类型
Morphological types of thyroid of the Chinese people

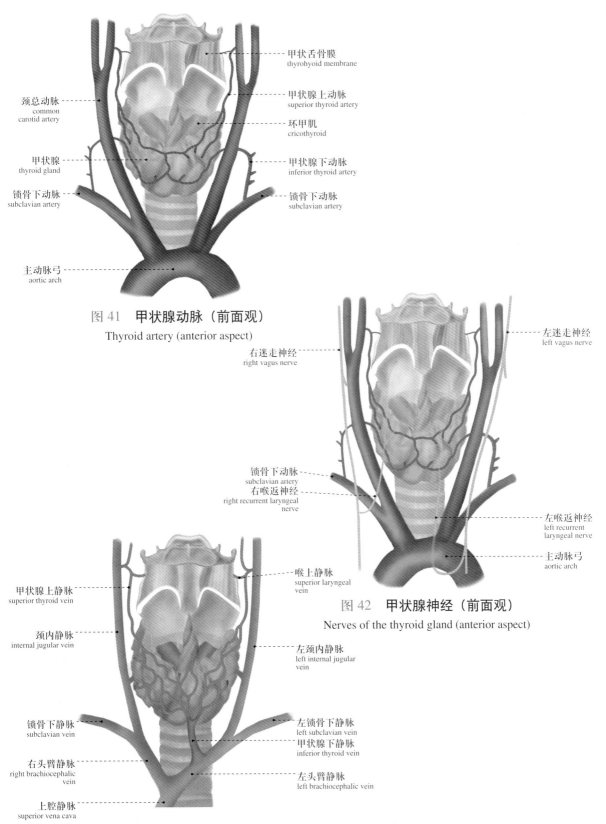

甲状舌骨膜
thyrohyoid membrane

颈总动脉
common
carotid artery

甲状腺上动脉
superior thyroid artery

环甲肌
cricothyroid

甲状腺
thyroid gland

甲状腺下动脉
inferior thyroid artery

锁骨下动脉
subclavian artery

锁骨下动脉
subclavian artery

主动脉弓
aortic arch

图 41 甲状腺动脉（前面观）
Thyroid artery (anterior aspect)

左迷走神经
left vagus nerve

右迷走神经
right vagus nerve

锁骨下动脉
subclavian artery
右喉返神经
right recurrent laryngeal
nerve

左喉返神经
left recurrent
laryngeal nerve

主动脉弓
aortic arch

喉上静脉
superior laryngeal
vein

图 42 甲状腺神经（前面观）
Nerves of the thyroid gland (anterior aspect)

甲状腺上静脉
superior thyroid vein

颈内静脉
internal jugular vein

左颈内静脉
left internal jugular
vein

锁骨下静脉
subclavian vein

左锁骨下静脉
left subclavian vein
甲状腺下静脉
inferior thyroid vein

右头臂静脉
right brachiocephalic
vein

左头臂静脉
left brachiocephalic
vein

上腔静脉
superior vena cava

图 43 甲状腺静脉（前面观）
Veins of the thyroid gland (anterior aspect)

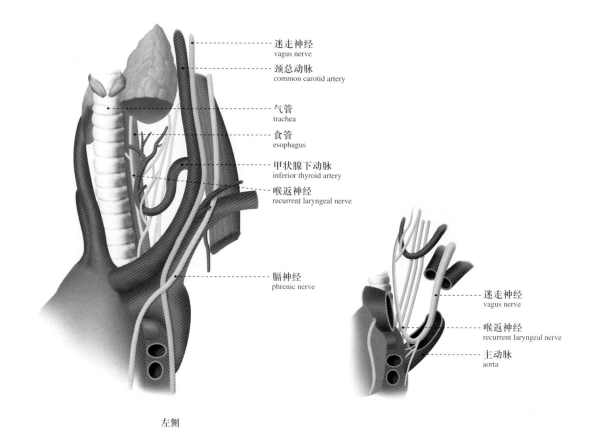

迷走神经
vagus nerve

颈总动脉
common carotid artery

气管
trachea

食管
esophagus

甲状腺下动脉
inferior thyroid artery

喉返神经
recurrent laryngeal nerve

膈神经
phrenic nerve

迷走神经
vagus nerve

喉返神经
recurrent laryngeal nerve

主动脉
aorta

左侧

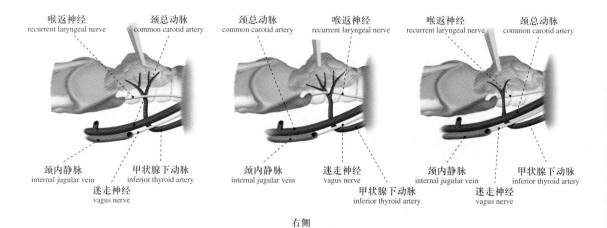

喉返神经
recurrent laryngeal nerve

颈总动脉
common carotid artery

颈总动脉
common carotid artery

喉返神经
recurrent laryngeal nerve

喉返神经
recurrent laryngeal nerve

颈总动脉
common carotid artery

颈内静脉
internal jugular vein

甲状腺下动脉
inferior thyroid artery

颈内静脉
internal jugular vein

迷走神经
vagus nerve

颈内静脉
internal jugular vein

甲状腺下动脉
inferior thyroid artery

迷走神经
vagus nerve

甲状腺下动脉
inferior thyroid artery

迷走神经
vagus nerve

右侧

图 44　甲状腺下动脉与喉返神经的关系

Relationship between the inferior thyroid artery and recurrent laryngeal nerve

第四节

胸锁乳突区及颈根部

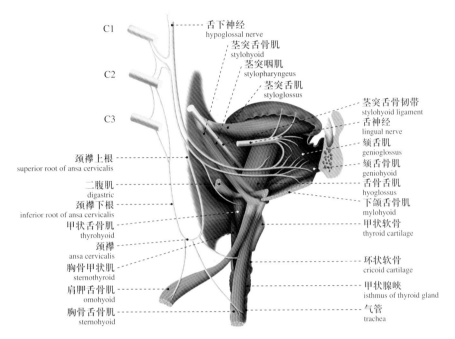

C1
C2
C3

舌下神经
hypoglossal nerve
茎突舌骨肌
stylohyoid
茎突咽肌
stylopharyngeus
茎突舌肌
styloglossus
茎突舌骨韧带
stylohyoid ligament
舌神经
lingual nerve
颏舌肌
genioglossus
颏舌骨肌
geniohyoid
舌骨舌肌
hyoglossus
下颌舌骨肌
mylohyoid
甲状软骨
thyroid cartilage
环状软骨
cricoid cartilage
甲状腺峡
isthmus of thyroid gland
气管
trachea

颈襻上根
superior root of ansa cervicalis
二腹肌
digastric
颈襻下根
inferior root of ansa cervicalis
甲状舌骨肌
thyrohyoid
颈襻
ansa cervicalis
胸骨甲状肌
sternothyroid
肩胛舌骨肌
omohyoid
胸骨舌骨肌
sternohyoid

图 45　颈襻及支配的肌肉
Ansa cervicalis and innervation of muscle

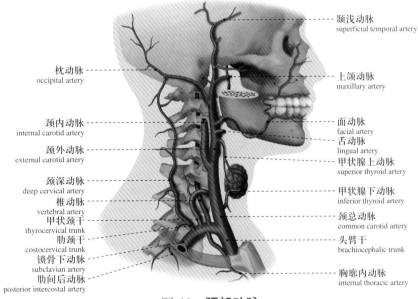

颞浅动脉
superficial temporal artery
枕动脉
occipital artery
上颌动脉
maxillary artery
颈内动脉
internal carotid artery
面动脉
facial artery
颈外动脉
external carotid artery
舌动脉
lingual artery
颈深动脉
deep cervical artery
甲状腺上动脉
superior thyroid artery
椎动脉
vertebral artery
甲状腺下动脉
inferior thyroid artery
甲状颈干
thyrocervical trunk
颈总动脉
common carotid artery
肋颈干
costocervical trunk
头臂干
brachiocephalic trunk
锁骨下动脉
subclavian artery
肋间后动脉
posterior intercostal artery
胸廓内动脉
internal thoracic artery

图 46　颈部动脉
Cervical artery

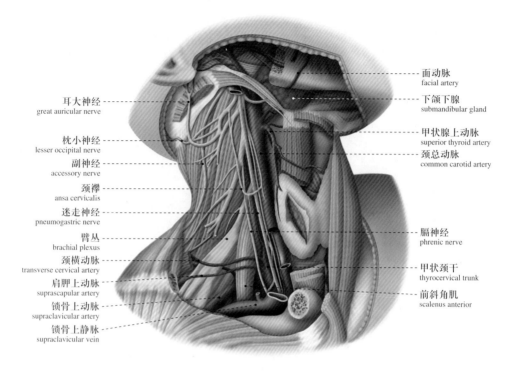

耳大神经
great auricular nerve

枕小神经
lesser occipital nerve

副神经
accessory nerve

颈襻
ansa cervicalis

迷走神经
pneumogastric nerve

臂丛
brachial plexus

颈横动脉
transverse cervical artery

肩胛上动脉
suprascapular artery

锁骨上动脉
supraclavicular artery

锁骨上静脉
supraclavicular vein

面动脉
facial artery

下颌下腺
submandibular gland

甲状腺上动脉
superior thyroid artery

颈总动脉
common carotid artery

膈神经
phrenic nerve

甲状颈干
thyrocervical trunk

前斜角肌
scalenus anterior

图 47　颈外侧区及其结构
Lateral cervical region and its structure

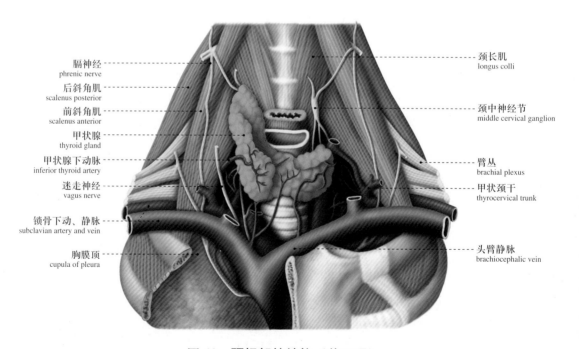

膈神经
phrenic nerve

后斜角肌
scalenus posterior

前斜角肌
scalenus anterior

甲状腺
thyroid gland

甲状腺下动脉
inferior thyroid artery

迷走神经
vagus nerve

锁骨下动、静脉
subclavian artery and vein

胸膜顶
cupula of pleura

颈长肌
longus colli

颈中神经节
middle cervical ganglion

臂丛
brachial plexus

甲状颈干
thyrocervical trunk

头臂静脉
brachiocephalic vein

图 48　颈根部的结构（前面观）
Structure of the root of neck (anterior aspect)

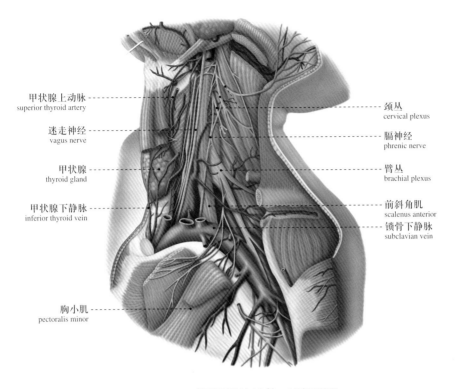

甲状腺上动脉
superior thyroid artery

迷走神经
vagus nerve

甲状腺
thyroid gland

甲状腺下静脉
inferior thyroid vein

胸小肌
pectoralis minor

颈丛
cervical plexus

膈神经
phrenic nerve

臂丛
brachial plexus

前斜角肌
scalenus anterior

锁骨下静脉
subclavian vein

图 49　颈根部的结构（侧面观）
Structure of the root of neck (lateral aspect)

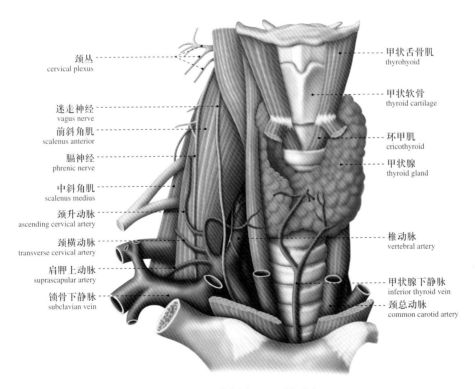

颈丛
cervical plexus

迷走神经
vagus nerve

前斜角肌
scalenus anterior

膈神经
phrenic nerve

中斜角肌
scalenus medius

颈升动脉
ascending cervical artery

颈横动脉
transverse cervical artery

肩胛上动脉
suprascapular artery

锁骨下静脉
subclavian vein

甲状舌骨肌
thyrohyoid

甲状软骨
thyroid cartilage

环甲肌
cricothyroid

甲状腺
thyroid gland

椎动脉
vertebral artery

甲状腺下静脉
inferior thyroid vein

颈总动脉
common carotid artery

图 50　前斜角肌及其毗邻
Scalenus anterior and its neighbourhood

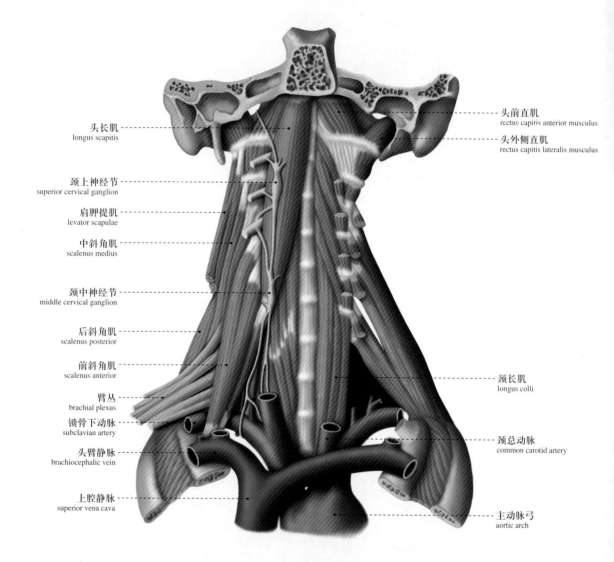

头长肌
longus scapitis

颈上神经节
superior cervical ganglion

肩胛提肌
levator scapulae

中斜角肌
scalenus medius

颈中神经节
middle cervical ganglion

后斜角肌
scalenus posterior

前斜角肌
scalenus anterior

臂丛
brachial plexus

锁骨下动脉
subclavian artery

头臂静脉
brachiocephalic vein

上腔静脉
superior vena cava

头前直肌
rectus capitis anterior musculus

头外侧直肌
rectus capitis lateralis musculus

颈长肌
longus colli

颈总动脉
common carotid artery

主动脉弓
aortic arch

图 51　颈根部的结构
Structure of the root of neck

第五节

颈外侧区

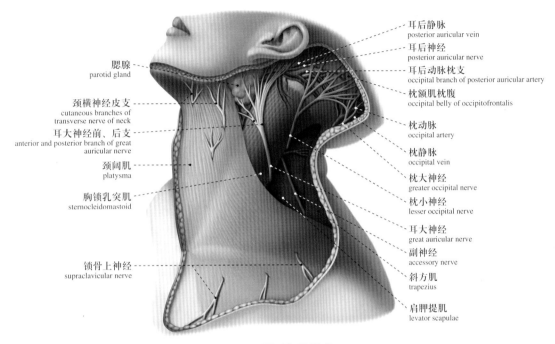

腮腺 parotid gland	耳后静脉 posterior auricular vein
颈横神经皮支 cutaneous branches of transverse nerve of neck	耳后神经 posterior auricular nerve
耳大神经前、后支 anterior and posterior branch of great auricular nerve	耳后动脉枕支 occipital branch of posterior auricular artery
颈阔肌 platysma	枕额肌枕腹 occipital belly of occipitofrontalis
胸锁乳突肌 sternocleidomastoid	枕动脉 occipital artery
锁骨上神经 supraclavicular nerve	枕静脉 occipital vein

枕大神经 greater occipital nerve
枕小神经 lesser occipital nerve
耳大神经 great auricular nerve
副神经 accessory nerve
斜方肌 trapezius
肩胛提肌 levator scapulae

图 52　颈部浅层结构 1
Neck superficial structure 1

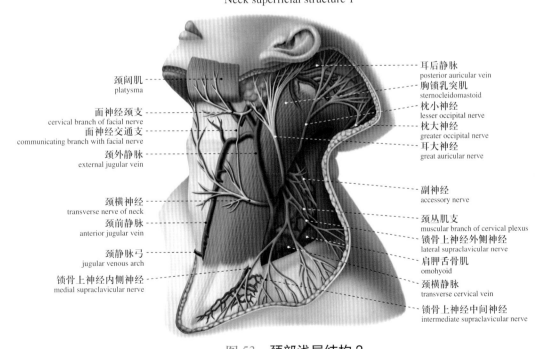

颈阔肌 platysma
面神经颈支 cervical branch of facial nerve
面神经交通支 communicating branch with facial nerve
颈外静脉 external jugular vein
颈横神经 transverse nerve of neck
颈前静脉 anterior jugular vein
颈静脉弓 jugular venous arch
锁骨上神经内侧神经 medial supraclavicular nerve

耳后静脉 posterior auricular vein
胸锁乳突肌 sternocleidomastoid
枕小神经 lesser occipital nerve
枕大神经 greater occipital nerve
耳大神经 great auricular nerve
副神经 accessory nerve
颈丛肌支 muscular branch of cervical plexus
锁骨上神经外侧神经 lateral supraclavicular nerve
肩胛舌骨肌 omohyoid
颈横静脉 transverse cervical vein
锁骨上神经中间神经 intermediate supraclavicular nerve

图 53　颈部浅层结构 2
Neck superficial structure 2

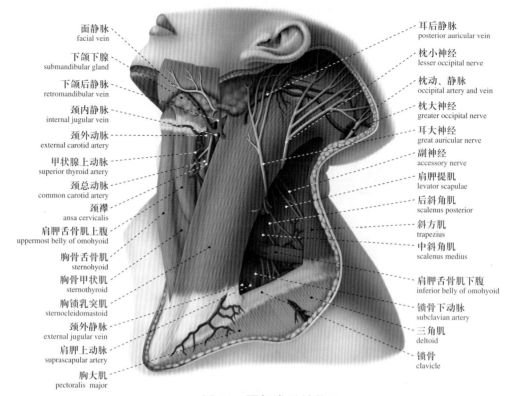

面静脉
facial vein

下颌下腺
submandibular gland

下颌后静脉
retromandibular vein

颈内静脉
internal jugular vein

颈外动脉
external carotid artery

甲状腺上动脉
superior thyroid artery

颈总动脉
common carotid artery

颈襻
ansa cervicalis

肩胛舌骨肌上腹
uppermost belly of omohyoid

胸骨舌骨肌
sternohyoid

胸骨甲状肌
sternothyroid

胸锁乳突肌
sternocleidomastoid

颈外静脉
external jugular vein

肩胛上动脉
suprascapular artery

胸大肌
pectoralis major

耳后静脉
posterior auricular vein

枕小神经
lesser occipital nerve

枕动、静脉
occipital artery and vein

枕大神经
greater occipital nerve

耳大神经
great auricular nerve

副神经
accessory nerve

肩胛提肌
levator scapulae

后斜角肌
scalenus posterior

斜方肌
trapezius

中斜角肌
scalenus medius

肩胛舌骨肌下腹
inferior belly of omohyoid

锁骨下动脉
subclavian artery

三角肌
deltoid

锁骨
clavicle

图 54 颈部浅层结构 3

Neck superficial structure 3

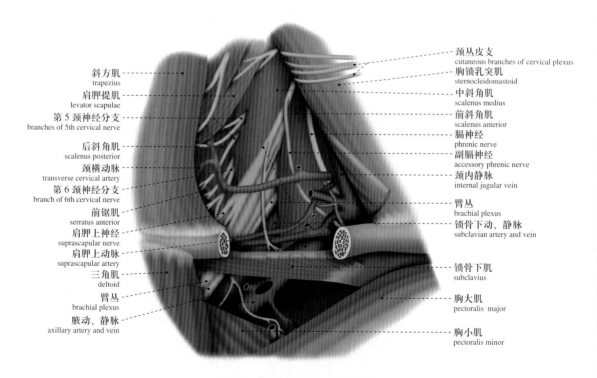

斜方肌
trapezius

肩胛提肌
levator scapulae

第 5 颈神经分支
branches of 5th cervical nerve

后斜角肌
scalenus posterior

颈横动脉
transverse cervical artery

第 6 颈神经分支
branch of 6th cervical nerve

前锯肌
serratus anterior

肩胛上神经
suprascapular nerve

肩胛上动脉
suprascapular artery

三角肌
deltoid

臂丛
brachial plexus

腋动、静脉
axillary artery and vein

颈丛皮支
cutaneous branches of cervical plexus

胸锁乳突肌
sternocleidomastoid

中斜角肌
scalenus medius

前斜角肌
scalenus anterior

膈神经
phrenic nerve

副膈神经
accessory phrenic nerve

颈内静脉
internal jugular vein

臂丛
brachial plexus

锁骨下动、静脉
subclavian artery and vein

锁骨下肌
subclavius

胸大肌
pectoralis major

胸小肌
pectoralis minor

图 55 锁骨上三角及其结构

Supraclavicular triangle and its structure

第六节

颈部淋巴回流

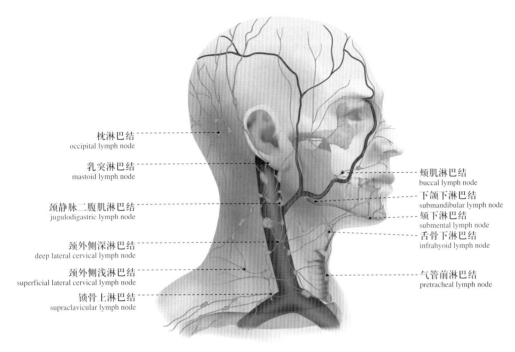

枕淋巴结
occipital lymph node

乳突淋巴结
mastoid lymph node

颈静脉二腹肌淋巴结
jugulodigastric lymph node

颈外侧深淋巴结
deep lateral cervical lymph node

颈外侧浅淋巴结
superficial lateral cervical lymph node

锁骨上淋巴结
supraclavicular lymph node

颊肌淋巴结
buccal lymph node

下颌下淋巴结
submandibular lymph node

颏下淋巴结
submental lymph node

舌骨下淋巴结
infrahyoid lymph node

气管前淋巴结
pretracheal lymph node

图 56　头颈部淋巴管和淋巴结（侧面观）
Lymphatic vessels and lymph nodes of the head and neck (lateral aspect)

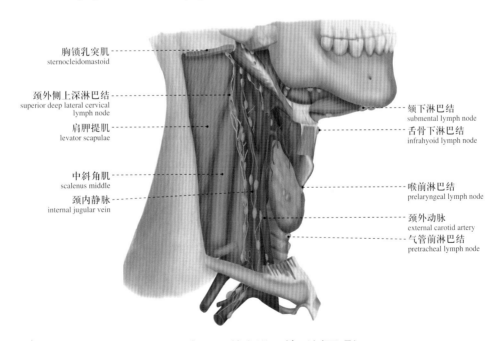

胸锁乳突肌
sternocleidomastoid

颈外侧上深淋巴结
superior deep lateral cervical
lymph node

肩胛提肌
levator scapulae

中斜角肌
scalenus middle

颈内静脉
internal jugular vein

颏下淋巴结
submental lymph node

舌骨下淋巴结
infrahyoid lymph node

喉前淋巴结
prelaryngeal lymph node

颈外动脉
external carotid artery

气管前淋巴结
pretracheal lymph node

图 57　颈部淋巴管和淋巴结（侧面观）
Lymphatic vessels and lymph nodes of the neck (lateral aspect)

第一节

表面解剖

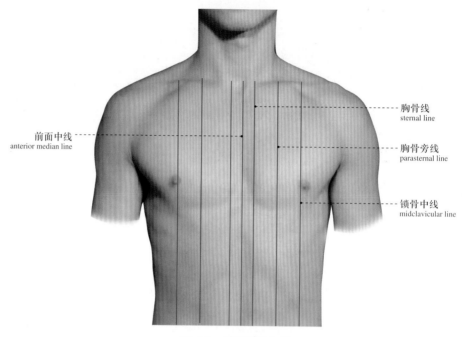

图 58　胸部标志线
Reference lines of the thorax

胸骨线
sternal line

前面中线
anterior median line

胸骨旁线
parasternal line

锁骨中线
midclavicular line

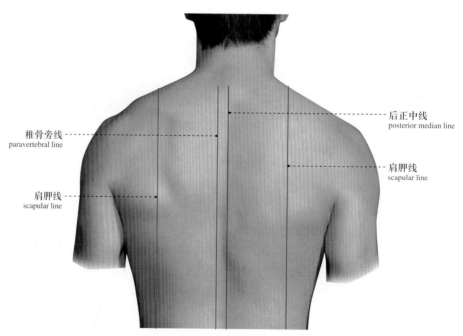

图 59　背部标志线
Reference lines of the back

后正中线
posterior median line

椎骨旁线
paravertebral line

肩胛线
scapular line

肩胛线
scapular line

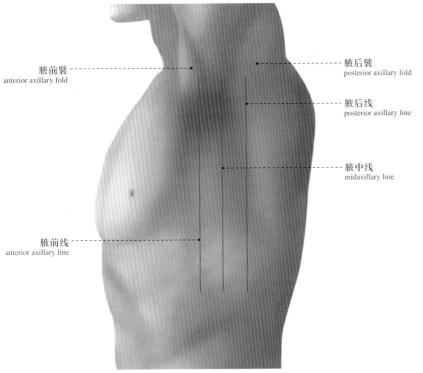

腋前襞
anterior axillary fold

腋后襞
posterior axillary fold

腋后线
posterior axillary line

腋中线
midaxillary line

腋前线
anterior axillary line

图 60　腋部标志线
Reference lines of the axillary

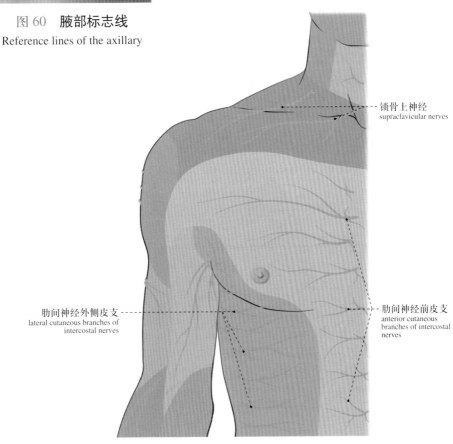

锁骨上神经
supraclavicular nerves

肋间神经外侧皮支
lateral cutaneous branches of
intercostal nerves

肋间神经前皮支
anterior cutaneous
branches of intercostal
nerves

图 61　胸壁皮神经（前面观）
Cutaneous nerves of chest wall (anterior aspect)

胸 壁

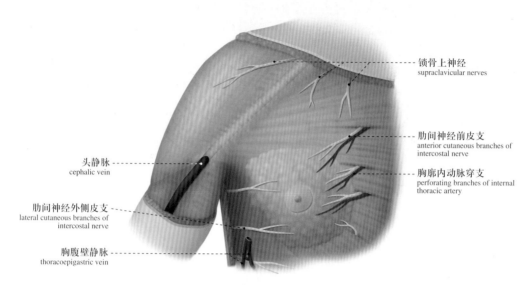

锁骨上神经
supraclavicular nerves

肋间神经前皮支
anterior cutaneous branches of intercostal nerve

胸廓内动脉穿支
perforating branches of internal thoracic artery

头静脉
cephalic vein

肋间神经外侧皮支
lateral cutaneous branches of intercostal nerve

胸腹壁静脉
thoracoepigastric vein

图 62　胸前、外侧区的皮神经及血管分支
Cutaneous nerve and blood vessel branches of the regiones pectoris anterior and lateral

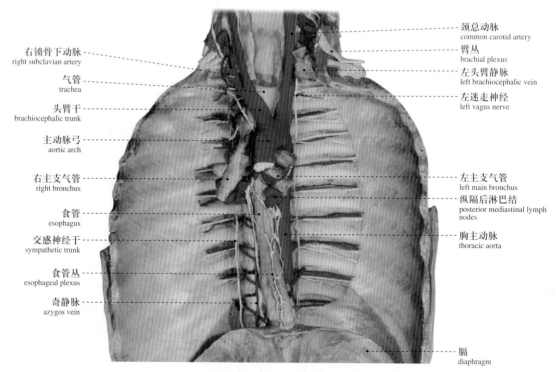

右锁骨下动脉
right subclavian artery

气管
trachea

头臂干
brachiocephalic trunk

主动脉弓
aortic arch

右主支气管
right bronchus

食管
esophagus

交感神经干
sympathetic trunk

食管丛
esophageal plexus

奇静脉
azygos vein

颈总动脉
common carotid artery

臂丛
brachial plexus

左头臂静脉
left brachiocephalic vein

左迷走神经
left vagus nerve

左主支气管
left main bronchus

纵隔后淋巴结
posterior mediastinal lymph nodes

胸主动脉
thoracic aorta

膈
diaphragm

图 63　胸廓内血管、神经和淋巴结
Internal thoracic vessels, nerves and lymph nodes

人体局部解剖图谱

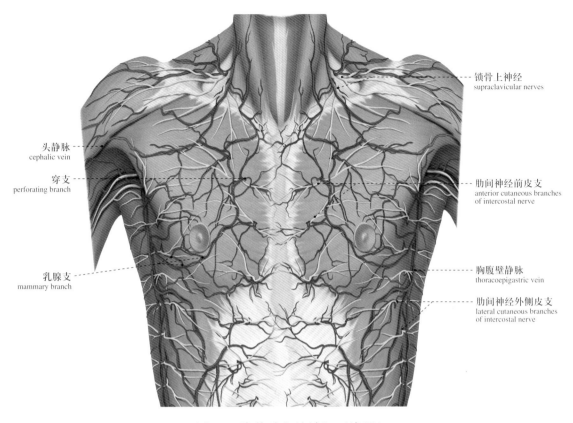

锁骨上神经
supraclavicular nerves

头静脉
cephalic vein

穿支
perforating branch

肋间神经前皮支
anterior cutaneous branches
of intercostal nerve

乳腺支
mammary branch

胸腹壁静脉
thoracoepigastric vein

肋间神经外侧皮支
lateral cutaneous branches
of intercostal nerve

图 64　胸前壁血管神经（浅层）
Blood vessels and nerves of the anterior thoracic wall (superficial layer)

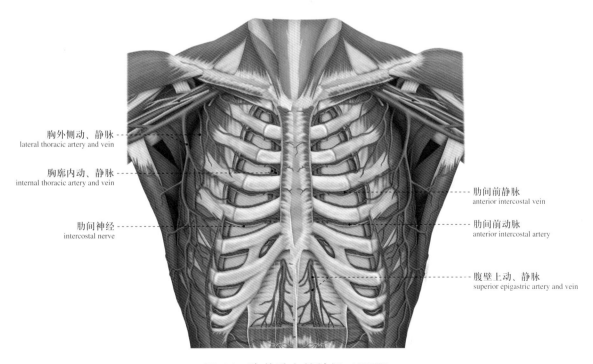

胸外侧动、静脉
lateral thoracic artery and vein

胸廓内动、静脉
internal thoracic artery and vein

肋间神经
intercostal nerve

肋间前静脉
anterior intercostal vein

肋间前动脉
anterior intercostal artery

腹壁上动、静脉
superior epigastric artery and vein

图 65　胸前壁血管神经（深层）
Blood vessels and nerves of anterior thoracic wall (deep layer)

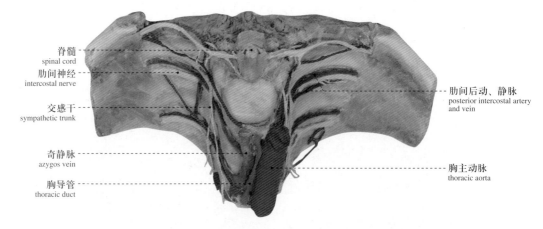

脊髓
spinal cord

肋间神经
intercostal nerve

交感干
sympathetic trunk

奇静脉
azygos vein

胸导管
thoracic duct

肋间后动、静脉
posterior intercostal artery
and vein

胸主动脉
thoracic aorta

图 66　肋间后动、静脉和肋间神经
Posterior intercostal artery, vein and intercostal nerve

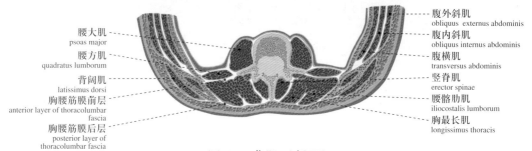

腰大肌
psoas major

腰方肌
quadratus lumborum

背阔肌
latissimus dorsi

胸腰筋膜前层
anterior layer of thoracolumbar
fascia

胸腰筋膜后层
posterior layer of
thoracolumbar fascia

腹外斜肌
obliquus externus abdominis

腹内斜肌
obliquus internus abdominis

腹横肌
transversus abdominis

竖脊肌
erector spinae

腰髂肋肌
iliocostalis lumborum

胸最长肌
longissimus thoracis

图 67　背肌（断面）
Muscles of the back (section)

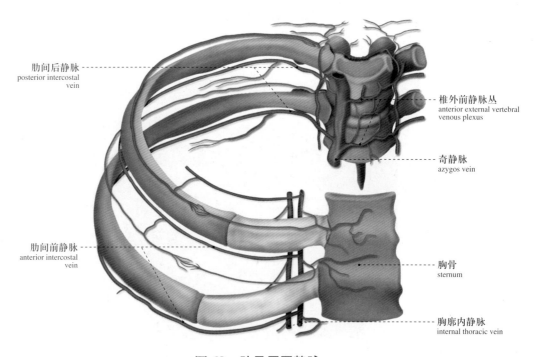

肋间后静脉
posterior intercostal
vein

肋间前静脉
anterior intercostal
vein

椎外前静脉丛
anterior external vertebral
venous plexus

奇静脉
azygos vein

胸骨
sternum

胸廓内静脉
internal thoracic vein

图 68　肋骨周围静脉
Veins around the ribs

人体局部解剖图谱

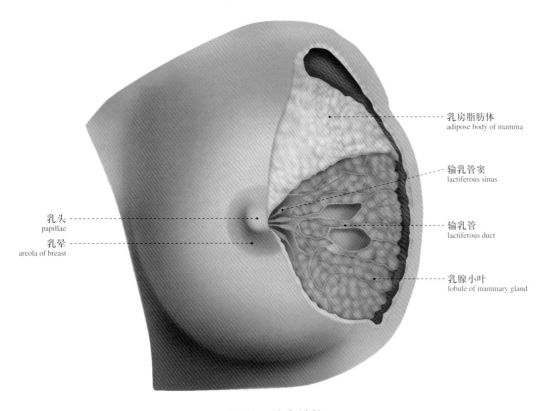

乳房脂肪体
adipose body of mamma

输乳管窦
lactiferous sinus

输乳管
lactiferous duct

乳腺小叶
lobule of mammary gland

乳头
papillae

乳晕
areola of breast

图 69　乳房结构
Mamma structure

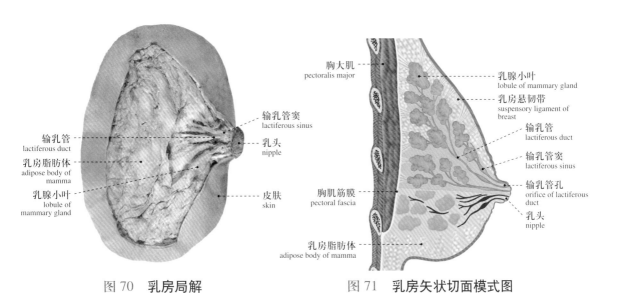

输乳管窦
lactiferous sinus

乳头
nipple

输乳管
lactiferous duct

乳房脂肪体
adipose body of mamma

乳腺小叶
lobule of mammary gland

皮肤
skin

胸大肌
pectoralis major

乳腺小叶
lobule of mammary gland

乳房悬韧带
suspensory ligament of breast

输乳管
lactiferous duct

输乳管窦
lactiferous sinus

输乳管孔
orifice of lactiferous duct

乳头
nipple

胸肌筋膜
pectoral fascia

乳房脂肪体
adipose body of mamma

图 70　乳房局解
Topography of the mamma

图 71　乳房矢状切面模式图
Diagram of the sagittal section of the mamma

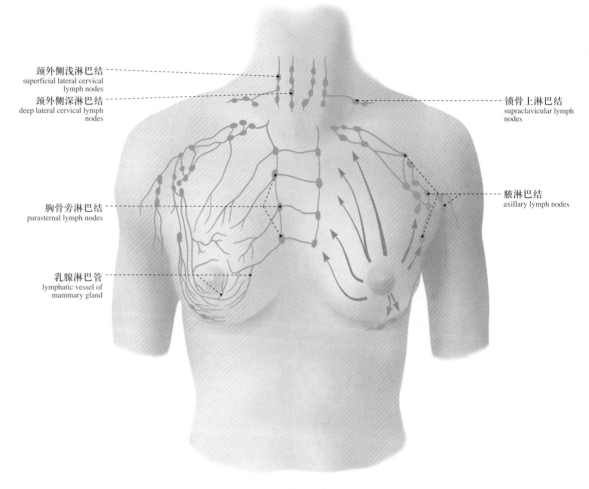

颈外侧浅淋巴结
superficial lateral cervical
lymph nodes

颈外侧深淋巴结
deep lateral cervical lymph
nodes

锁骨上淋巴结
supraclavicular lymph
nodes

胸骨旁淋巴结
parasternal lymph nodes

腋淋巴结
axillary lymph nodes

乳腺淋巴管
lymphatic vessel of
mammary gland

图 72　女性乳房淋巴
Lymph of the female breast

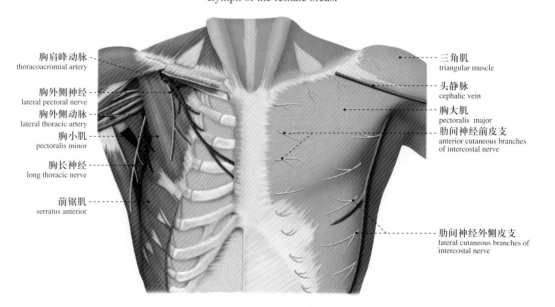

胸肩峰动脉
thoracoacromial artery

胸外侧神经
lateral pectoral nerve

胸外侧动脉
lateral thoracic artery

胸小肌
pectoralis minor

胸长神经
long thoracic nerve

前锯肌
serratus anterior

三角肌
triangular muscle

头静脉
cephalic vein

胸大肌
pectoralis major

肋间神经前皮支
anterior cutaneous branches
of intercostal nerve

肋间神经外侧皮支
lateral cutaneous branches of
intercostal nerve

图 73　胸壁的结构
Structure of the chest wall

第三节

膈 肌

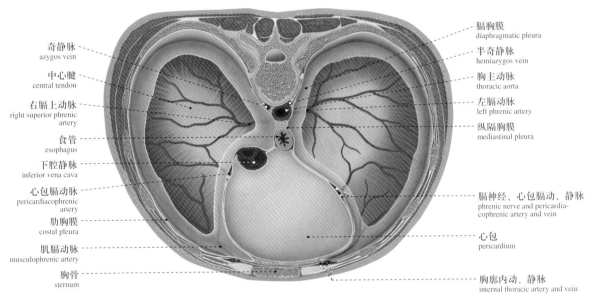

奇静脉 azygos vein
中心腱 central tendon
右膈上动脉 right superior phrenic artery
食管 esophagus
下腔静脉 inferior vena cava
心包膈动脉 pericardiacophrenic artery
肋胸膜 costal pleura
肌膈动脉 musculophrenic artery
胸骨 sternum

膈胸膜 diaphragmatic pleura
半奇静脉 hemiazygos vein
胸主动脉 thoracic aorta
左膈动脉 left phrenic artery
纵隔胸膜 mediastinal pleura
膈神经、心包膈动、静脉 phrenic nerve and pericardia-cophrenic artery and vein
心包 pericardium
胸廓内动、静脉 internal thoracic artery and vein

图 74 膈的动脉（上面观）
Arteries of the diaphragm (superior aspect)

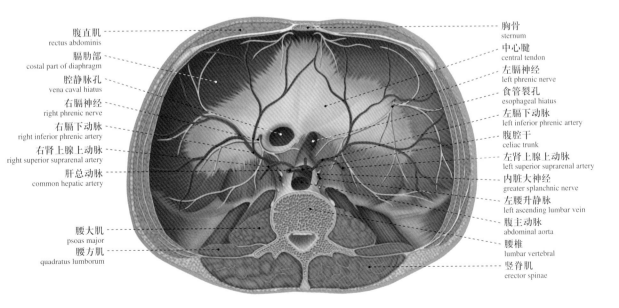

腹直肌 rectus abdominis
膈肋部 costal part of diaphragm
腔静脉孔 vena caval hiatus
右膈神经 right phrenic nerve
右膈下动脉 right inferior phrenic artery
右肾上腺上动脉 right superior suprarenal artery
肝总动脉 common hepatic artery
腰大肌 psoas major
腰方肌 quadratus lumborum

胸骨 sternum
中心腱 central tendon
左膈神经 left phrenic nerve
食管裂孔 esophageal hiatus
左膈下动脉 left inferior phrenic artery
腹腔干 celiac trunk
左肾上腺上动脉 left superior suprarenal artery
内脏大神经 greater splanchnic nerve
左腰升静脉 left ascending lumbar vein
腹主动脉 abdominal aorta
腰椎 lumbar vertebral
竖脊肌 erector spinae

图 75 膈的动脉和神经（下面观）
Arteries and nerves of the diaphragm (inferior aspect)

第四节

胸膜及肺体表投影

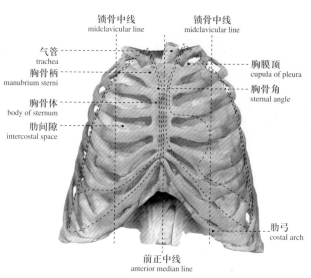

锁骨中线 midclavicular line
锁骨中线 midclavicular line
气管 trachea
胸骨柄 manubrium sterni
胸骨体 body of sternum
肋间隙 intercostal space
胸膜顶 cupula of pleura
胸骨角 sternal angle
肋弓 costal arch
前正中线 anterior median line

图 76　胸膜及肺体表投影（前面观）
The body surface projection of the pleura and the lung
(anterior aspect)

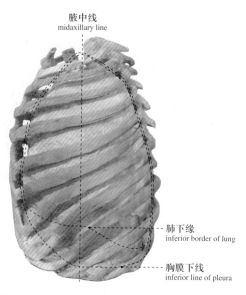

腋中线 midaxillary line
肺下缘 inferior border of lung
胸膜下线 inferior line of pleura

图 77　胸膜及肺体表投影（左侧面观）
The body surface projection of the pleura and the
lung (left lateral aspect)

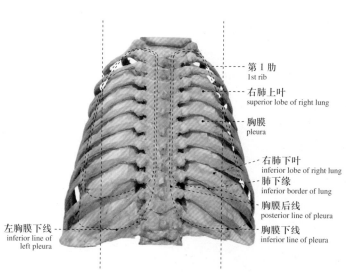

第 1 肋 1st rib
右肺上叶 superior lobe of right lung
胸膜 pleura
右肺下叶 inferior lobe of right lung
肺下缘 inferior border of lung
胸膜后线 posterior line of pleura
胸膜下线 inferior line of pleura
左胸膜下线 inferior line of left pleura

图 78　胸膜及肺体表投影（后面观）
The body surface projection of the pleura and the lung
(posterior aspect)

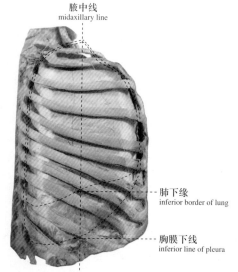

腋中线 midaxillary line
肺下缘 inferior border of lung
胸膜下线 inferior line of pleura

图 79　胸膜及肺体表投影（右侧面观）
The body surface projection of the pleura and the
lung (right lateral aspect)

第五节

肺

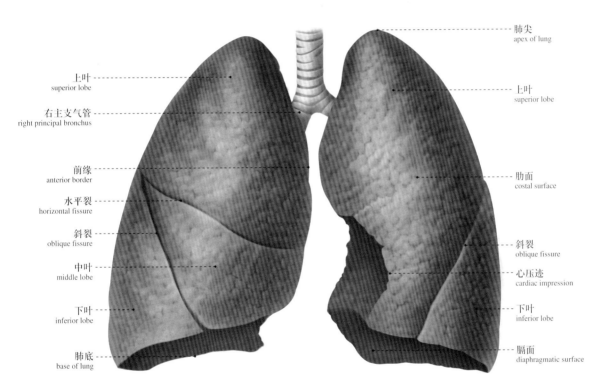

上叶
superior lobe

右主支气管
right principal bronchus

前缘
anterior border

水平裂
horizontal fissure

斜裂
oblique fissure

中叶
middle lobe

下叶
inferior lobe

肺底
base of lung

肺尖
apex of lung

上叶
superior lobe

肋面
costal surface

斜裂
oblique fissure

心压迹
cardiac impression

下叶
inferior lobe

膈面
diaphragmatic surface

图 80　气管、支气管和肺（前面观）
The trachea, bronchi and lungs (anterior aspect)

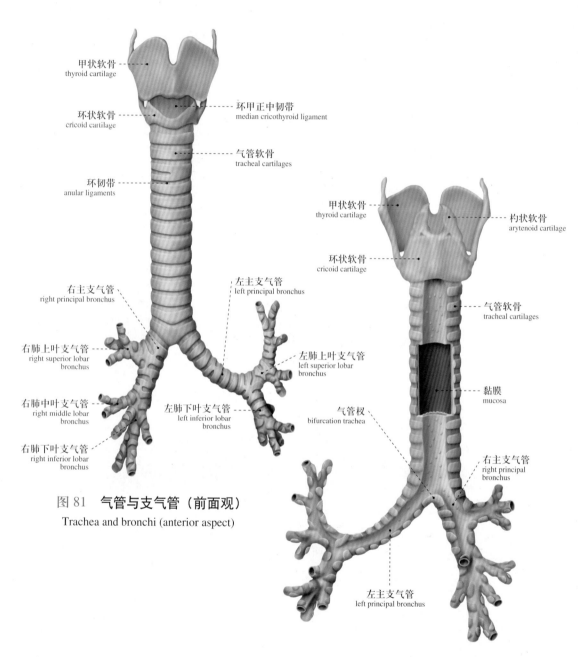

甲状软骨
thyroid cartilage

环状软骨
cricoid cartilage

环甲正中韧带
median cricothyroid ligament

气管软骨
tracheal cartilages

环韧带
anular ligaments

右主支气管
right principal bronchus

左主支气管
left principal bronchus

右肺上叶支气管
right superior lobar bronchus

左肺上叶支气管
left superior lobar bronchus

右肺中叶支气管
right middle lobar bronchus

左肺下叶支气管
left inferior lobar bronchus

右肺下叶支气管
right inferior lobar bronchus

图 81　气管与支气管（前面观）
Trachea and bronchi (anterior aspect)

甲状软骨
thyroid cartilage

杓状软骨
arytenoid cartilage

环状软骨
cricoid cartilage

气管软骨
tracheal cartilages

黏膜
mucosa

气管杈
bifurcation trachea

右主支气管
right principal bronchus

左主支气管
left principal bronchus

图 82　气管与支气管（后面观）
Trachea and bronchi (posterior aspect)

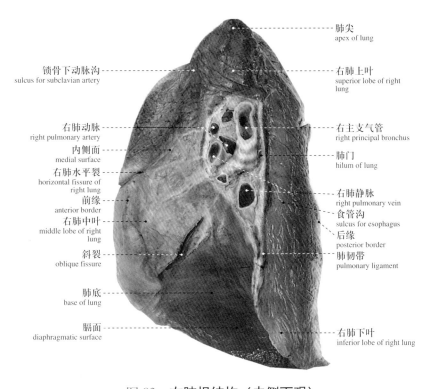

肺尖
apex of lung

锁骨下动脉沟
sulcus for subclavian artery

右肺上叶
superior lobe of right lung

右肺动脉
right pulmonary artery

右主支气管
right principal bronchus

内侧面
medial surface

肺门
hilum of lung

右肺水平裂
horizontal fissure of right lung

前缘
anterior border

右肺静脉
right pulmonary vein

食管沟
sulcus for esophagus

右肺中叶
middle lobe of right lung

后缘
posterior border

斜裂
oblique fissure

肺韧带
pulmonary ligament

肺底
base of lung

膈面
diaphragmatic surface

右肺下叶
inferior lobe of right lung

图 83 右肺根结构（内侧面观）
Structure of the right lung root (medial aspect)

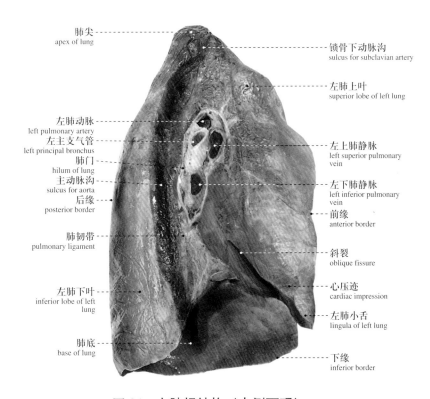

肺尖
apex of lung

锁骨下动脉沟
sulcus for subclavian artery

左肺上叶
superior lobe of left lung

左肺动脉
left pulmonary artery

左主支气管
left principal bronchus

肺门
hilum of lung

左上肺静脉
left superior pulmonary vein

主动脉沟
sulcus for aorta

后缘
posterior border

左下肺静脉
left inferior pulmonary vein

前缘
anterior border

肺韧带
pulmonary ligament

斜裂
oblique fissure

心压迹
cardiac impression

左肺下叶
inferior lobe of left lung

左肺小舌
lingula of left lung

肺底
base of lung

下缘
inferior border

图 84 左肺根结构（内侧面观）
Structure of the left lung root (medial aspect)

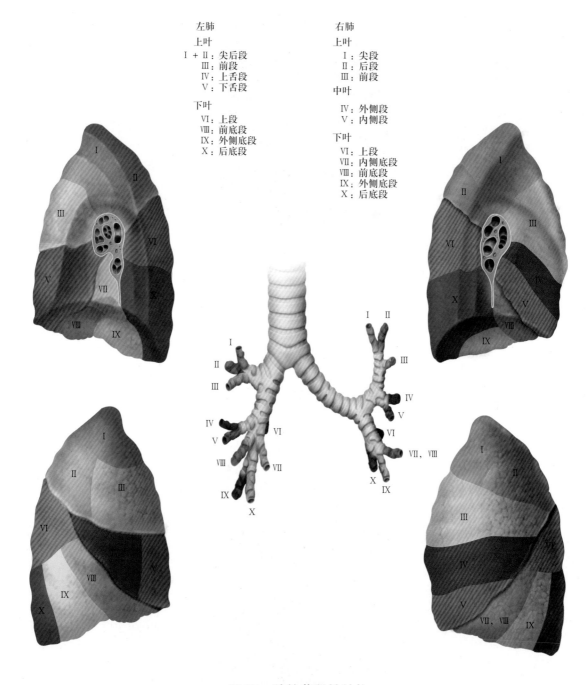

左肺
上叶
I + II：尖后段
III：前段
IV：上舌段
V：下舌段

下叶
VI：上段
VIII：前底段
IX：外侧底段
X：后底段

右肺
上叶
I：尖段
II：后段
III：前段
中叶
IV：外侧段
V：内侧段
下叶
VI：上段
VII：内侧底段
VIII：前底段
IX：外侧底段
X：后底段

图 85　肺的节段性结构
Segmental architecture of the lungs

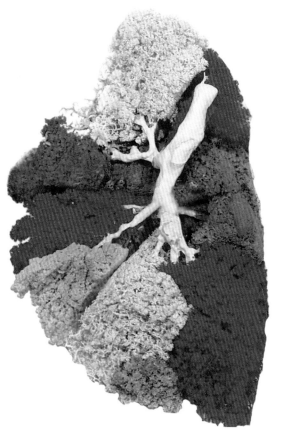

图 86　支气管肺段铸型（内面观）
Cast of the bronchopulmonary segments (medial aspect)

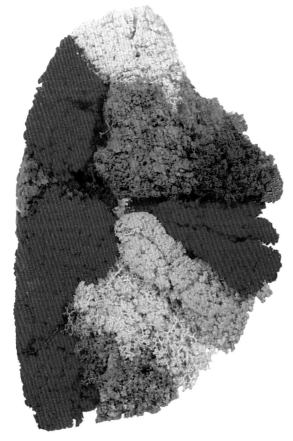

图 87　支气管肺段铸型（外面观）
Cast of the bronchopulmonary segments (lateral aspect)

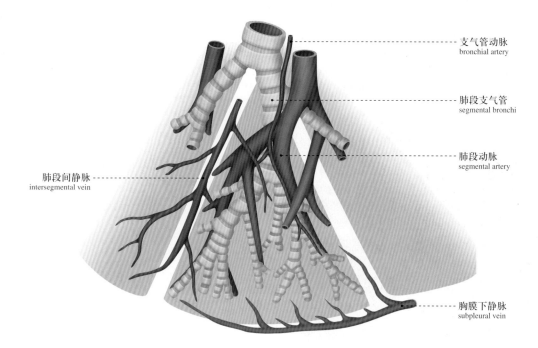

支气管动脉
bronchial artery

肺段支气管
segmental bronchi

肺段动脉
segmental artery

肺段间静脉
intersegmental vein

胸膜下静脉
subpleural vein

图 88　肺段内结构与肺段间静脉（模式图）
Structure of the lung segment and intersegmental vein (diagram)

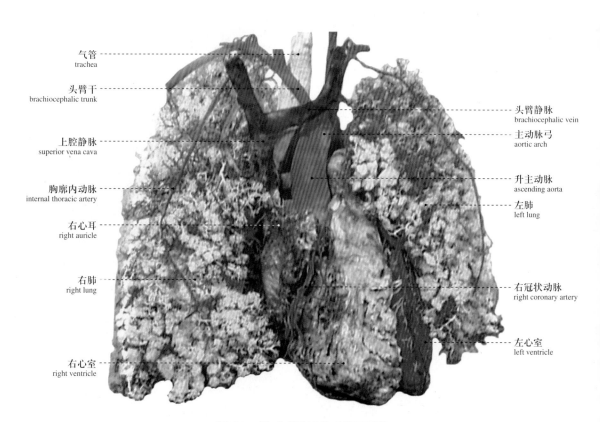

气管
trachea

头臂干
brachiocephalic trunk

上腔静脉
superior vena cava

胸廓内动脉
internal thoracic artery

右心耳
right auricle

右肺
right lung

右心室
right ventricle

头臂静脉
brachiocephalic vein

主动脉弓
aortic arch

升主动脉
ascending aorta

左肺
left lung

右冠状动脉
right coronary artery

左心室
left ventricle

图 89　肺血管铸型（前面观）
Cast of the blood vessels of the lung (anterior aspect)

第六节

纵 隔

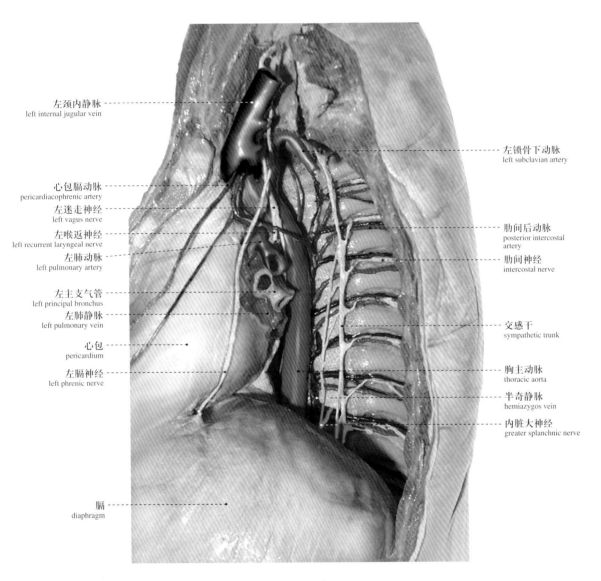

左颈内静脉
left internal jugular vein

左锁骨下动脉
left subclavian artery

心包膈动脉
pericardiacophrenic artery

左迷走神经
left vagus nerve

左喉返神经
left recurrent laryngeal nerve

肋间后动脉
posterior intercostal artery

左肺动脉
left pulmonary artery

肋间神经
intercostal nerve

左主支气管
left principal bronchus

左肺静脉
left pulmonary vein

交感干
sympathetic trunk

心包
pericardium

胸主动脉
thoracic aorta

左膈神经
left phrenic nerve

半奇静脉
hemiazygos vein

内脏大神经
greater splanchnic nerve

膈
diaphragm

图 90　纵隔（左面观）

Mediastinum (left aspect)

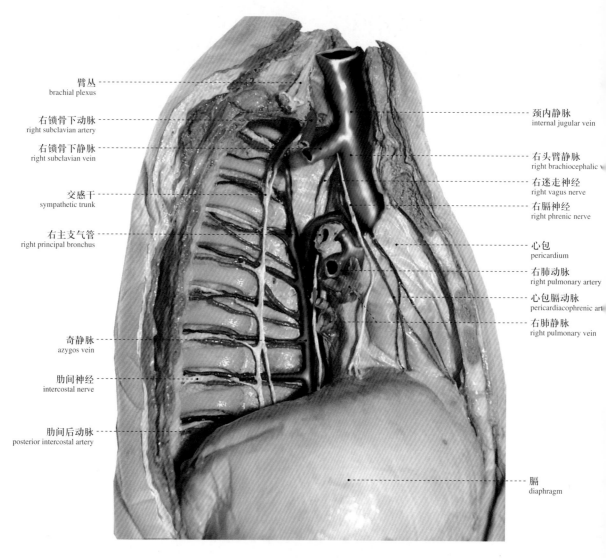

臂丛
brachial plexus

右锁骨下动脉
right subclavian artery

右锁骨下静脉
right subclavian vein

交感干
sympathetic trunk

右主支气管
right principal bronchus

奇静脉
azygos vein

肋间神经
intercostal nerve

肋间后动脉
posterior intercostal artery

颈内静脉
internal jugular vein

右头臂静脉
right brachiocephalic v

右迷走神经
right vagus nerve

右膈神经
right phrenic nerve

心包
pericardium

右肺动脉
right pulmonary artery

心包膈动脉
pericardiacophrenic art

右肺静脉
right pulmonary vein

膈
diaphragm

图 91　纵隔（右面观）
Mediastinum (right aspect)

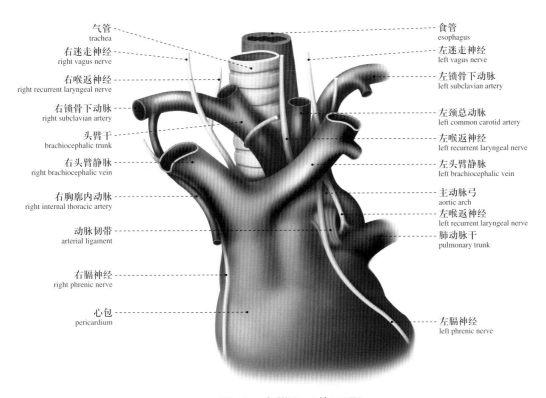

气管 trachea	食管 esophagus
右迷走神经 right vagus nerve	左迷走神经 left vagus nerve
右喉返神经 right recurrent laryngeal nerve	左锁骨下动脉 left subclavian artery
右锁骨下动脉 right subclavian artery	左颈总动脉 left common carotid artery
头臂干 brachiocephalic trunk	左喉返神经 left recurrent laryngeal nerve
右头臂静脉 right brachiocephalic vein	左头臂静脉 left brachiocephalic vein
右胸廓内动脉 right internal thoracic artery	主动脉弓 aortic arch
动脉韧带 arterial ligament	左喉返神经 left recurrent laryngeal nerve
	肺动脉干 pulmonary trunk
右膈神经 right phrenic nerve	
心包 pericardium	左膈神经 left phrenic nerve

图 92 上纵隔（前面观）
Superior mediastinum (anterior aspect)

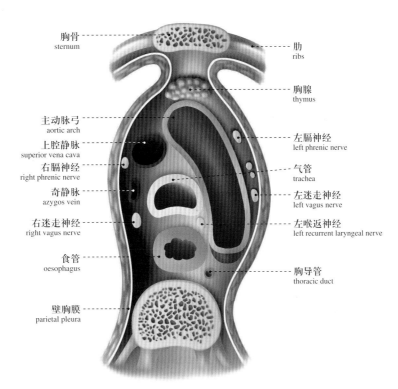

胸骨 sternum	肋 ribs
	胸腺 thymus
主动脉弓 aortic arch	左膈神经 left phrenic nerve
上腔静脉 superior vena cava	气管 trachea
右膈神经 right phrenic nerve	左迷走神经 left vagus nerve
奇静脉 azygos vein	左喉返神经 left recurrent laryngeal nerve
右迷走神经 right vagus nerve	
食管 oesophagus	胸导管 thoracic duct
壁胸膜 parietal pleura	

图 93 上纵隔（下面观，第 4 胸椎水平断面）
Superior mediastinum (inferior aspect, 4th thoracic horizontal section)

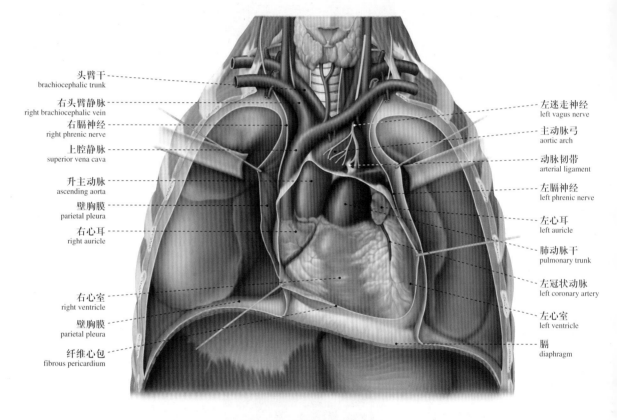

头臂干
brachiocephalic trunk

右头臂静脉
right brachiocephalic vein

右膈神经
right phrenic nerve

上腔静脉
superior vena cava

升主动脉
ascending aorta

壁胸膜
parietal pleura

右心耳
right auricle

右心室
right ventricle

壁胸膜
parietal pleura

纤维心包
fibrous pericardium

左迷走神经
left vagus nerve

主动脉弓
aortic arch

动脉韧带
arterial ligament

左膈神经
left phrenic nerve

左心耳
left auricle

肺动脉干
pulmonary trunk

左冠状动脉
left coronary artery

左心室
left ventricle

膈
diaphragm

图 94 纵隔（前面观）
Mediastinum (anterior aspect)

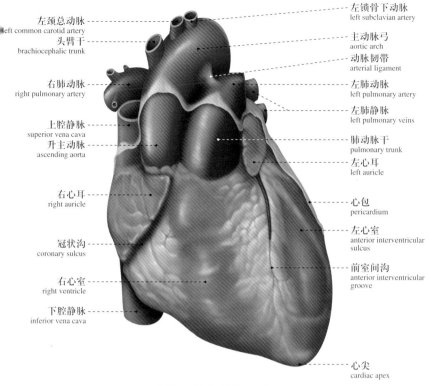

左颈总动脉
left common carotid artery

头臂干
brachiocephalic trunk

右肺动脉
right pulmonary artery

上腔静脉
superior vena cava

升主动脉
ascending aorta

右心耳
right auricle

冠状沟
coronary sulcus

右心室
right ventricle

下腔静脉
inferior vena cava

左锁骨下动脉
left subclavian artery

主动脉弓
aortic arch

动脉韧带
arterial ligament

左肺动脉
left pulmonary artery

左肺静脉
left pulmonary veins

肺动脉干
pulmonary trunk

左心耳
left auricle

心包
pericardium

左心室
anterior interventricular sulcus

前室间沟
anterior interventricular groove

心尖
cardiac apex

图 95　心脏的形状和结构（前面观）
Shape and structure of the heart (anterior aspect)

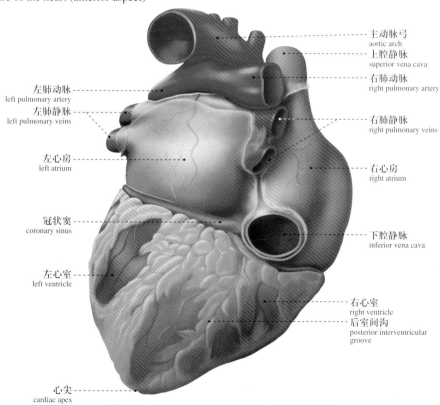

左肺动脉
left pulmonary artery

左肺静脉
left pulmonary veins

左心房
left atrium

冠状窦
coronary sinus

左心室
left ventricle

心尖
cardiac apex

主动脉弓
aortic arch

上腔静脉
superior vena cava

右肺动脉
right pulmonary artery

右肺静脉
right pulmonary veins

右心房
right atrium

下腔静脉
inferior vena cava

右心室
right ventricle

后室间沟
posterior interventricular groove

图 96　心脏的形状和结构（后下面观）
Shape and structure of the heart (posteroinferior aspect)

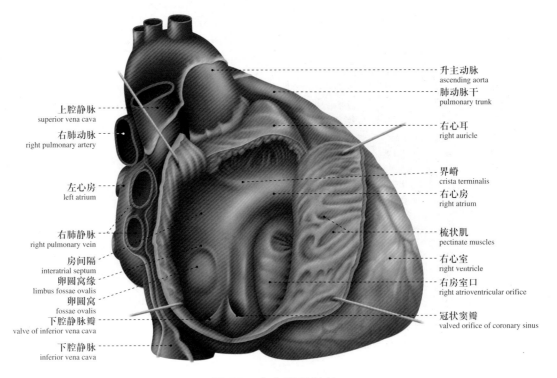

升主动脉
ascending aorta

肺动脉干
pulmonary trunk

右心耳
right auricle

界嵴
crista terminalis

右心房
right atrium

梳状肌
pectinate muscles

右心室
right ventricle

右房室口
right atrioventricular orifice

冠状窦瓣
valved orifice of coronary sinus

上腔静脉
superior vena cava

右肺动脉
right pulmonary artery

左心房
left atrium

右肺静脉
right pulmonary vein

房间隔
interatrial septum

卵圆窝缘
limbus fossae ovalis

卵圆窝
fossae ovalis

下腔静脉瓣
valve of inferior vena cava

下腔静脉
inferior vena cava

图 97　右心房的结构
Structure of right atrium

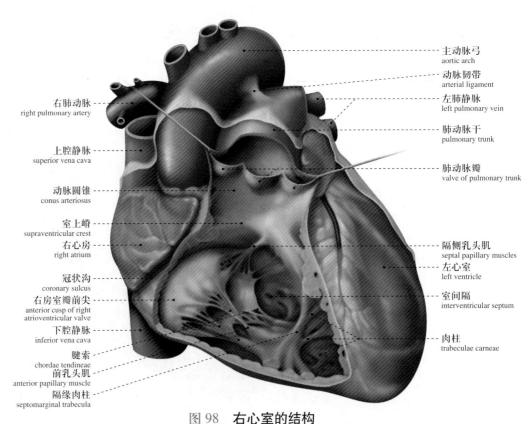

主动脉弓
aortic arch

动脉韧带
arterial ligament

左肺静脉
left pulmonary vein

肺动脉干
pulmonary trunk

肺动脉瓣
valve of pulmonary trunk

隔侧乳头肌
septal papillary muscles

左心室
left ventricle

室间隔
interventricular septum

肉柱
trabeculae carneae

右肺动脉
right pulmonary artery

上腔静脉
superior vena cava

动脉圆锥
conus arteriosus

室上嵴
supraventricular crest

右心房
right atrium

冠状沟
coronary sulcus

右房室瓣前尖
anterior cusp of right
atrioventricular valve

下腔静脉
inferior vena cava

腱索
chordae tendineae

前乳头肌
anterior papillary muscle

隔缘肉柱
septomarginal trabecula

图 98　右心室的结构
Structure of right ventricular

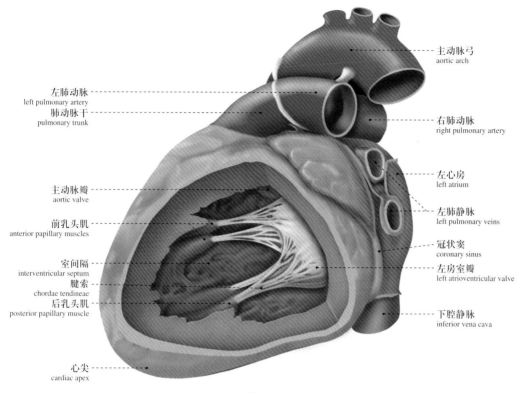

主动脉弓
aortic arch

左肺动脉
left pulmonary artery

肺动脉干
pulmonary trunk

右肺动脉
right pulmonary artery

左心房
left atrium

主动脉瓣
aortic valve

左肺静脉
left pulmonary veins

前乳头肌
anterior papillary muscles

冠状窦
coronary sinus

室间隔
interventricular septum

左房室瓣
left atrioventricular valve

腱索
chordae tendineae

后乳头肌
posterior papillary muscle

下腔静脉
inferior vena cava

心尖
cardiac apex

图 99 左心室的结构
Structure of left ventricular

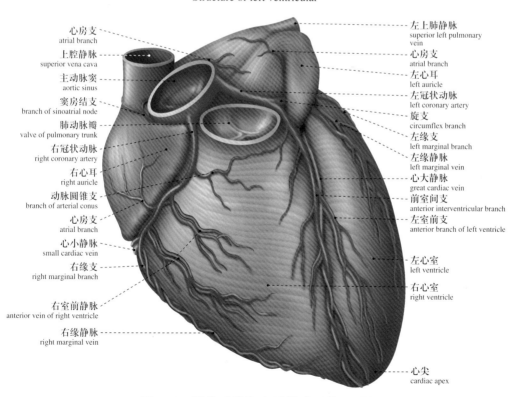

心房支
atrial branch

左上肺静脉
superior left pulmonary vein

上腔静脉
superior vena cava

心房支
atrial branch

主动脉窦
aortic sinus

左心耳
left auricle

窦房结支
branch of sinoatrial node

左冠状动脉
left coronary artery

肺动脉瓣
valve of pulmonary trunk

旋支
circumflex branch

右冠状动脉
right coronary artery

左缘支
left marginal branch

右心耳
right auricle

左缘静脉
left marginal vein

动脉圆锥支
branch of arterial conus

心大静脉
great cardiac vein

心房支
atrial branch

前室间支
anterior interventricular branch

心小静脉
small cardiac vein

左室前支
anterior branch of left ventricle

右缘支
right marginal branch

左心室
left ventricle

右室前静脉
anterior vein of right ventricle

右心室
right ventricle

右缘静脉
right marginal vein

心尖
cardiac apex

图 100 冠状动脉和心脏静脉（前面观）
Coronary arteries and cardiac veins (anterior aspect)

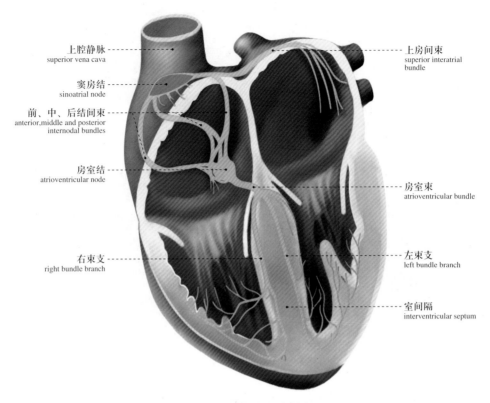

上腔静脉
superior vena cava

窦房结
sinoatrial node

前、中、后结间束
anterior,middle and posterior
internodal bundles

房室结
atrioventricular node

右束支
right bundle branch

上房间束
superior interatrial
bundle

房室束
atrioventricular bundle

左束支
left bundle branch

室间隔
interventricular septum

图 101　心传导系统（前面观）

Conduction system of heart (anterior aspect)

主动脉弓
aortic arch

上腔静脉
superior vena cava

窦房结
sinoatrial node

左束支
left bundle branch

房室束
atrioventricular bundle

房室结
atrioventricular node

浦肯野纤维
Purkinje fibers

肺动脉干
pulmonary trunk

室间隔
interventricular septum

右束支
right bundle branch

右心室
right ventricle

隔缘肉柱
septomarginal trabecula

前乳头肌
anterior papillary muscle

图 102　心传导系统（右侧面观）

Conduction system of heart (right lateral aspect)

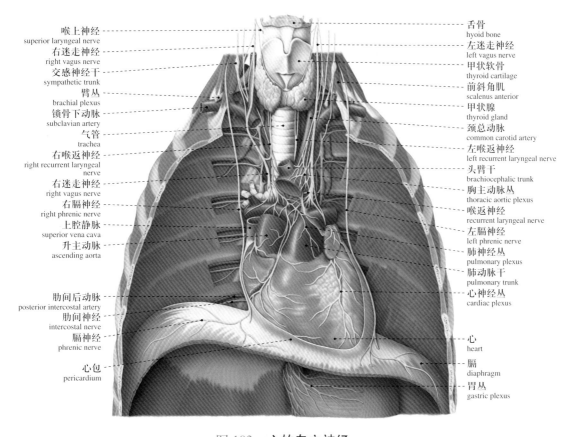

喉上神经
superior laryngeal nerve
右迷走神经
right vagus nerve
交感神经干
sympathetic trunk
臂丛
brachial plexus
锁骨下动脉
subclavian artery
气管
trachea
右喉返神经
right recurrent laryngeal
nerve
右迷走神经
right vagus nerve
右膈神经
right phrenic nerve
上腔静脉
superior vena cava
升主动脉
ascending aorta
肋间后动脉
posterior intercostal artery
肋间神经
intercostal nerve
膈神经
phrenic nerve
心包
pericardium

舌骨
hyoid bone
左迷走神经
left vagus nerve
甲状软骨
thyroid cartilage
前斜角肌
scalenus anterior
甲状腺
thyroid gland
颈总动脉
common carotid artery
左喉返神经
left recurrent laryngeal nerve
头臂干
brachiocephalic trunk
胸主动脉丛
thoracic aortic plexus
喉返神经
recurrent laryngeal nerve
左膈神经
left phrenic nerve
肺神经丛
pulmonary plexus
肺动脉干
pulmonary trunk
心神经丛
cardiac plexus
心
heart
膈
diaphragm
胃丛
gastric plexus

图 103　心的自主神经

Autonomic nerves of the heart

主动脉
aorta
上腔静脉
superior vena cava
主动脉瓣听诊区
aortic auscultation area
主动脉瓣
aortic valve
三尖瓣
tricuspid valve
三尖瓣听诊区
tricuspid auscultation
area

肺动脉瓣听诊区
pulmonary auscultation area
肺动脉干
pulmonary trunk
肺动脉瓣
valve of pulmonary trunk
二尖瓣
mitral valve
二尖瓣听诊区
mitral auscultation area

图 104　心瓣膜的体表投影

Surface projection of the valves of the heart

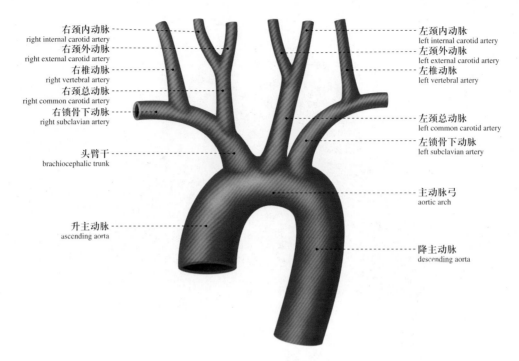

右颈内动脉
right internal carotid artery
右颈外动脉
right external carotid artery
右椎动脉
right vertebral artery
右颈总动脉
right common carotid artery
右锁骨下动脉
right subclavian artery
头臂干
brachiocephalic trunk
升主动脉
ascending aorta

左颈内动脉
left internal carotid artery
左颈外动脉
left external carotid artery
左椎动脉
left vertebral artery
左颈总动脉
left common carotid artery
左锁骨下动脉
left subclavian artery
主动脉弓
aortic arch
降主动脉
descending aorta

图 105　主动脉弓及其分支
Aortic arch and its branches

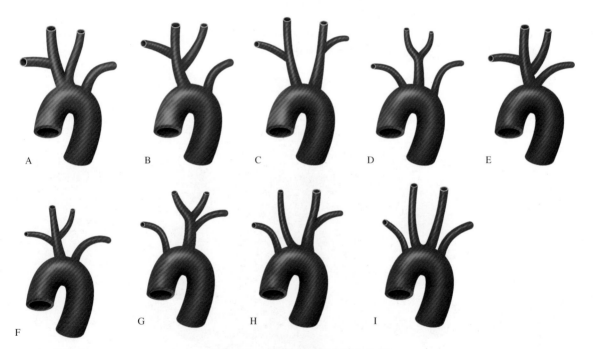

图 106　主动脉弓主要分支变异
Variation of the main branch of the aortic arch

A. 右头臂干与左颈总动脉共干（13%）；B. 左颈总动脉由右头臂干发出（9%）；C. 左、右 2 条头臂干（＜1%）；D. 两侧颈总动脉共干（＜0.1%）；E. 右头臂干与左颈总、左锁骨下动脉共干，形成 1 条头臂动脉干（＜0.1%）；F. 左、右颈总动脉共干并发出右锁骨下动脉（＜0.1%）；G. 左、右颈总动脉共干并发出左锁骨下动脉（＜0.1%）；H. 左头臂干形成，右颈总动脉、右锁骨下动脉独立起自主动脉弓（＜0.1%）；I. 无头臂干，各分支独立起自主动脉弓（＜0.1%）

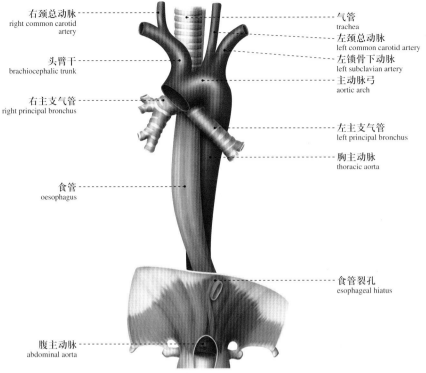

右颈总动脉
right common carotid artery

头臂干
brachiocephalic trunk

右主支气管
right principal bronchus

食管
oesophagus

腹主动脉
abdominal aorta

气管
trachea

左颈总动脉
left common carotid artery

左锁骨下动脉
left subclavian artery

主动脉弓
aortic arch

左主支气管
left principal bronchus

胸主动脉
thoracic aorta

食管裂孔
esophageal hiatus

图 107　食管与胸主动脉（前面观）
Esophagus and thoracic aorta (anterior aspect)

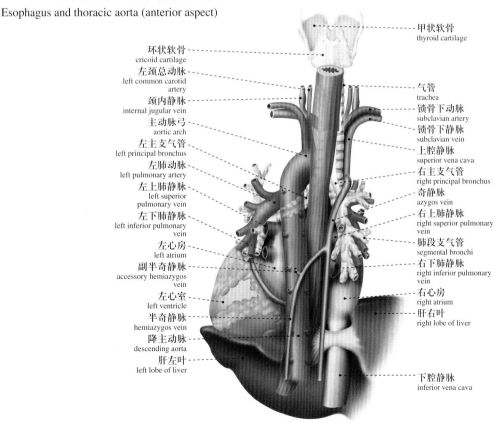

环状软骨
cricoid cartilage

左颈总动脉
left common carotid artery

颈内静脉
internal jugular vein

主动脉弓
aortic arch

左主支气管
left principal bronchus

左肺动脉
left pulmonary artery

左上肺静脉
left superior pulmonary vein

左下肺静脉
left inferior pulmonary vein

左心房
left atrium

副半奇静脉
accessory hemiazygos vein

左心室
left ventricle

半奇静脉
hemiazygos vein

降主动脉
descending aorta

肝左叶
left lobe of liver

甲状软骨
thyroid cartilage

气管
trachea

锁骨下动脉
subclavian artery

锁骨下静脉
subclavian vein

上腔静脉
superior vena cava

右主支气管
right principal bronchus

奇静脉
azygos vein

右上肺静脉
right superior pulmonary vein

肺段支气管
segmental bronchi

右下肺静脉
right inferior pulmonary vein

右心房
right atrium

肝右叶
right lobe of liver

下腔静脉
inferior vena cava

图 108　食管周围血管（后面观）
Vascular around esophageal (posterior aspect)

第七节

胸部断面

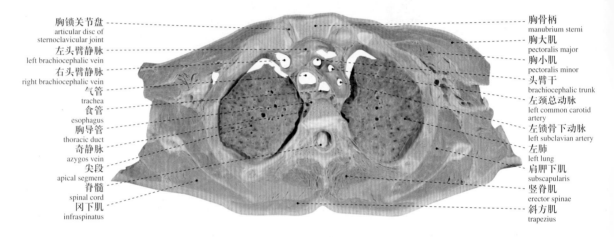

胸锁关节盘
articular disc of
sternoclavicular joint
左头臂静脉
left brachiocephalic vein
右头臂静脉
right brachiocephalic vein
气管
trachea
食管
esophagus
胸导管
thoracic duct
奇静脉
azygos vein
尖段
apical segment
脊髓
spinal cord
冈下肌
infraspinatus

胸骨柄
manubrium sterni
胸大肌
pectoralis major
胸小肌
pectoralis minor
头臂干
brachiocephalic trunk
左颈总动脉
left common carotid
artery
左锁骨下动脉
left subclavian artery
左肺
left lung
肩胛下肌
subscapularis
竖脊肌
erector spinae
斜方肌
trapezius

图 109　胸部水平断面 1

Horizontal section of the thorax 1

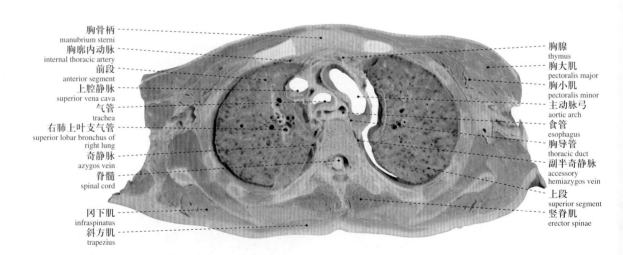

胸骨柄
manubrium sterni
胸廓内动脉
internal thoracic artery
前段
anterior segment
上腔静脉
superior vena cava
气管
trachea
右肺上叶支气管
superior lobar bronchus of
right lung
奇静脉
azygos vein
脊髓
spinal cord
冈下肌
infraspinatus
斜方肌
trapezius

胸腺
thymus
胸大肌
pectoralis major
胸小肌
pectoralis minor
主动脉弓
aortic arch
食管
esophagus
胸导管
thoracic duct
副半奇静脉
accessory
hemiazygos vein
上段
superior segment
竖脊肌
erector spinae

图 110　胸部水平断面 2

Horizontal section of the thorax 2

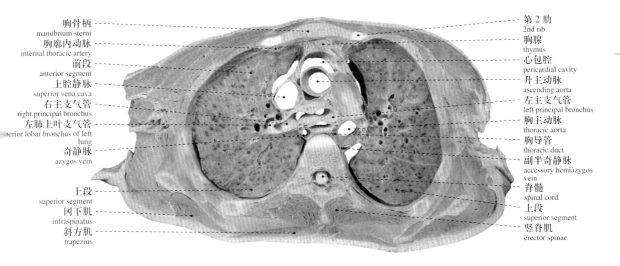

胸骨柄
manubrium sterni
胸廓内动脉
internal thoracic artery
前段
anterior segment
上腔静脉
superior vena cava
右主支气管
right principal bronchus
左肺上叶支气管
superior lobar bronchus of left lung
奇静脉
azygos vein
上段
superior segment
冈下肌
infraspinatus
斜方肌
trapezius

第 2 肋
2nd rib
胸腺
thymus
心包腔
pericardial cavity
升主动脉
ascending aorta
左主支气管
left principal bronchus
胸主动脉
thoracic aorta
胸导管
thoracic duct
副半奇静脉
accessory hemiazygos vein
脊髓
spinal cord
上段
superior segment
竖脊肌
erector spinae

图 111　胸部水平断面 3
Horizontal section of the thorax 3

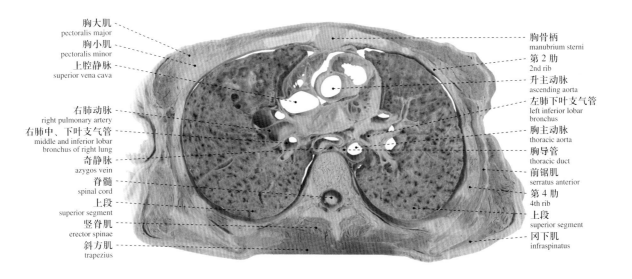

胸大肌
pectoralis major
胸小肌
pectoralis minor
上腔静脉
superior vena cava
右肺动脉
right pulmonary artery
右肺中、下叶支气管
middle and inferior lobar bronchus of right lung
奇静脉
azygos vein
脊髓
spinal cord
上段
superior segment
竖脊肌
erector spinae
斜方肌
trapezius

胸骨柄
manubrium sterni
第 2 肋
2nd rib
升主动脉
ascending aorta
左肺下叶支气管
left inferior lobar bronchus
胸主动脉
thoracic aorta
胸导管
thoracic duct
前锯肌
serratus anterior
第 4 肋
4th rib
上段
superior segment
冈下肌
infraspinatus

图 112　胸部水平断面 4
Horizontal section of the thorax 4

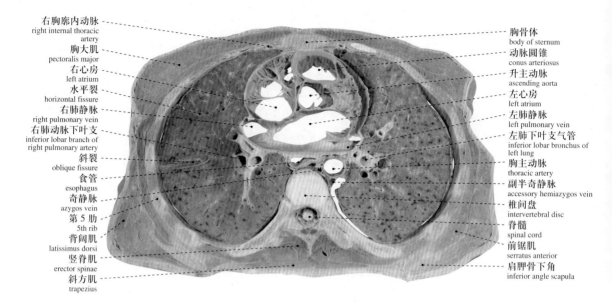

右胸廓内动脉 right internal thoracic artery
胸大肌 pectoralis major
右心房 left atrium
水平裂 horizontal fissure
右肺静脉 right pulmonary vein
右肺动脉下叶支 inferior lobar branch of right pulmonary artery
斜裂 oblique fissure
食管 esophagus
奇静脉 azygos vein
第 5 肋 5th rib
背阔肌 latissimus dorsi
竖脊肌 erector spinae
斜方肌 trapezius

胸骨体 body of sternum
动脉圆锥 conus arteriosus
升主动脉 ascending aorta
左心房 left atrium
左肺静脉 left pulmonary vein
左肺下叶支气管 inferior lobar bronchus of left lung
胸主动脉 thoracic artery
副半奇静脉 accessory hemiazygos vein
椎间盘 intervertebral disc
脊髓 spinal cord
前锯肌 serratus anterior
肩胛骨下角 inferior angle scapula

图 113　胸部水平断面 5

Horizontal section of the thorax 5

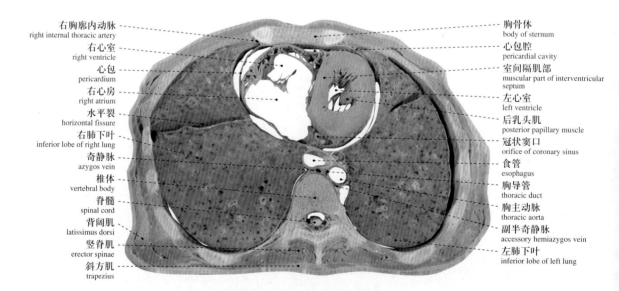

右胸廓内动脉 right internal thoracic artery
右心室 right ventricle
心包 pericardium
右心房 right atrium
水平裂 horizontal fissure
右肺下叶 inferior lobe of right lung
奇静脉 azygos vein
椎体 vertebral body
脊髓 spinal cord
背阔肌 latissimus dorsi
竖脊肌 erector spinae
斜方肌 trapezius

胸骨体 body of sternum
心包腔 pericardial cavity
室间隔肌部 muscular part of interventricular septum
左心室 left ventricle
后乳头肌 posterior papillary muscle
冠状窦口 orifice of coronary sinus
食管 esophagus
胸导管 thoracic duct
胸主动脉 thoracic aorta
副半奇静脉 accessory hemiazygos vein
左肺下叶 inferior lobe of left lung

图 114　胸部水平断面 6

Horizontal section of the thorax 6

第一节

腹部分区及常用手术切口

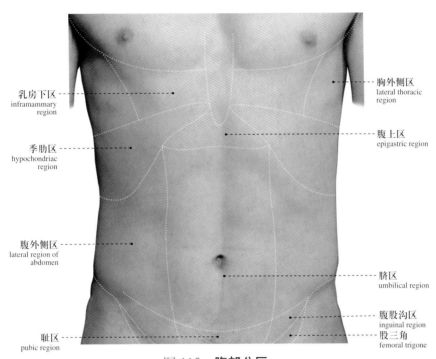

乳房下区
inframammary region

季肋区
hypochondriac region

腹外侧区
lateral region of abdomen

耻区
pubic region

胸外侧区
lateral thoracic region

腹上区
epigastric region

脐区
umbilical region

腹股沟区
inguinal region

股三角
femoral trigone

图 115　腹部分区
Regions of the abdomen

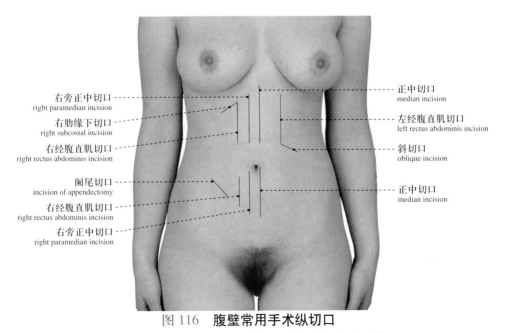

右旁正中切口
right paramedian incision

右肋缘下切口
right subcostal incision

右经腹直肌切口
right rectus abdominis incision

阑尾切口
incision of appendectomy

右经腹直肌切口
right rectus abdominis incision

右旁正中切口
right paramedian incision

正中切口
median incision

左经腹直肌切口
left rectus abdominis incision

斜切口
oblique incision

正中切口
median incision

图 116　腹壁常用手术纵切口
Common vertical surgical incision of the abdominal wall

腹前外侧壁

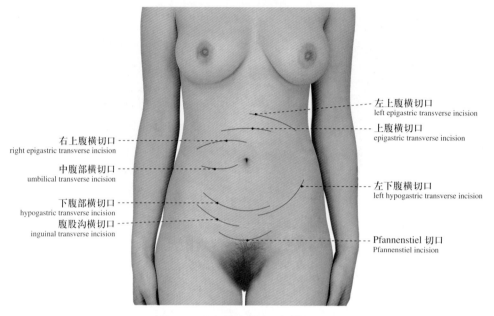

左上腹横切口
left epigastric transverse incision

上腹横切口
epigastric transverse incision

右上腹横切口
right epigastric transverse incision

中腹部横切口
umbilical transverse incision

左下腹横切口
left hypogastric transverse incision

下腹部横切口
hypogastric transverse incision

腹股沟横切口
inguinal transverse incision

Pfannenstiel 切口
Pfannenstiel incision

图 117　腹壁常用手术横切口
Common transverse surgical incision of the abdominal wall

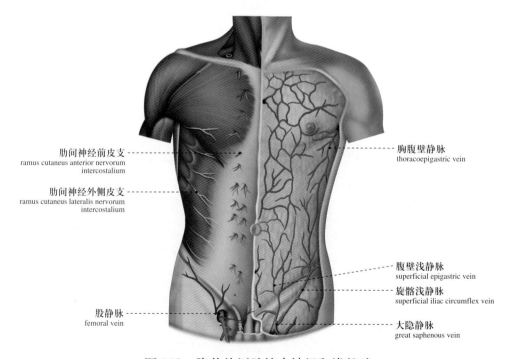

肋间神经前皮支
ramus cutaneus anterior nervorum intercostalium

肋间神经外侧皮支
ramus cutaneus lateralis nervorum intercostalium

股静脉
femoral vein

胸腹壁静脉
thoracoepigastric vein

腹壁浅静脉
superficial epigastric vein

旋髂浅静脉
superficial iliac circumflex vein

大隐静脉
great saphenous vein

图 118　腹前外侧壁的皮神经和浅静脉
Cutaneous nerves and superficial veins of the anterolateral abdominal wall

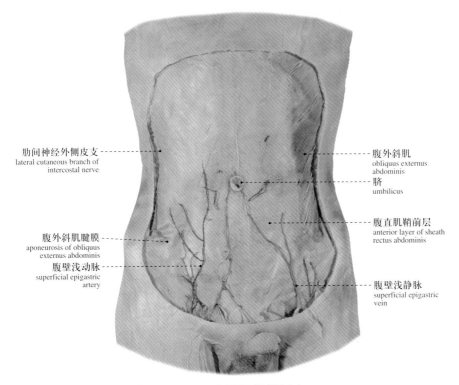

肋间神经外侧皮支
lateral cutaneous branch of
intercostal nerve

腹外斜肌
obliquus externus
abdominis

脐
umbilicus

腹外斜肌腱膜
aponeurosis of obliquus
externus abdominis

腹壁浅动脉
superficial epigastric
artery

腹直肌鞘前层
anterior layer of sheath
rectus abdominis

腹壁浅静脉
superficial epigastric
vein

图 119 腹部局部解剖 1
Topography of the abdomen 1

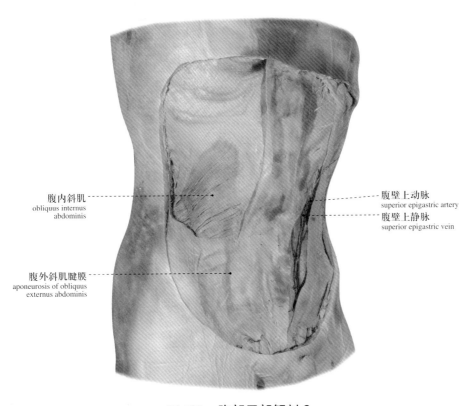

腹内斜肌
obliquus internus
abdominis

腹外斜肌腱膜
aponeurosis of obliquus
externus abdominis

腹壁上动脉
superior epigastric artery

腹壁上静脉
superior epigastric vein

图 120 腹部局部解剖 2
Topography of the abdomen 2

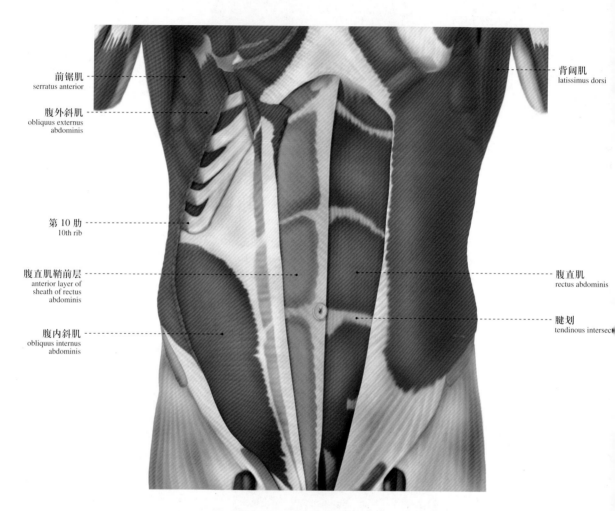

前锯肌
serratus anterior

背阔肌
latissimus dorsi

腹外斜肌
obliquus externus
abdominis

第 10 肋
10th rib

腹直肌鞘前层
anterior layer of
sheath of rectus
abdominis

腹直肌
rectus abdominis

腱划
tendinous intersec

腹内斜肌
obliquus internus
abdominis

图 121　腹肌（前面观）
Muscles of the abdomen (anterior aspect)

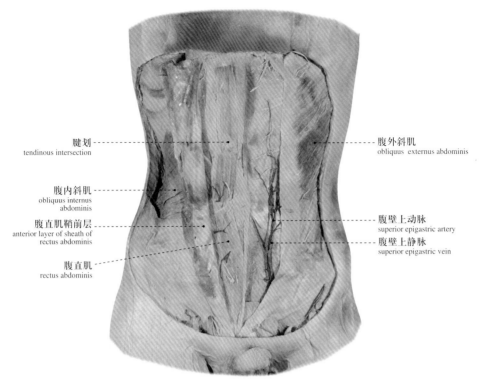

腱划
tendinous intersection

腹外斜肌
obliquus externus abdominis

腹内斜肌
obliquus internus
abdominis

腹直肌鞘前层
anterior layer of sheath of
rectus abdominis

腹壁上动脉
superior epigastric artery

腹壁上静脉
superior epigastric vein

腹直肌
rectus abdominis

图 122　腹部局部解剖 3
Topography of the abdomen 3

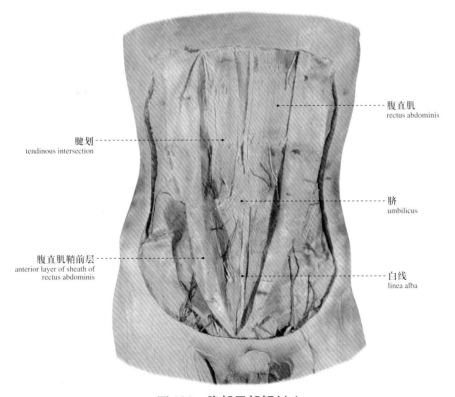

腹直肌
rectus abdominis

腱划
tendinous intersection

脐
umbilicus

腹直肌鞘前层
anterior layer of sheath of
rectus abdominis

白线
linea alba

图 123　腹部局部解剖 4
Topography of the abdomen 4

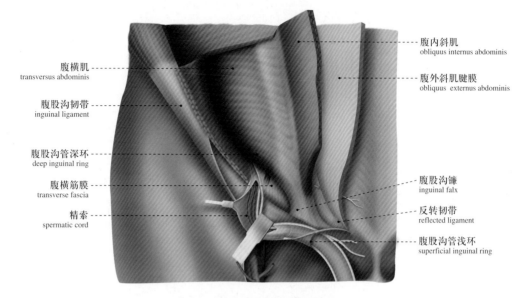

腹横肌
transversus abdominis

腹股沟韧带
inguinal ligament

腹股沟管深环
deep inguinal ring

腹横筋膜
transverse fascia

精索
spermatic cord

腹内斜肌
obliquus internus abdominis

腹外斜肌腱膜
obliquus externus abdominis

腹股沟镰
inguinal falx

反转韧带
reflected ligament

腹股沟管浅环
superficial inguinal ring

图 124　腹股沟区的深层结构
Deep structure of the inguinal region

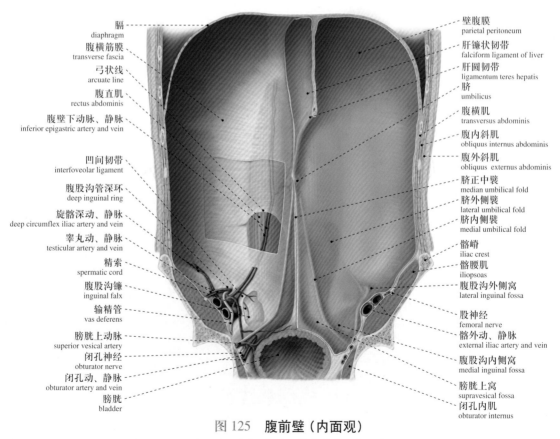

膈
diaphragm

腹横筋膜
transverse fascia

弓状线
arcuate line

腹直肌
rectus abdominis

腹壁下动脉、静脉
inferior epigastric artery and vein

凹间韧带
interfoveolar ligament

腹股沟管深环
deep inguinal ring

旋髂深动、静脉
deep circumflex iliac artery and vein

睾丸动、静脉
testicular artery and vein

精索
spermatic cord

腹股沟镰
inguinal falx

输精管
vas deferens

膀胱上动脉
superior vesical artery

闭孔神经
obturator nerve

闭孔动、静脉
obturator artery and vein

膀胱
bladder

壁腹膜
parietal peritoneum

肝镰状韧带
falciform ligament of liver

肝圆韧带
ligamentum teres hepatis

脐
umbilicus

腹横肌
transversus abdominis

腹内斜肌
obliquus internus abdominis

腹外斜肌
obliquus externus abdominis

脐正中襞
median umbilical fold

脐外侧襞
lateral umbilical fold

脐内侧襞
medial umbilical fold

髂嵴
iliac crest

髂腰肌
iliopsoas

腹股沟外侧窝
lateral inguinal fossa

股神经
femoral nerve

髂外动、静脉
external iliac artery and vein

腹股沟内侧窝
medial inguinal fossa

膀胱上窝
supravesical fossa

闭孔内肌
obturator internus

图 125　腹前壁（内面观）
Anterior abdominal wall (inferior aspect)

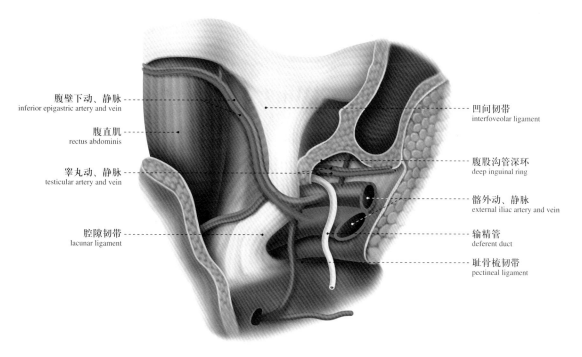

腹壁下动、静脉
inferior epigastric artery and vein

腹直肌
rectus abdominis

睾丸动、静脉
testicular artery and vein

腔隙韧带
lacunar ligament

凹间韧带
interfoveolar ligament

腹股沟管深环
deep inguinal ring

髂外动、静脉
external iliac artery and vein

输精管
deferent duct

耻骨梳韧带
pectineal ligament

图 126　腹股沟区（内面观）
Inguinal region (inferior aspect)

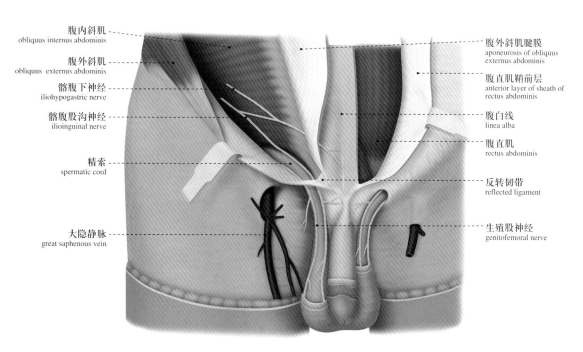

腹内斜肌
obliquus internus abdominis

腹外斜肌
obliquus externus abdominis

髂腹下神经
iliohypogastric nerve

髂腹股沟神经
ilioinguinal nerve

精索
spermatic cord

大隐静脉
great saphenous vein

腹外斜肌腱膜
aponeurosis of obliquus externus abdominis

腹直肌鞘前层
anterior layer of sheath of rectus abdominis

腹白线
linea alba

腹直肌
rectus abdominis

反转韧带
reflected ligament

生殖股神经
genitofemoral nerve

图 127　腹股沟管（外面观）
Inguinal canal (outside aspect)

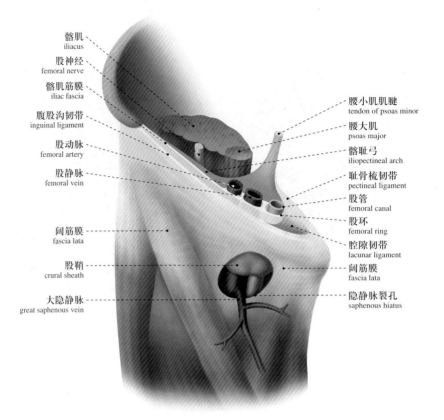

髂肌
iliacus

股神经
femoral nerve

髂肌筋膜
iliac fascia

腹股沟韧带
inguinal ligament

股动脉
femoral artery

股静脉
femoral vein

阔筋膜
fascia lata

股鞘
crural sheath

大隐静脉
great saphenous vein

腰小肌肌腱
tendon of psoas minor

腰大肌
psoas major

髂耻弓
iliopectineal arch

耻骨梳韧带
pectineal ligament

股管
femoral canal

股环
femoral ring

腔隙韧带
lacunar ligament

阔筋膜
fascia lata

隐静脉裂孔
saphenous hiatus

图 128　**股鞘**

Femoral sheath

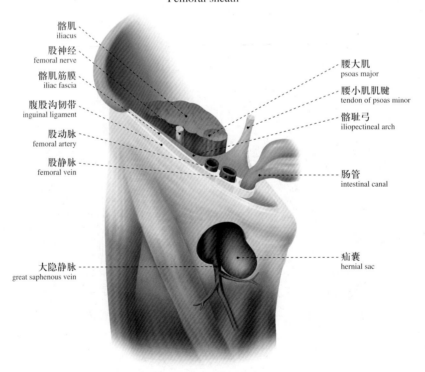

髂肌
iliacus

股神经
femoral nerve

髂肌筋膜
iliac fascia

腹股沟韧带
inguinal ligament

股动脉
femoral artery

股静脉
femoral vein

大隐静脉
great saphenous vein

腰大肌
psoas major

腰小肌肌腱
tendon of psoas minor

髂耻弓
iliopectineal arch

肠管
intestinal canal

疝囊
hernial sac

图 129　**股疝**

Femoral hernia

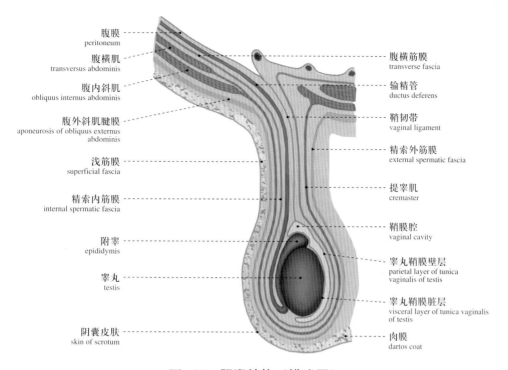

腹膜
peritoneum

腹横肌
transversus abdominis

腹内斜肌
obliquus internus abdominis

腹外斜肌腱膜
aponeurosis of obliquus externus abdominis

浅筋膜
superficial fascia

精索内筋膜
internal spermatic fascia

附睾
epididymis

睾丸
testis

阴囊皮肤
skin of scrotum

腹横筋膜
transverse fascia

输精管
ductus deferens

鞘韧带
vaginal ligament

精索外筋膜
external spermatic fascia

提睾肌
cremaster

鞘膜腔
vaginal cavity

睾丸鞘膜壁层
parietal layer of tunica vaginalis of testis

睾丸鞘膜脏层
visceral layer of tunica vaginalis of testis

肉膜
dartos coat

图 130　阴囊结构（模式图）
Structure of the scrotum (diagram)

腹膜腔
peritoneal cavity

鞘韧带
vaginal ligament

鞘膜腔
cavity of tunica vaginalis

睾丸系带
testicular lace

图 131　睾丸下降
Orchiocatabasis

67

第三节

结肠上区

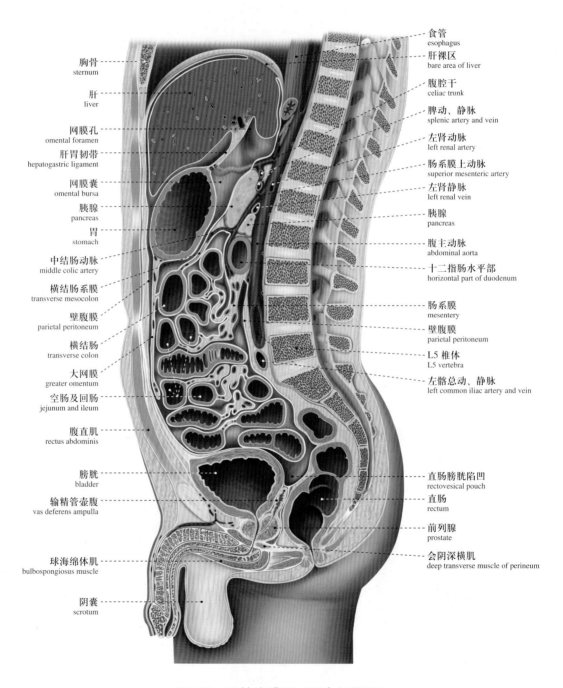

胸骨
sternum

肝
liver

网膜孔
omental foramen

肝胃韧带
hepatogastric ligament

网膜囊
omental bursa

胰腺
pancreas

胃
stomach

中结肠动脉
middle colic artery

横结肠系膜
transverse mesocolon

壁腹膜
parietal peritoneum

横结肠
transverse colon

大网膜
greater omentum

空肠及回肠
jejunum and ileum

腹直肌
rectus abdominis

膀胱
bladder

输精管壶腹
vas deferens ampulla

球海绵体肌
bulbospongiosus muscle

阴囊
scrotum

食管
esophagus

肝裸区
bare area of liver

腹腔干
celiac trunk

脾动、静脉
splenic artery and vein

左肾动脉
left renal artery

肠系膜上动脉
superior mesenteric artery

左肾静脉
left renal vein

胰腺
pancreas

腹主动脉
abdominal aorta

十二指肠水平部
horizontal part of duodenum

肠系膜
mesentery

壁腹膜
parietal peritoneum

L5 椎体
L5 vertebra

左髂总动、静脉
left common iliac artery and vein

直肠膀胱陷凹
rectovesical pouch

直肠
rectum

前列腺
prostate

会阴深横肌
deep transverse muscle of perineum

图 132　男性腹膜腔（正中矢状断）
Male peritoneal cavity (median sagittal aspect)

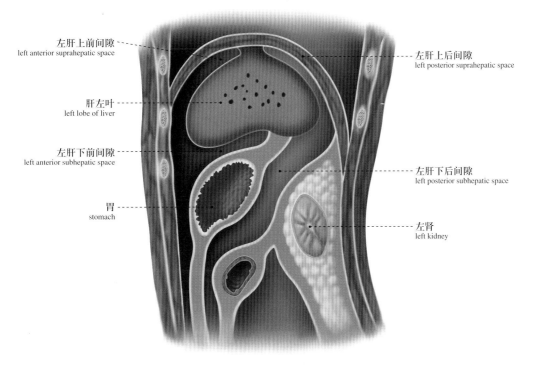

左肝上前间隙
left anterior suprahepatic space

肝左叶
left lobe of liver

左肝下前间隙
left anterior subhepatic space

胃
stomach

左肝上后间隙
left posterior suprahepatic space

左肝下后间隙
left posterior subhepatic space

左肾
left kidney

A

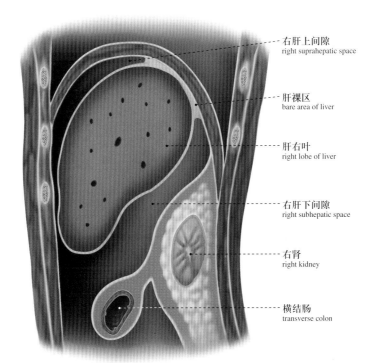

右肝上间隙
right suprahepatic space

肝裸区
bare area of liver

肝右叶
right lobe of liver

右肝下间隙
right subhepatic space

右肾
right kidney

横结肠
transverse colon

B

图 133　结肠上区的间隙
Space of superior region of colon
A. 肝左侧；B. 肝右侧

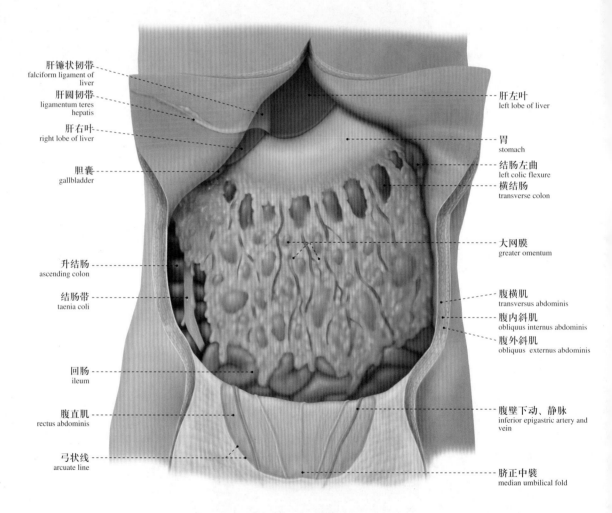

肝镰状韧带
falciform ligament of liver

肝圆韧带
ligamentum teres hepatis

肝右叶
right lobe of liver

胆囊
gallbladder

升结肠
ascending colon

结肠带
taenia coli

回肠
ileum

腹直肌
rectus abdominis

弓状线
arcuate line

肝左叶
left lobe of liver

胃
stomach

结肠左曲
left colic flexure

横结肠
transverse colon

大网膜
greater omentum

腹横肌
transversus abdominis

腹内斜肌
obliquus internus abdominis

腹外斜肌
obliquus externus abdominis

腹壁下动、静脉
inferior epigastric artery and vein

脐正中襞
median umbilical fold

图 134　网膜
Omentum

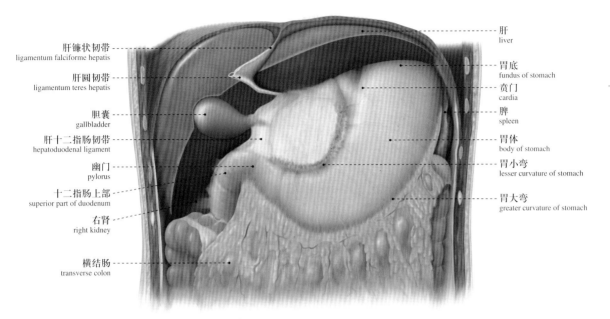

肝镰状韧带
ligamentum falciforme hepatis

肝圆韧带
ligamentum teres hepatis

胆囊
gallbladder

肝十二指肠韧带
hepatoduodenal ligament

幽门
pylorus

十二指肠上部
superior part of duodenum

右肾
right kidney

横结肠
transverse colon

肝
liver

胃底
fundus of stomach

贲门
cardia

脾
spleen

胃体
body of stomach

胃小弯
lesser curvature of stomach

胃大弯
greater curvature of stomach

图 135　结肠上区
Superior region of colon

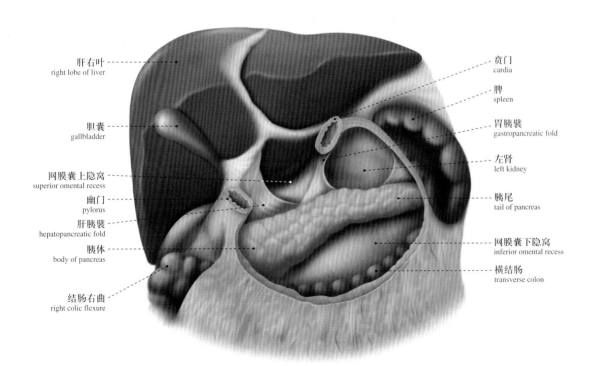

肝右叶
right lobe of liver

胆囊
gallbladder

网膜囊上隐窝
superior omental recess

幽门
pylorus

肝胰襞
hepatopancreatic fold

胰体
body of pancreas

结肠右曲
right colic flexure

贲门
cardia

脾
spleen

胃胰襞
gastropancreatic fold

左肾
left kidney

胰尾
tail of pancreas

网膜囊下隐窝
inferior omental recess

横结肠
transverse colon

图 136　胃胰襞和肝胰襞
Gastropancreatic fold and hepatopancreatic fold

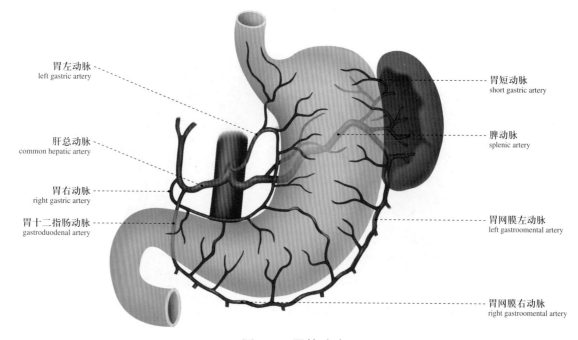

左胃动脉
left gastric artery

肝总动脉
common hepatic artery

胃右动脉
right gastric artery

胃十二指肠动脉
gastroduodenal artery

胃短动脉
short gastric artery

脾动脉
splenic artery

胃网膜左动脉
left gastroomental artery

胃网膜右动脉
right gastroomental artery

图 137　胃的动脉
Gastric arteries

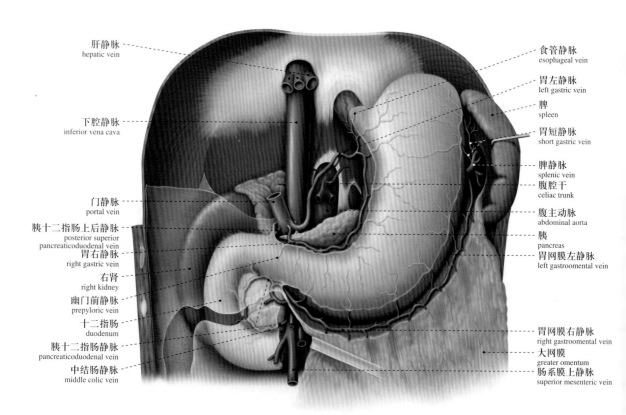

肝静脉
hepatic vein

下腔静脉
inferior vena cava

门静脉
portal vein

胰十二指肠上后静脉
posterior superior pancreaticoduodenal vein

胃右静脉
right gastric vein

右肾
right kidney

幽门前静脉
prepyloric vein

十二指肠
duodenum

胰十二指肠静脉
pancreaticoduodenal vein

中结肠静脉
middle colic vein

食管静脉
esophageal vein

胃左静脉
left gastric vein

脾
spleen

胃短静脉
short gastric vein

脾静脉
splenic vein

腹腔干
celiac trunk

腹主动脉
abdominal aorta

胰
pancreas

胃网膜左静脉
left gastroomental vein

胃网膜右静脉
right gastroomental vein

大网膜
greater omentum

肠系膜上静脉
superior mesenteric vein

图 138　胃的静脉
Gastric veins

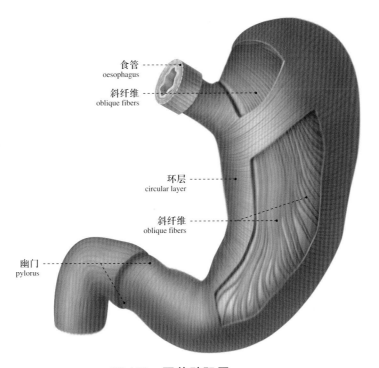

食管
oesophagus

斜纤维
oblique fibers

环层
circular layer

斜纤维
oblique fibers

幽门
pylorus

图 139　**胃前壁肌层**
Muscle layer of the anterior wall of the stomach

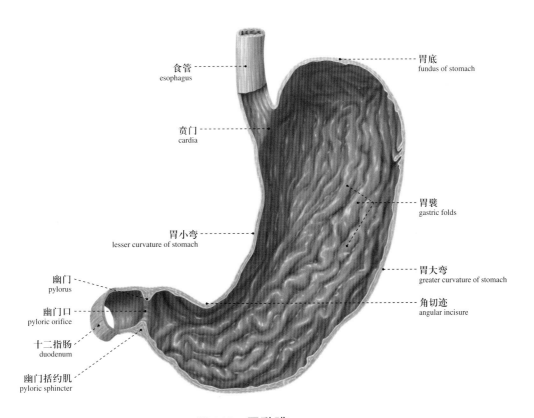

食管
esophagus

贲门
cardia

胃小弯
lesser curvature of stomach

幽门
pylorus

幽门口
pyloric orifice

十二指肠
duodenum

幽门括约肌
pyloric sphincter

胃底
fundus of stomach

胃襞
gastric folds

胃大弯
greater curvature of stomach

角切迹
angular incisure

图 140　**胃黏膜**
Mucous membrane of the stomach

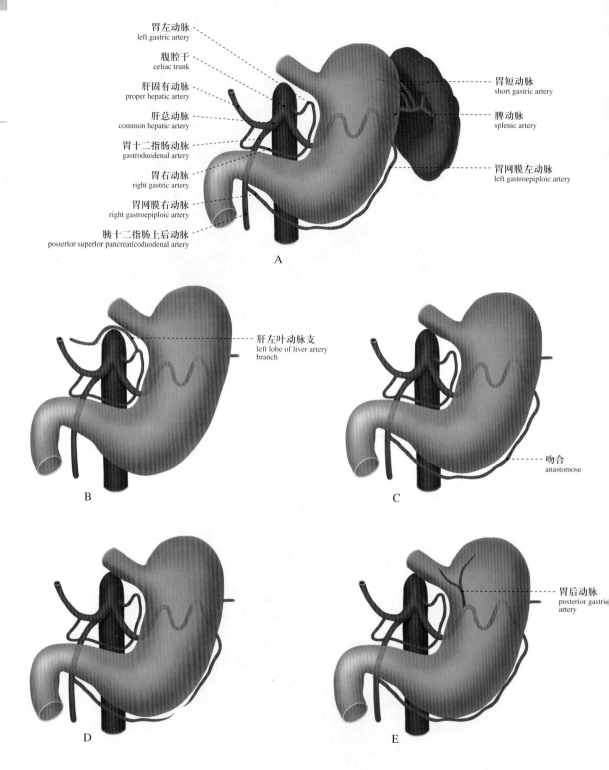

胃左动脉
left gastric artery

腹腔干
celiac trunk

肝固有动脉
proper hepatic artery

肝总动脉
common hepatic artery

胃十二指肠动脉
gastroduodenal artery

胃右动脉
right gastric artery

胃网膜右动脉
right gastroepiploic artery

胰十二指肠上后动脉
posterior superior pancreaticoduodenal artery

胃短动脉
short gastric artery

脾动脉
splenic artery

胃网膜左动脉
left gastroepiploic artery

A

肝左叶动脉支
left lobe of liver artery branch

B

吻合
anastomose

C

D

E

胃后动脉
posterior gastric artery

图 141　胃的动脉变异

Variations of the gastric arteries

A. 在胃小弯和胃大弯吻合成动脉弓；B. 胃左动脉参与肝左叶的血供；C. 在胃大弯胃网膜左、右动脉之间吻合；D. 在胃大弯胃网膜左、右动脉不吻合；E. 辅助的胃后动脉起自脾动脉，营养胃后壁

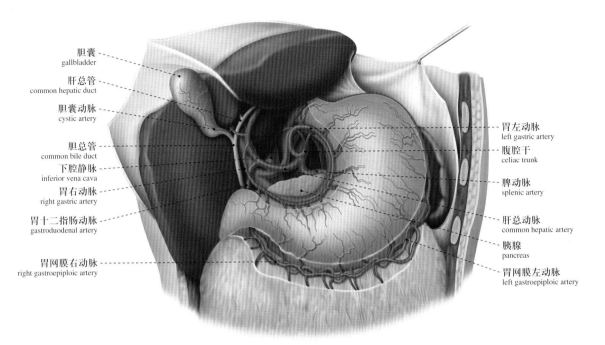

胆囊
gallbladder

肝总管
common hepatic duct

胆囊动脉
cystic artery

胆总管
common bile duct

下腔静脉
inferior vena cava

胃右动脉
right gastric artery

胃十二指肠动脉
gastroduodenal artery

胃网膜右动脉
right gastroepiploic artery

胃左动脉
left gastric artery

腹腔干
celiac trunk

脾动脉
splenic artery

肝总动脉
common hepatic artery

胰腺
pancreas

胃网膜左动脉
left gastroepiploic artery

图 142　腹腔干及其分支（胃前面观）
Celiac trunk and its branches (anterior aspect of stomach)

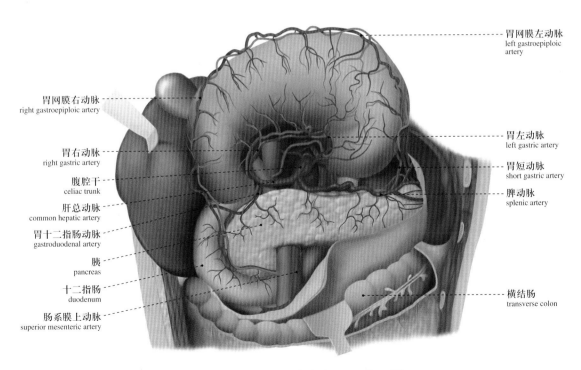

胃网膜右动脉
right gastroepiploic artery

胃右动脉
right gastric artery

腹腔干
celiac trunk

肝总动脉
common hepatic artery

胃十二指肠动脉
gastroduodenal artery

胰
pancreas

十二指肠
duodenum

肠系膜上动脉
superior mesenteric artery

胃网膜左动脉
left gastroepiploic artery

胃左动脉
left gastric artery

胃短动脉
short gastric artery

脾动脉
splenic artery

横结肠
transverse colon

图 143　腹腔干及其分支（胃后面观）
Celiac trunk and its branches (posterior aspect of stomach)

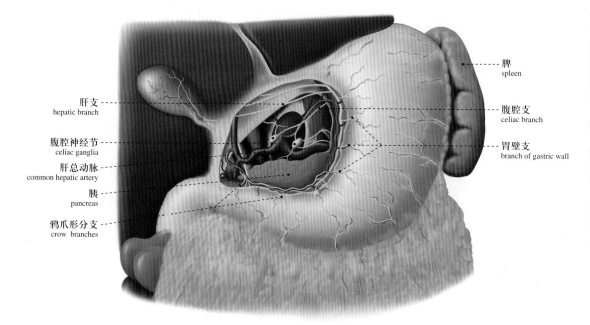

肝支
hepatic branch

腹腔神经节
celiac ganglia

肝总动脉
common hepatic artery

胰
pancreas

鸦爪形分支
crow branches

脾
spleen

腹腔支
celiac branch

胃壁支
branch of gastric wall

图 144　胃的迷走神经（胃前面观）
Gastric vagus nerve (anterior aspect of stomach)

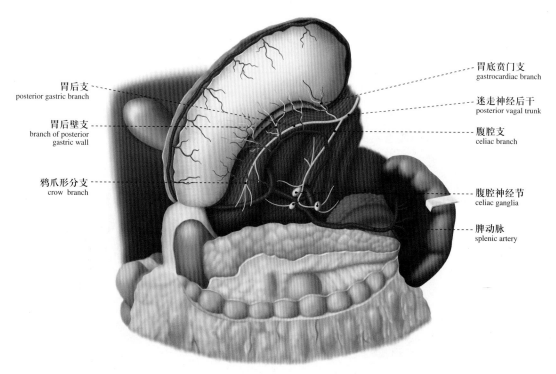

胃后支
posterior gastric branch

胃后壁支
branch of posterior gastric wall

鸦爪形分支
crow branch

胃底贲门支
gastrocardiac branch

迷走神经后干
posterior vagal trunk

腹腔支
celiac branch

腹腔神经节
celiac ganglia

脾动脉
splenic artery

图 145　胃的迷走神经（胃后面观）
Gastric vagus nerve (posterior aspect of stomach)

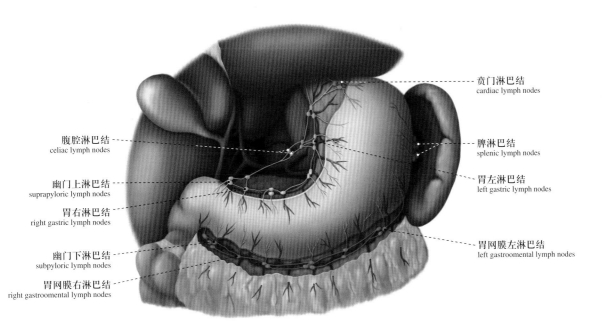

贲门淋巴结
cardiac lymph nodes

脾淋巴结
splenic lymph nodes

胃左淋巴结
left gastric lymph nodes

胃网膜左淋巴结
left gastroomental lymph nodes

腹腔淋巴结
celiac lymph nodes

幽门上淋巴结
suprapyloric lymph nodes

胃右淋巴结
right gastric lymph nodes

幽门下淋巴结
subpyloric lymph nodes

胃网膜右淋巴结
right gastroomental lymph nodes

图 146　胃的淋巴（胃前面观）
Gastric lymph (anterior aspect of stomach)

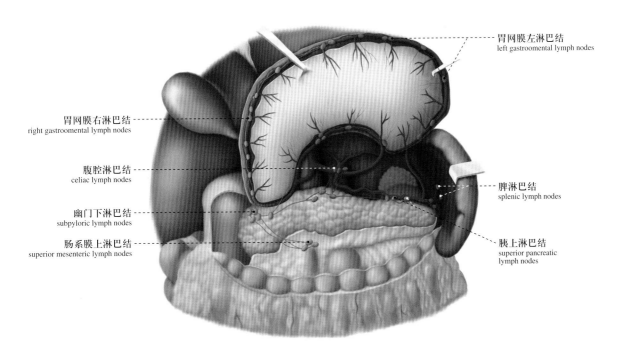

胃网膜左淋巴结
left gastroomental lymph nodes

胃网膜右淋巴结
right gastroomental lymph nodes

腹腔淋巴结
celiac lymph nodes

幽门下淋巴结
subpyloric lymph nodes

肠系膜上淋巴结
superior mesenteric lymph nodes

脾淋巴结
splenic lymph nodes

胰上淋巴结
superior pancreatic lymph nodes

图 147　胃的淋巴（胃后面观）
Gastric lymph (posterior aspect of stomach)

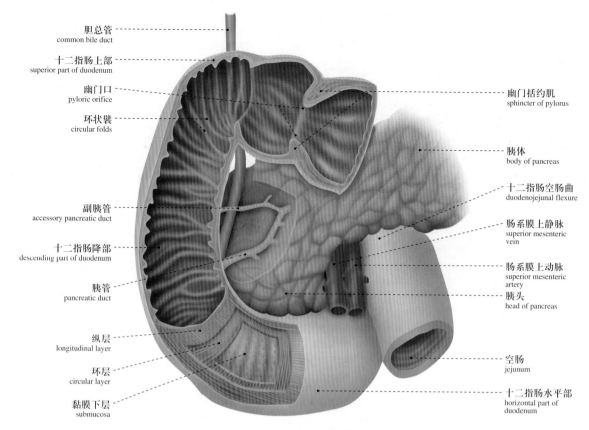

胆总管
common bile duct

十二指肠上部
superior part of duodenum

幽门口
pyloric orifice

环状襞
circular folds

副胰管
accessory pancreatic duct

十二指肠降部
descending part of duodenum

胰管
pancreatic duct

纵层
longitudinal layer

环层
circular layer

黏膜下层
submucosa

幽门括约肌
sphincter of pylorus

胰体
body of pancreas

十二指肠空肠曲
duodenojejunal flexure

肠系膜上静脉
superior mesenteric vein

肠系膜上动脉
superior mesenteric artery

胰头
head of pancreas

空肠
jejunum

十二指肠水平部
horizontal part of duodenum

图 148　十二指肠的结构
Structure of the duodenum

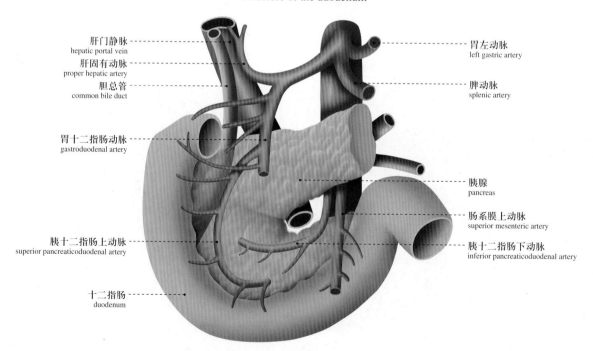

肝门静脉
hepatic portal vein

肝固有动脉
proper hepatic artery

胆总管
common bile duct

胃十二指肠动脉
gastroduodenal artery

胰十二指肠上动脉
superior pancreaticoduodenal artery

十二指肠
duodenum

胃左动脉
left gastric artery

脾动脉
splenic artery

胰腺
pancreas

肠系膜上动脉
superior mesenteric artery

胰十二指肠下动脉
inferior pancreaticoduodenal artery

图 149　十二指肠的动脉
Duodenal arteries

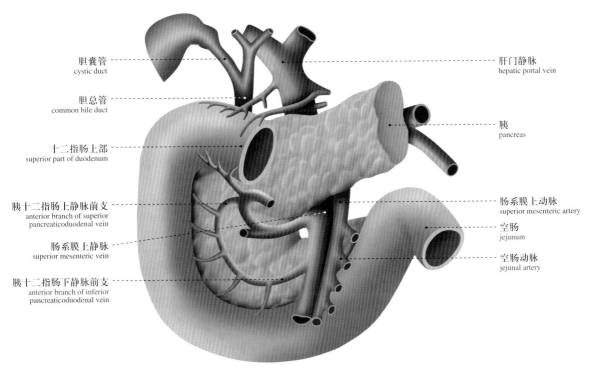

胆囊管
cystic duct

胆总管
common bile duct

十二指肠上部
superior part of duodenum

胰十二指肠上静脉前支
anterior branch of superior
pancreaticoduodenal vein

肠系膜上静脉
superior mesenteric vein

胰十二指肠下静脉前支
anterior branch of inferior
pancreaticoduodenal vein

肝门静脉
hepatic portal vein

胰
pancreas

肠系膜上动脉
superior mesenteric artery

空肠
jejunum

空肠动脉
jejunal artery

图 150 十二指肠的静脉（前面观）
Duodenal veins (anterior aspect)

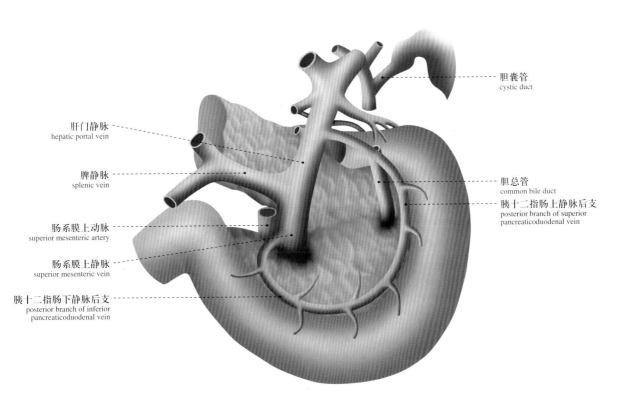

肝门静脉
hepatic portal vein

脾静脉
splenic vein

肠系膜上动脉
superior mesenteric artery

肠系膜上静脉
superior mesenteric vein

胰十二指肠下静脉后支
posterior branch of inferior
pancreaticoduodenal vein

胆囊管
cystic duct

胆总管
common bile duct

胰十二指肠上静脉后支
posterior branch of superior
pancreaticoduodenal vein

图 151 十二指肠的静脉（后面观）
Duodenal veins (posterior aspect)

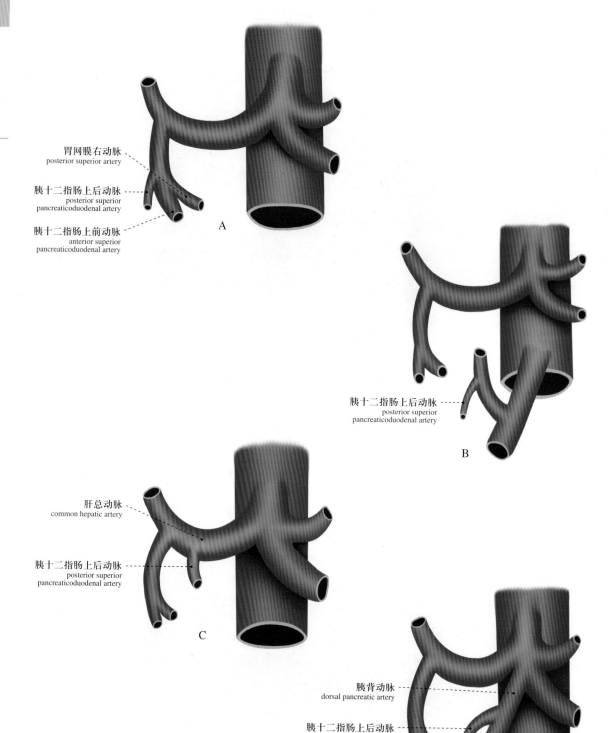

胃网膜右动脉
posterior superior artery

胰十二指肠上后动脉
posterior superior
pancreaticoduodenal artery

胰十二指肠上前动脉
anterior superior
pancreaticoduodenal artery

A

胰十二指肠上后动脉
posterior superior
pancreaticoduodenal artery

B

肝总动脉
common hepatic artery

胰十二指肠上后动脉
posterior superior
pancreaticoduodenal artery

C

胰背动脉
dorsal pancreatic artery

胰十二指肠上后动脉
posterior superior
pancreaticoduodenal artery

D

图 152　胰十二指肠上后动脉的起源变异

Genetic variations of the posterior superior pancreaticoduodenal artery

A. 胰十二指肠上后动脉起自胃十二指肠动脉，为常见型；B. 起自迷走肝右动脉；C. 起自肝总动脉；D. 起自胰背动脉

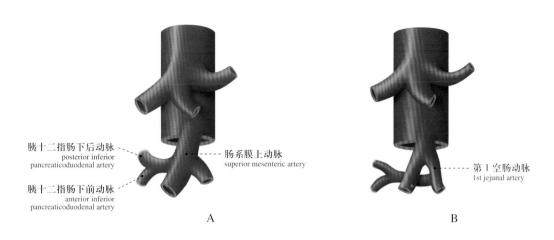

胰十二指肠下后动脉
posterior inferior
pancreaticoduodenal artery

胰十二指肠下前动脉
anterior inferior
pancreaticoduodenal artery

肠系膜上动脉
superior mesenteric artery

A

第 1 空肠动脉
1st jejunal artery

B

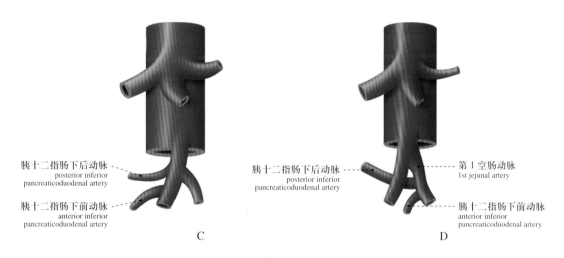

胰十二指肠下后动脉
posterior inferior
pancreaticoduodenal artery

胰十二指肠下前动脉
anterior inferior
pancreaticoduodenal artery

C

胰十二指肠下后动脉
posterior inferior
pancreaticoduodenal artery

第 1 空肠动脉
1st jejunal artery

胰十二指肠下前动脉
anterior inferior
pancreaticoduodenal artery

D

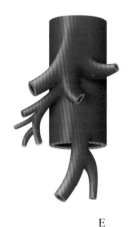

E

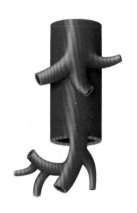

F

图 153　胰十二指肠下前、下后动脉的起源变异

Genetic variations of the anterior inferior and posterior inferior pancreaticoduodenal artery

A. 胰十二指肠下前、下后动脉共干起自肠系膜上动脉；B. 胰十二指肠下动脉共干起自第 1 空肠动脉；C. 分别起自肠
系膜上动脉；D. 分别起自第 1 空肠动脉；E. 分别起自胰背动脉；F. 分别起自迷走肝右动脉

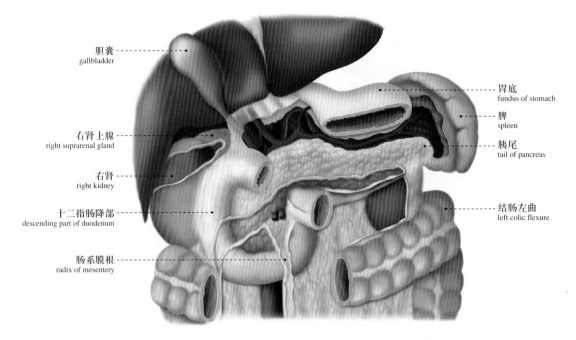

胆囊
gallbladder

右肾上腺
right suprarenal gland

右肾
right kidney

十二指肠降部
descending part of duodenum

肠系膜根
radix of mesentery

胃底
fundus of stomach

脾
spleen

胰尾
tail of pancreas

结肠左曲
left colic flexure

图 154　十二指肠和胰（前面观）
Duodenum and pancreas (anterior aspect)

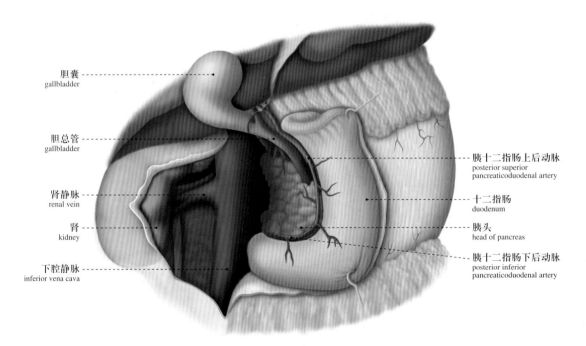

胆囊
gallbladder

胆总管
gallbladder

肾静脉
renal vein

肾
kidney

下腔静脉
inferior vena cava

胰十二指肠上后动脉
posterior superior
pancreaticoduodenal artery

十二指肠
duodenum

胰头
head of pancreas

胰十二指肠下后动脉
posterior inferior
pancreaticoduodenal artery

图 155　十二指肠和胰头的毗邻
Neighbourhood of the duodenum and pancreatic head

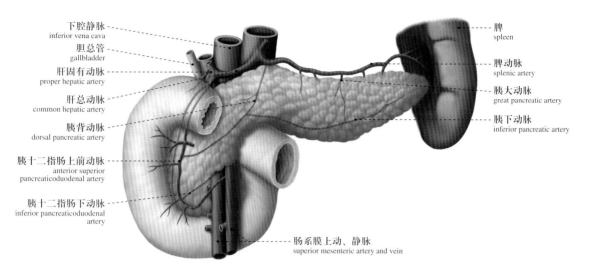

下腔静脉
inferior vena cava

胆总管
gallbladder

肝固有动脉
proper hepatic artery

肝总动脉
common hepatic artery

胰背动脉
dorsal pancreatic artery

胰十二指肠上前动脉
anterior superior
pancreaticoduodenal artery

胰十二指肠下动脉
inferior pancreaticoduodenal
artery

脾
spleen

脾动脉
splenic artery

胰大动脉
great pancreatic artery

胰下动脉
inferior pancreatic artery

肠系膜上动、静脉
superior mesenteric artery and vein

图 156　十二指肠、胰和脾的动脉（前面观）
Arteries of duodenum, pancreas and spleen (anterior aspect)

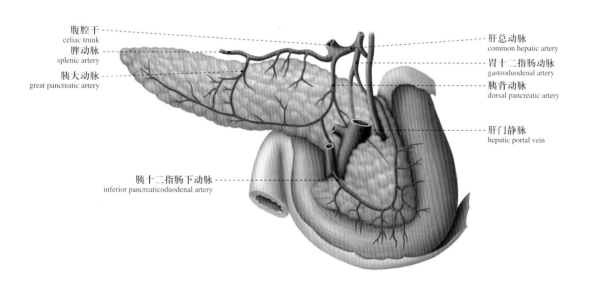

腹腔干
celiac trunk

脾动脉
splenic artery

胰大动脉
great pancreatic artery

肝总动脉
common hepatic artery

胃十二指肠动脉
gastroduodenal artery

胰背动脉
dorsal pancreatic artery

肝门静脉
hepatic portal vein

胰十二指肠下动脉
inferior pancreaticoduodenal artery

图 157　十二指肠、胰和脾的动脉（后面观）
Arteries of duodenum, pancreas and spleen (posterior aspect)

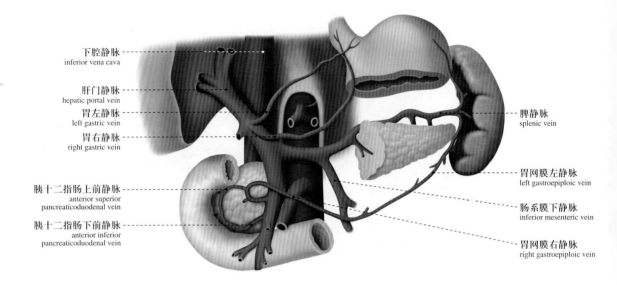

下腔静脉
inferior vena cava

肝门静脉
hepatic portal vein

胃左静脉
left gastric vein

胃右静脉
right gastric vein

胰十二指肠上前静脉
anterior superior
pancreaticoduodenal vein

胰十二指肠下前静脉
anterior inferior
pancreaticoduodenal vein

脾静脉
splenic vein

胃网膜左静脉
left gastroepiploic vein

肠系膜下静脉
inferior mesenteric vein

胃网膜右静脉
right gastroepiploic vein

图 158　十二指肠、胰和脾的静脉（前面观）
Veins of duodenum, pancreas and spleen（anterior aspect）

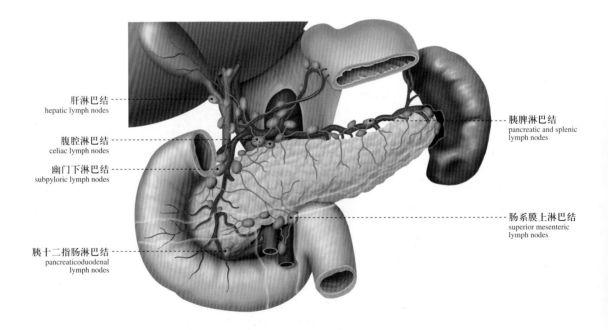

肝淋巴结
hepatic lymph nodes

腹腔淋巴结
celiac lymph nodes

幽门下淋巴结
subpyloric lymph nodes

胰十二指肠淋巴结
pancreaticoduodenal
lymph nodes

胰脾淋巴结
pancreatic and splenic
lymph nodes

肠系膜上淋巴结
superior mesenteric
lymph nodes

图 159　十二指肠、胰和脾的淋巴（前面观）
Lymphs of duodenum, pancreas and spleen (anterior aspect)

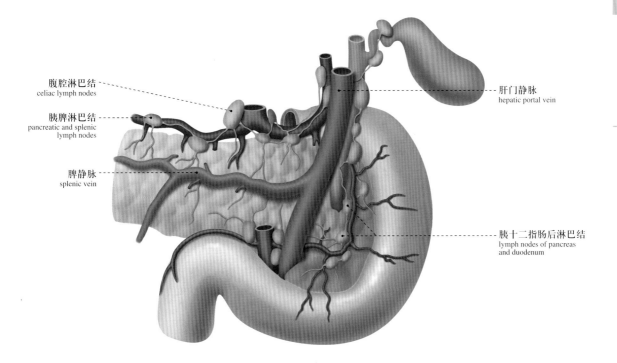

腹腔淋巴结
celiac lymph nodes

胰脾淋巴结
pancreatic and splenic
lymph nodes

脾静脉
splenic vein

肝门静脉
hepatic portal vein

胰十二指肠后淋巴结
lymph nodes of pancreas
and duodenum

图 160 **十二指肠、胰和脾的淋巴（后面观）**
Lymphs of duodenum, pancreas and spleen (posterior aspect)

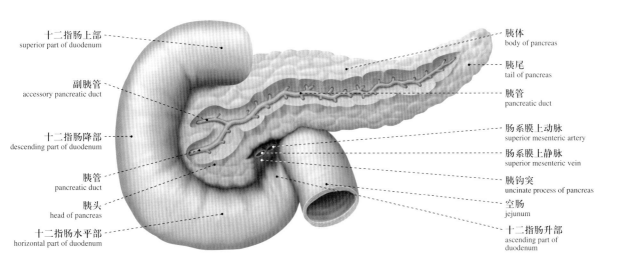

十二指肠上部
superior part of duodenum

副胰管
accessory pancreatic duct

十二指肠降部
descending part of duodenum

胰管
pancreatic duct

胰头
head of pancreas

十二指肠水平部
horizontal part of duodenum

胰体
body of pancreas

胰尾
tail of pancreas

胰管
pancreatic duct

肠系膜上动脉
superior mesenteric artery

肠系膜上静脉
superior mesenteric vein

胰钩突
uncinate process of pancreas

空肠
jejunum

十二指肠升部
ascending part of
duodenum

图 161 **胰的构造**
Structure of the pancreas

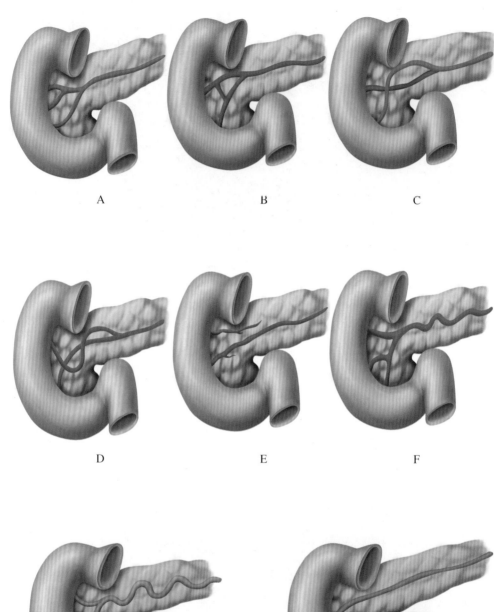

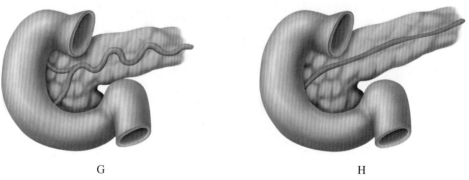

图 162　胰管的变异
Variation of pancreatic duct

A. 双副胰管；B. 吻合胰管；C. 交叉胰管；D. 双胰管交叉；E. 双胰管并行；F. 双胰管；G. 弯曲胰管；H. 副胰管缺失

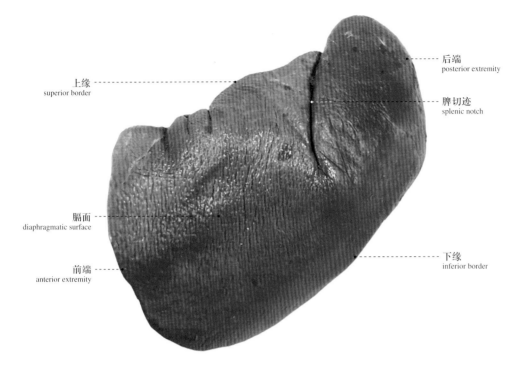

上缘
superior border

后端
posterior extremity

脾切迹
splenic notch

膈面
diaphragmatic surface

前端
anterior extremity

下缘
inferior border

图 163 脾（膈面观）
Spleen (diaphragmatic aspect)

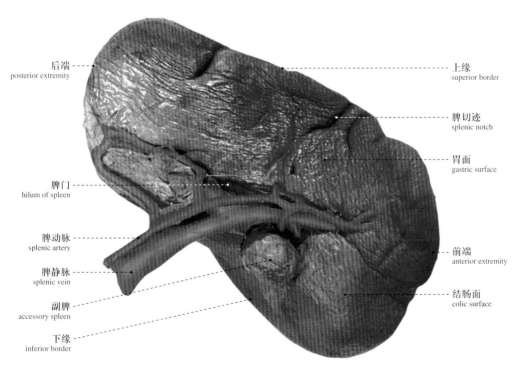

后端
posterior extremity

脾门
hilum of spleen

脾动脉
splenic artery

脾静脉
splenic vein

副脾
accessory spleen

下缘
inferior border

上缘
superior border

脾切迹
splenic notch

胃面
gastric surface

前端
anterior extremity

结肠面
colic surface

图 164 脾（脏面观）
Spleen (visceral aspect)

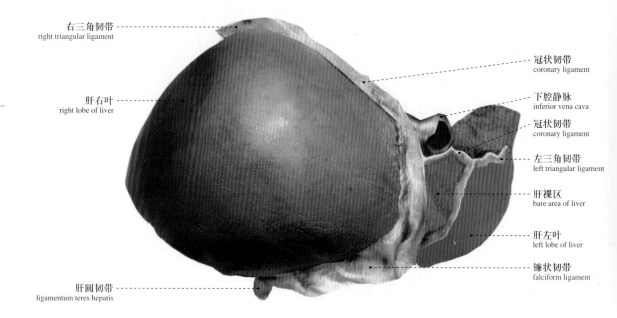

右三角韧带
right triangular ligament

冠状韧带
coronary ligament

肝右叶
right lobe of liver

下腔静脉
inferior vena cava

冠状韧带
coronary ligament

左三角韧带
left triangular ligament

肝裸区
bare area of liver

肝左叶
left lobe of liver

镰状韧带
falciform ligament

肝圆韧带
ligamentum teres hepatis

图 165　肝的膈面
Diaphragmatic surface of the liver

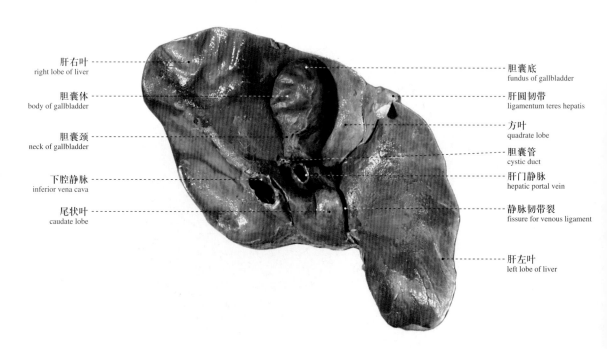

肝右叶
right lobe of liver

胆囊底
fundus of gallbladder

胆囊体
body of gallbladder

肝圆韧带
ligamentum teres hepatis

胆囊颈
neck of gallbladder

方叶
quadrate lobe

下腔静脉
inferior vena cava

胆囊管
cystic duct

尾状叶
caudate lobe

肝门静脉
hepatic portal vein

静脉韧带裂
fissure for venous ligament

肝左叶
left lobe of liver

图 166　肝的脏面
Visceral surface of the liver

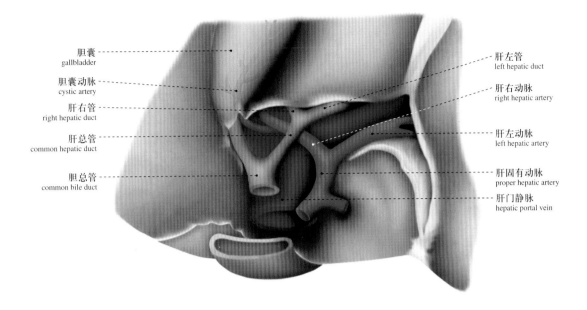

胆囊
gallbladder

胆囊动脉
cystic artery

肝右管
right hepatic duct

肝总管
common hepatic duct

胆总管
common bile duct

肝左管
left hepatic duct

肝右动脉
right hepatic artery

肝左动脉
left hepatic artery

肝固有动脉
proper hepatic artery

肝门静脉
hepatic portal vein

图 167　第一肝门及其结构
First porta hepatis and its structure

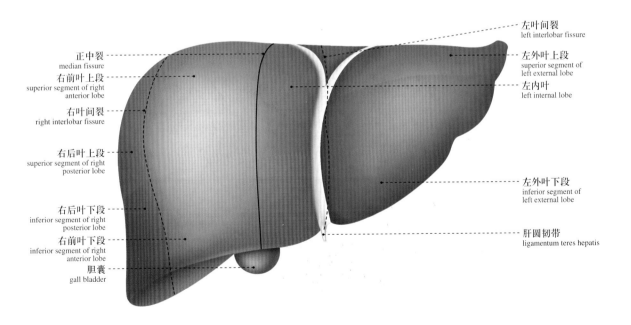

正中裂
median fissure

右前叶上段
superior segment of right anterior lobe

右叶间裂
right interlobar fissure

右后叶上段
superior segment of right posterior lobe

右后叶下段
inferior segment of right posterior lobe

右前叶下段
inferior segment of right anterior lobe

胆囊
gall bladder

左叶间裂
left interlobar fissure

左外叶上段
superior segment of left external lobe

左内叶
left internal lobe

左外叶下段
inferior segment of left external lobe

肝圆韧带
ligamentum teres hepatis

图 168　肝段及肝叶（前面观）
Hepatic segments and lobes (anterior aspect)

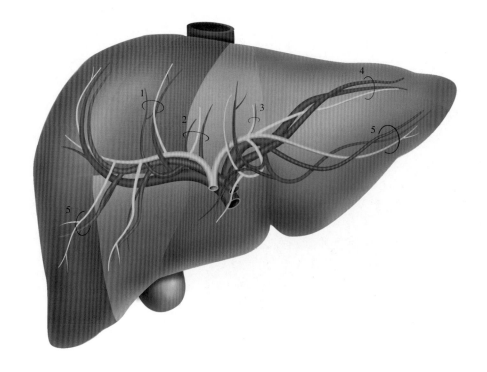

图 169　Glisson 系统在肝内的分布（前面观）

Distribution of Glisson system in the liver (anterior aspect)

1. 右前叶上支；2. 尾状叶右支；3. 尾状叶左支；4. 上段支；5. 下段支

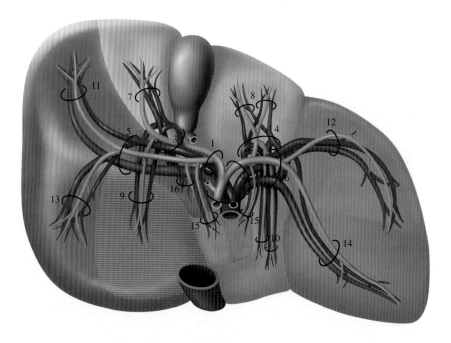

图 170　Glisson 系统在肝内的分布（下面观）

Distribution of Glisson system in the liver (inferior aspect)

1. 右支；2. 左支；3. 前段；4. 内侧段；5. 后段；6. 外侧段；7. 前上区；8. 内侧下区；9. 前上区；10. 内侧上区；11. 后下区；
12. 下外侧区；13. 后上区；14. 外侧区；15. 尾叶；16. 尾状突

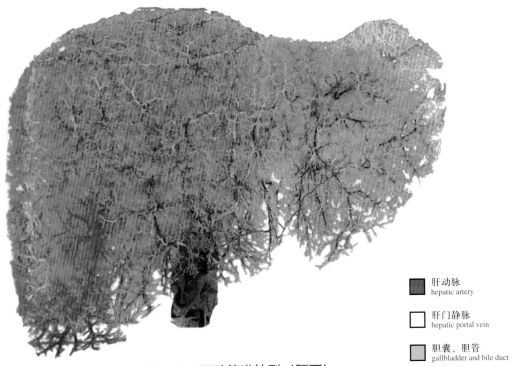

肝动脉
hepatic artery

肝门静脉
hepatic portal vein

胆囊、胆管
gallbladder and bile duct

图 171 肝脏管道铸型（膈面）
Cast of the hepatic duct (diaphragmatic aspect)

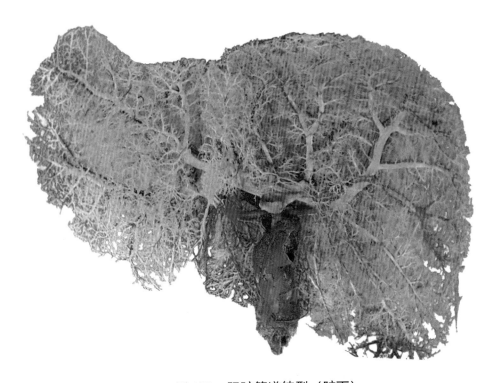

图 172 肝脏管道铸型（脏面）
Cast of the hepatic duct (visceral aspect)

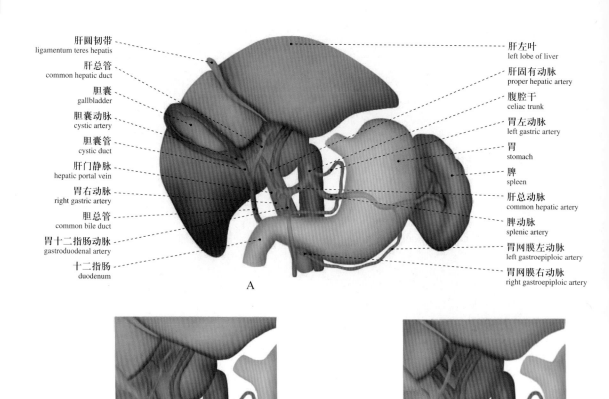

肝圆韧带
ligamentum teres hepatis

肝总管
common hepatic duct

胆囊
gallbladder

胆囊动脉
cystic artery

胆囊管
cystic duct

肝门静脉
hepatic portal vein

胃右动脉
right gastric artery

胆总管
common bile duct

胃十二指肠动脉
gastroduodenal artery

十二指肠
duodenum

肝左叶
left lobe of liver

肝固有动脉
proper hepatic artery

腹腔干
celiac trunk

胃左动脉
left gastric artery

胃
stomach

脾
spleen

肝总动脉
common hepatic artery

脾动脉
splenic artery

胃网膜左动脉
left gastroepiploic artery

胃网膜右动脉
right gastroepiploic artery

A

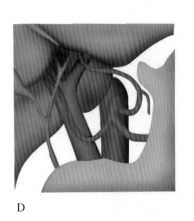

肝固有动脉右支
right branch of proper
hepatic artery

B

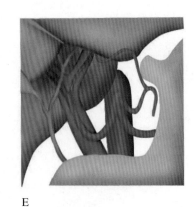

肝总动脉
common hepatic artery

C

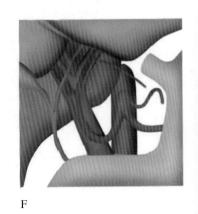

D   E   F

图 173　肝动脉的变异
Variation of the hepatic artery

A. 常见情况；B. 肠系膜上动脉参与肝右叶的血供；C. 肝总动脉起于肠系膜上动脉；D. 胃左动脉供应肝左叶；
E. 除肝固有动脉左支之外，胃左动脉的分支参与肝左叶的血供；F. 肝固有动脉的侧支供应胃小弯

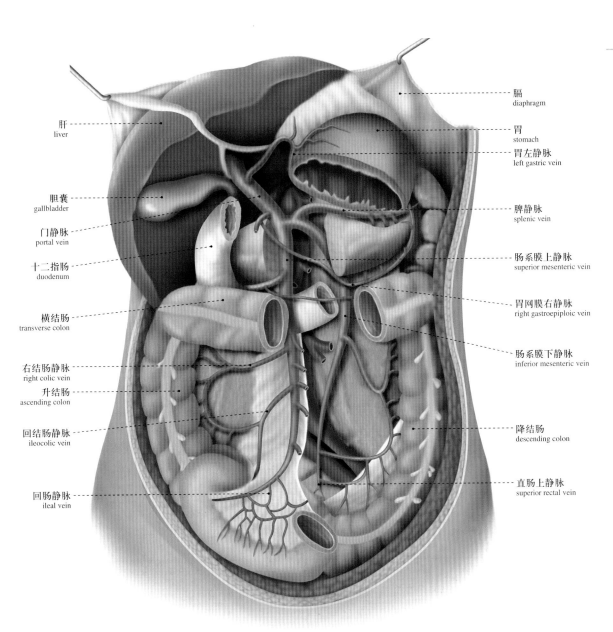

膈
diaphragm

肝
liver

胃
stomach

胃左静脉
left gastric vein

胆囊
gallbladder

脾静脉
splenic vein

门静脉
portal vein

十二指肠
duodenum

肠系膜上静脉
superior mesenteric vein

横结肠
transverse colon

胃网膜右静脉
right gastroepiploic vein

肠系膜下静脉
inferior mesenteric vein

右结肠静脉
right colic vein

升结肠
ascending colon

降结肠
descending colon

回结肠静脉
ileocolic vein

直肠上静脉
superior rectal vein

回肠静脉
ileal vein

图 174 肝门静脉及其属支
Hepatic portal vein and its branches

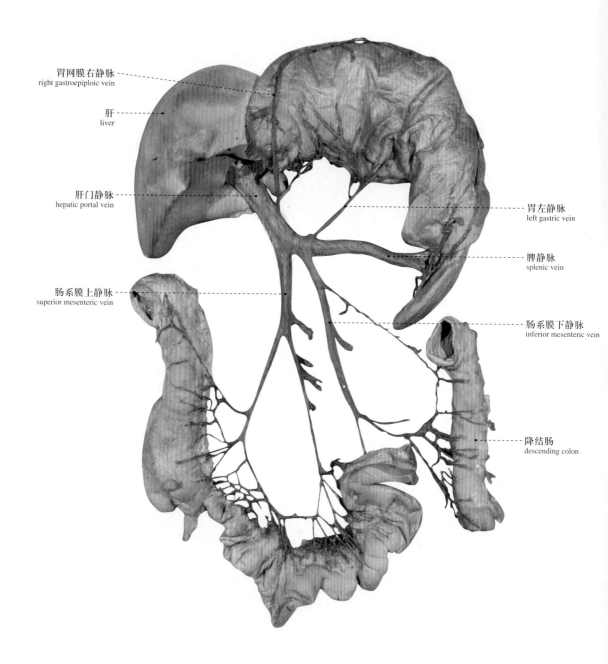

胃网膜右静脉
right gastroepiploic vein

肝
liver

肝门静脉
hepatic portal vein

肠系膜上静脉
superior mesenteric vein

胃左静脉
left gastric vein

脾静脉
splenic vein

肠系膜下静脉
inferior mesenteric vein

降结肠
descending colon

图 175　肝门静脉
Hepatic portal vein

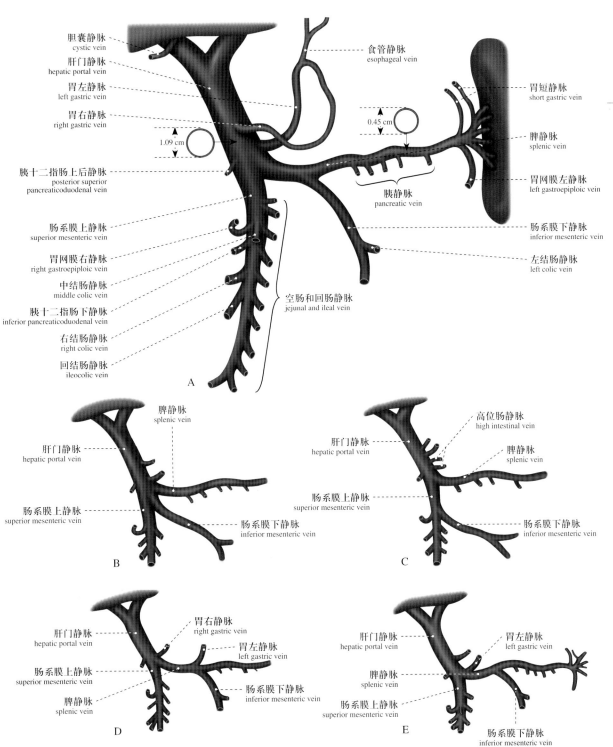

胆囊静脉
cystic vein

肝门静脉
hepatic portal vein

胃左静脉
left gastric vein

胃右静脉
right gastric vein

食管静脉
esophageal vein

胃短静脉
short gastric vein

0.45 cm

脾静脉
splenic vein

1.09 cm

胰十二指肠上后静脉
posterior superior
pancreaticoduodenal vein

胃网膜左静脉
left gastroepiploic vein

胰静脉
pancreatic vein

肠系膜上静脉
superior mesenteric vein

肠系膜下静脉
inferior mesenteric vein

胃网膜右静脉
right gastroepiploic vein

左结肠静脉
left colic vein

中结肠静脉
middle colic vein

胰十二指肠下静脉
inferior pancreaticoduodenal vein

右结肠静脉
right colic vein

空肠和回肠静脉
jejunal and ileal vein

回结肠静脉
ileocolic vein

A

脾静脉
splenic vein

肝门静脉
hepatic portal vein

肠系膜上静脉
superior mesenteric vein

肠系膜下静脉
inferior mesenteric vein

B

高位肠静脉
high intestinal vein

肝门静脉
hepatic portal vein

脾静脉
splenic vein

肠系膜上静脉
superior mesenteric vein

肠系膜下静脉
inferior mesenteric vein

C

肝门静脉
hepatic portal vein

胃右静脉
right gastric vein

胃左静脉
left gastric vein

肠系膜上静脉
superior mesenteric vein

肠系膜下静脉
inferior mesenteric vein

脾静脉
splenic vein

D

肝门静脉
hepatic portal vein

胃左静脉
left gastric vein

脾静脉
splenic vein

肠系膜上静脉
superior mesenteric vein

肠系膜下静脉
inferior mesenteric vein

E

图 176 肝门静脉的变异
Variations of hepatic portal vein

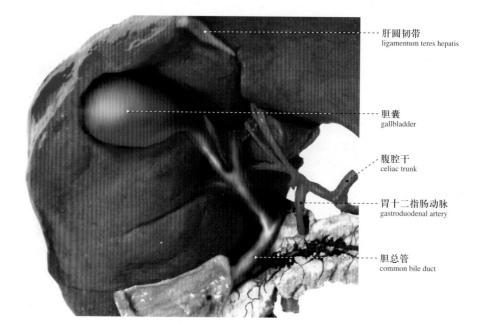

肝圆韧带
ligamentum teres hepatis

胆囊
gallbladder

腹腔干
celiac trunk

胃十二指肠动脉
gastroduodenal artery

胆总管
common bile duct

图 177　胆囊
Gallbladder

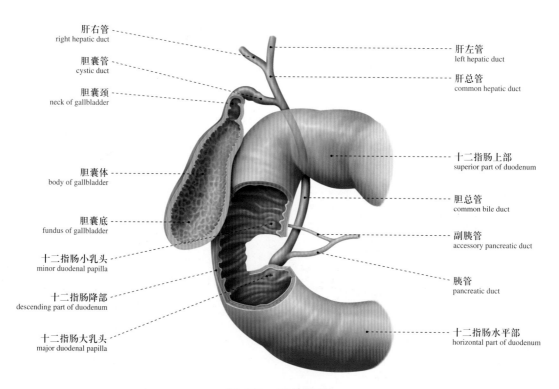

肝右管
right hepatic duct

胆囊管
cystic duct

胆囊颈
neck of gallbladder

胆囊体
body of gallbladder

胆囊底
fundus of gallbladder

十二指肠小乳头
minor duodenal papilla

十二指肠降部
descending part of duodenum

十二指肠大乳头
major duodenal papilla

肝左管
left hepatic duct

肝总管
common hepatic duct

十二指肠上部
superior part of duodenum

胆总管
common bile duct

副胰管
accessory pancreatic duct

胰管
pancreatic duct

十二指肠水平部
horizontal part of duodenum

图 178　肝外胆管
Extrahepatic bile ducts

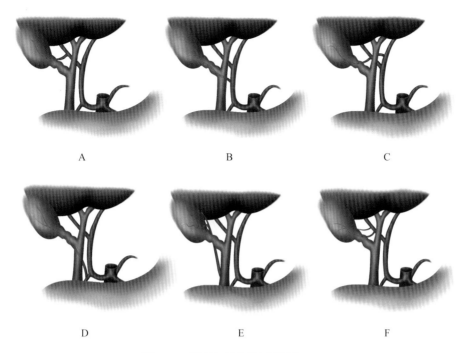

图 179　胆囊动脉常见类型
Common types of cystic artery

A. 正常型；B. 胆囊动脉起自肝固有动脉；C. 胆囊动脉起自肝左动脉；D. 双胆囊动脉（一支起自肝右动脉，
另一支起自胃十二指肠动脉）；E. 胆囊动脉起自副肝右动脉；F. 双胆囊动脉（二支均起自肝右动脉）

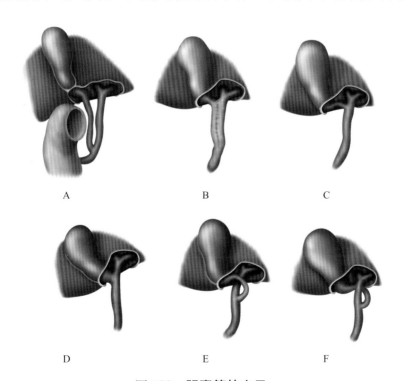

图 180　胆囊管的变异
Variations in cystic duct

A. 胆囊管和肝总管低位汇合；B. 胆囊管附着于肝总管；C. 胆囊管和肝总管高位汇合；D. 胆囊管非常短或缺如；
E. 胆囊管从前方盘旋于肝总管左侧；F. 胆囊管从后方盘旋于肝总管左侧

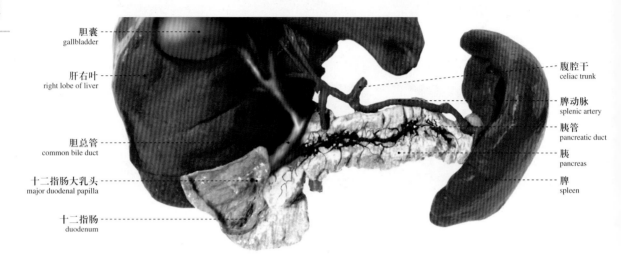

胆囊
gallbladder

肝右叶
right lobe of liver

胆总管
common bile duct

十二指肠大乳头
major duodenal papilla

十二指肠
duodenum

腹腔干
celiac trunk

脾动脉
splenic artery

胰管
pancreatic duct

胰
pancreas

脾
spleen

图 181　胰管
Pancreatic duct

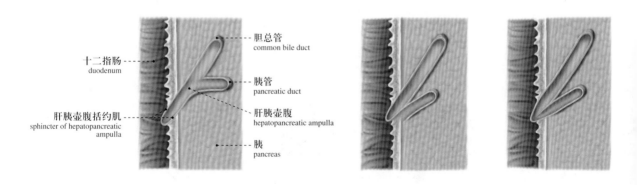

十二指肠
duodenum

肝胰壶腹括约肌
sphincter of hepatopancreatic ampulla

胆总管
common bile duct

胰管
pancreatic duct

肝胰壶腹
hepatopancreatic ampulla

胰
pancreas

图 182　胆总管和胰管结合处的变异
Variation of the common bile duct combined with the pancreatic duct

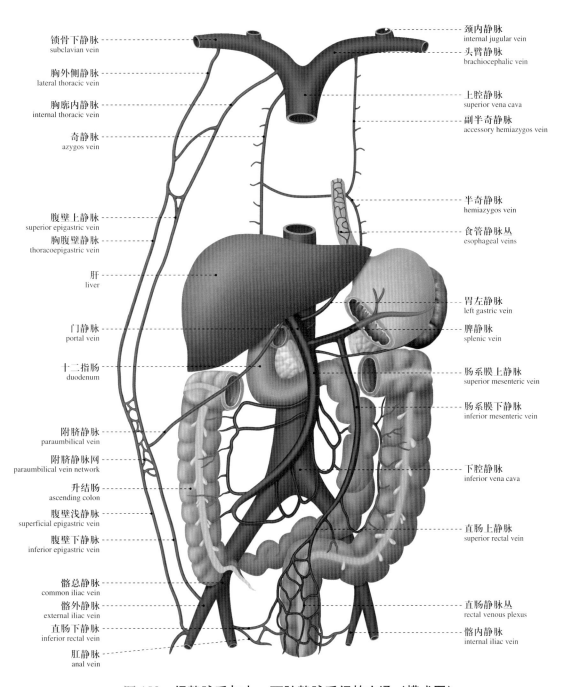

锁骨下静脉
subclavian vein

胸外侧静脉
lateral thoracic vein

胸廓内静脉
internal thoracic vein

奇静脉
azygos vein

腹壁上静脉
superior epigastric vein

胸腹壁静脉
thoracoepigastric vein

肝
liver

门静脉
portal vein

十二指肠
duodenum

附脐静脉
paraumbilical vein

附脐静脉网
paraumbilical vein network

升结肠
ascending colon

腹壁浅静脉
superficial epigastric vein

腹壁下静脉
inferior epigastric vein

髂总静脉
common iliac vein

髂外静脉
external iliac vein

直肠下静脉
inferior rectal vein

肛静脉
anal vein

颈内静脉
internal jugular vein

头臂静脉
brachiocephalic vein

上腔静脉
superior vena cava

副半奇静脉
accessory hemiazygos vein

半奇静脉
hemiazygos vein

食管静脉丛
esophageal veins

胃左静脉
left gastric vein

脾静脉
splenic vein

肠系膜上静脉
superior mesenteric vein

肠系膜下静脉
inferior mesenteric vein

下腔静脉
inferior vena cava

直肠上静脉
superior rectal vein

直肠静脉丛
rectal venous plexus

髂内静脉
internal iliac vein

图 183　门静脉系与上、下腔静脉系间的交通（模式图）

Transportation between portal vein and vena cava system (diagram)

第四节

结肠下区

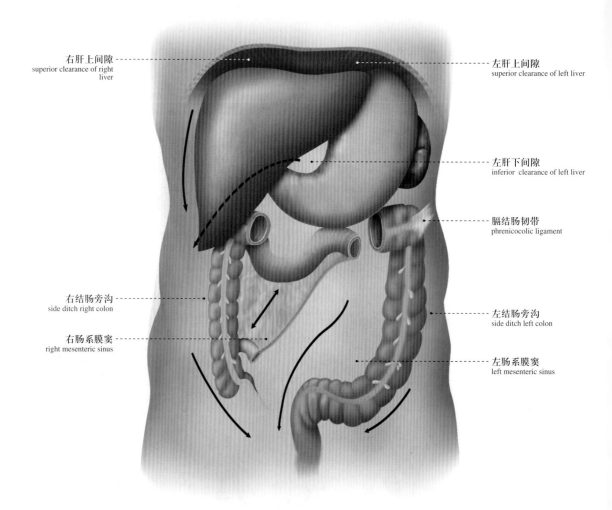

右肝上间隙
superior clearance of right
liver

左肝上间隙
superior clearance of left liver

左肝下间隙
inferior clearance of left liver

膈结肠韧带
phrenicocolic ligament

右结肠旁沟
side ditch right colon

右肠系膜窦
right mesenteric sinus

左结肠旁沟
side ditch left colon

左肠系膜窦
left mesenteric sinus

图 184 结肠下区的间隙及交通
Gap of the colon down region and traffic

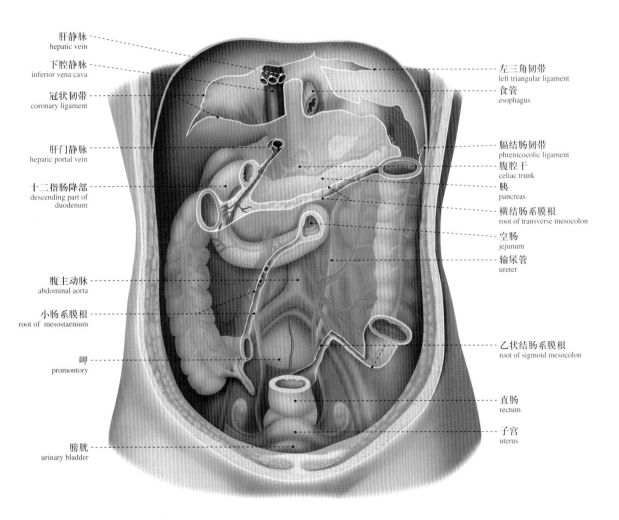

肝静脉
hepatic vein

下腔静脉
inferior vena cava

冠状韧带
coronary ligament

肝门静脉
hepatic portal vein

十二指肠降部
descending part of
duodenum

腹主动脉
abdominal aorta

小肠系膜根
root of mesostaenium

岬
promontory

膀胱
urinary bladder

左三角韧带
left triangular ligament

食管
esophagus

膈结肠韧带
phrenicocolic ligament

腹腔干
celiac trunk

胰
pancreas

横结肠系膜根
root of transverse mesocolon

空肠
jejunum

输尿管
ureter

乙状结肠系膜根
root of sigmoid mesocolon

直肠
rectum

子宫
uterus

图 185　腹后壁腹膜的配布
Arrangement of the peritoneum on the posterior abdominal wall

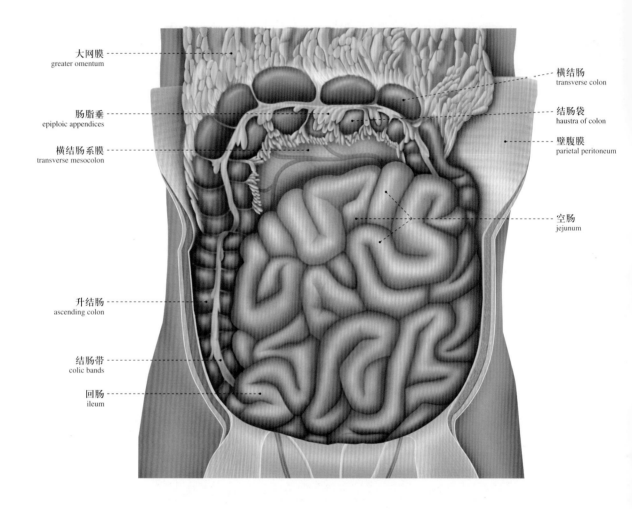

大网膜
greater omentum

肠脂垂
epiploic appendices

横结肠系膜
transverse mesocolon

升结肠
ascending colon

结肠带
colic bands

回肠
ileum

横结肠
transverse colon

结肠袋
haustra of colon

壁腹膜
parietal peritoneum

空肠
jejunum

图 186　小肠
Small intestine

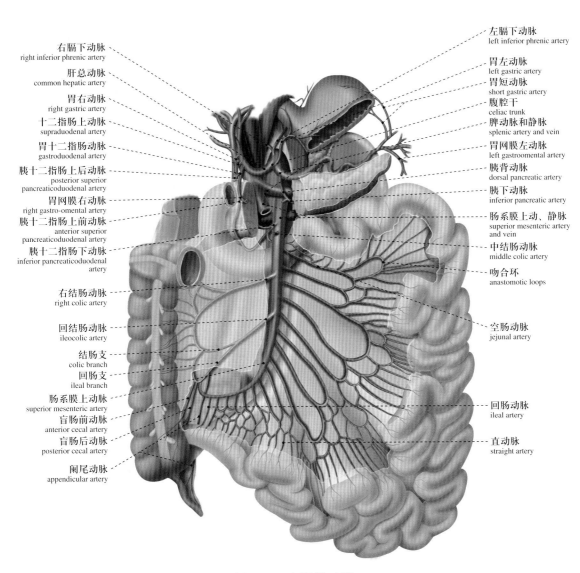

右膈下动脉
right inferior phrenic artery

肝总动脉
common hepatic artery

胃右动脉
right gastric artery

十二指肠上动脉
supraduodenal artery

胃十二指肠动脉
gastroduodenal artery

胰十二指肠上后动脉
posterior superior
pancreaticoduodenal artery

胃网膜右动脉
right gastro-omental artery

胰十二指肠上前动脉
anterior superior
pancreaticoduodenal artery

胰十二指肠下动脉
inferior pancreaticoduodenal
artery

右结肠动脉
right colic artery

回结肠动脉
ileocolic artery

结肠支
colic branch

回肠支
ileal branch

肠系膜上动脉
superior mesenteric artery

盲肠前动脉
anterior cecal artery

盲肠后动脉
posterior cecal artery

阑尾动脉
appendicular artery

左膈下动脉
left inferior phrenic artery

胃左动脉
left gastric artery

胃短动脉
short gastric artery

腹腔干
celiac trunk

脾动脉和静脉
splenic artery and vein

胃网膜左动脉
left gastroomental artery

胰背动脉
dorsal pancreatic artery

胰下动脉
inferior pancreatic artery

肠系膜上动、静脉
superior mesenteric artery
and vein

中结肠动脉
middle colic artery

吻合环
anastomotic loops

空肠动脉
jejunal artery

回肠动脉
ileal artery

直动脉
straight artery

图 187　小肠的动脉
Arteries of small intestine

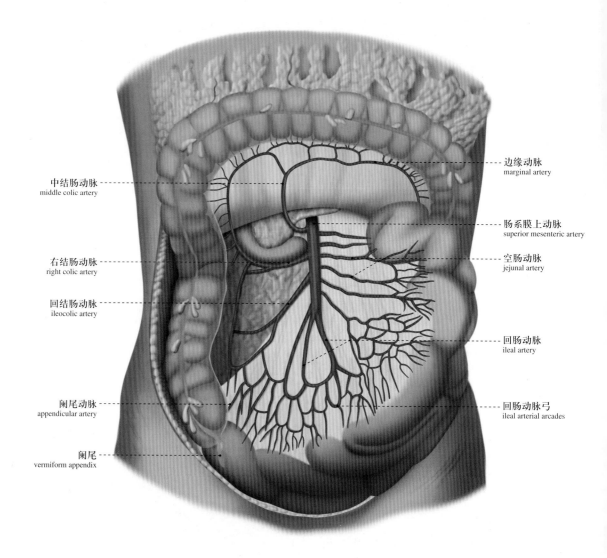

中结肠动脉
middle colic artery

右结肠动脉
right colic artery

回结肠动脉
ileocolic artery

阑尾动脉
appendicular artery

阑尾
vermiform appendix

边缘动脉
marginal artery

肠系膜上动脉
superior mesenteric artery

空肠动脉
jejunal artery

回肠动脉
ileal artery

回肠动脉弓
ileal arterial arcades

图 188　肠系膜上动脉及其分支
Superior mesenteric artery and its branches

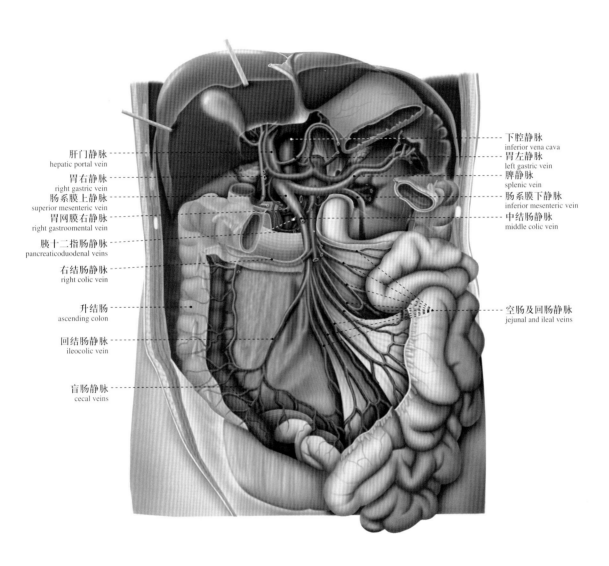

肝门静脉
hepatic portal vein

胃右静脉
right gastric vein

肠系膜上静脉
superior mesenteric vein

胃网膜右静脉
right gastroomental vein

胰十二指肠静脉
pancreaticoduodenal veins

右结肠静脉
right colic vein

升结肠
ascending colon

回结肠静脉
ileocolic vein

盲肠静脉
cecal veins

下腔静脉
inferior vena cava

胃左静脉
left gastric vein

脾静脉
splenic vein

肠系膜下静脉
inferior mesenteric vein

中结肠静脉
middle colic vein

空肠及回肠静脉
jejunal and ileal veins

图 189　肠系膜上静脉及其属支
Superior mesenteric vein and its tributaries

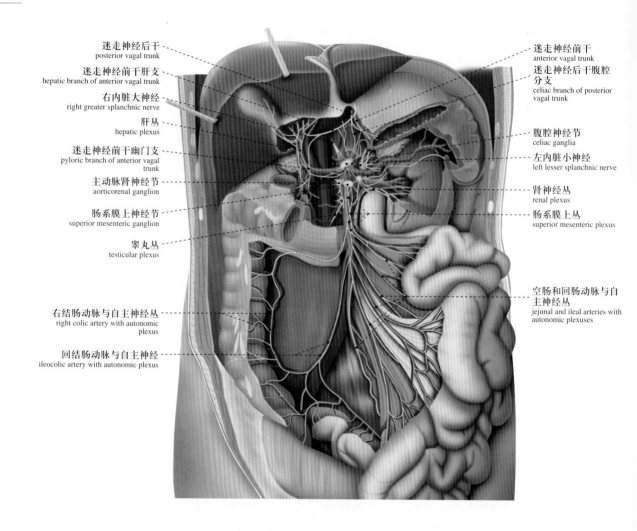

迷走神经后干
posterior vagal trunk

迷走神经前干肝支
hepatic branch of anterior vagal trunk

右内脏大神经
right greater splanchnic nerve

肝丛
hepatic plexus

迷走神经前干幽门支
pyloric branch of anterior vagal trunk

主动脉肾神经节
aorticorenal ganglion

肠系膜上神经节
superior mesenteric ganglion

睾丸丛
testicular plexus

右结肠动脉与自主神经丛
right colic artery with autonomic plexus

回结肠动脉与自主神经
ileocolic artery with autonomic plexus

迷走神经前干
anterior vagal trunk

迷走神经后干腹腔分支
celiac branch of posterior vagal trunk

腹腔神经节
celiac ganglia

左内脏小神经
left lesser splanchnic nerve

肾神经丛
renal plexus

肠系膜上丛
superior mesenteric plexus

空肠和回肠动脉与自主神经丛
jejunal and ileal arteries with autonomic plexuses

图 190　肠系膜上丛至小肠的自主神经分布
Autonomic distribution of the superior mesenteric plexus to the intestine

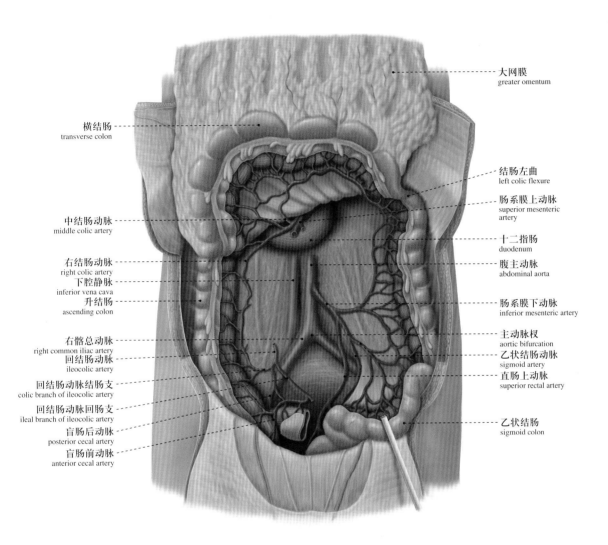

大网膜
greater omentum

横结肠
transverse colon

结肠左曲
left colic flexure

肠系膜上动脉
superior mesenteric artery

中结肠动脉
middle colic artery

十二指肠
duodenum

右结肠动脉
right colic artery

腹主动脉
abdominal aorta

下腔静脉
inferior vena cava

升结肠
ascending colon

肠系膜下动脉
inferior mesenteric artery

右髂总动脉
right common iliac artery

主动脉杈
aortic bifurcation

回结肠动脉
ileocolic artery

乙状结肠动脉
sigmoid artery

回结肠动脉结肠支
colic branch of ileocolic artery

直肠上动脉
superior rectal artery

回结肠动脉回肠支
ileal branch of ileocolic artery

盲肠后动脉
posterior cecal artery

乙状结肠
sigmoid colon

盲肠前动脉
anterior cecal artery

图 191　大肠的动脉
Arteries of the large intestine

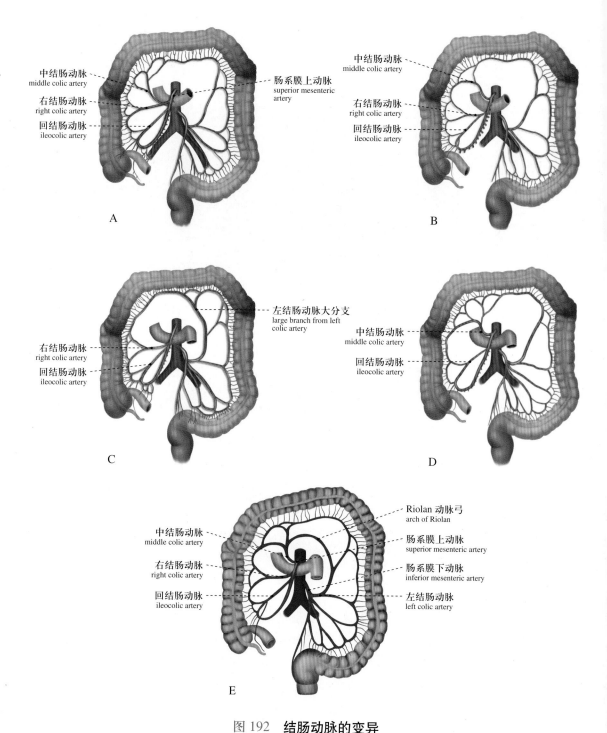

中结肠动脉
middle colic artery

右结肠动脉
right colic artery

回结肠动脉
ileocolic artery

肠系膜上动脉
superior mesenteric artery

A

中结肠动脉
middle colic artery

右结肠动脉
right colic artery

回结肠动脉
ileocolic artery

B

左结肠动脉大分支
large branch from left colic artery

右结肠动脉
right colic artery

回结肠动脉
ileocolic artery

C

中结肠动脉
middle colic artery

回结肠动脉
ileocolic artery

D

Riolan 动脉弓
arch of Riolan

肠系膜上动脉
superior mesenteric artery

肠系膜下动脉
inferior mesenteric artery

左结肠动脉
left colic artery

中结肠动脉
middle colic artery

右结肠动脉
right colic artery

回结肠动脉
ileocolic artery

E

图 192　结肠动脉的变异
Variations of the colic artery

A. 右结肠动脉和中结肠动脉共干；B. 右结肠动脉和回肠动脉共干；C. 中结肠动脉缺如；
D. 右结肠动脉缺如；E. 左结肠动脉与中结肠动脉之间形成 Riolan 动脉弓

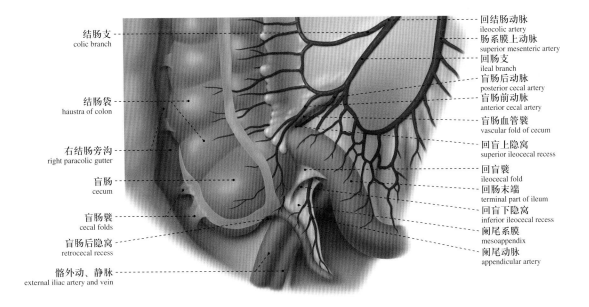

结肠支 colic branch
结肠袋 haustra of colon
右结肠旁沟 right paracolic gutter
盲肠 cecum
盲肠襞 cecal folds
盲肠后隐窝 retrocecal recess
髂外动、静脉 external iliac artery and vein

回结肠动脉 ileocolic artery
肠系膜上动脉 superior mesenteric artery
回肠支 ileal branch
盲肠后动脉 posterior cecal artery
盲肠前动脉 anterior cecal artery
盲肠血管襞 vascular fold of cecum
回盲上隐窝 superior ileocecal recess
回盲襞 ileocecal fold
回肠末端 terminal part of ileum
回盲下隐窝 inferior ileocecal recess
阑尾系膜 mesoappendix
阑尾动脉 appendicular artery

图 193　回肠末端、阑尾和盲肠的动脉

Arteries of the distal end of the ileum, vermiform appendix and cecum

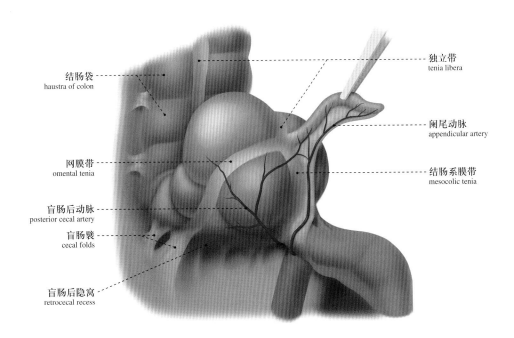

结肠袋 haustra of colon
网膜带 omental tenia
盲肠后动脉 posterior cecal artery
盲肠襞 cecal folds
盲肠后隐窝 retrocecal recess

独立带 tenia libera
阑尾动脉 appendicular artery
结肠系膜带 mesocolic tenia

图 194　阑尾动脉

Appendix artery

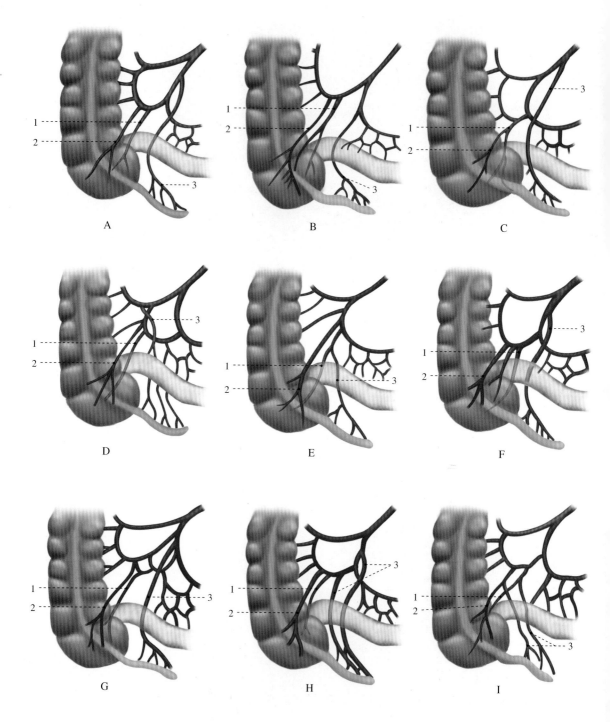

图 195　盲肠动脉和阑尾动脉的变异

Variations of the colic and the appendix arteries

1. 盲肠后动脉 posterior cecal artery；2. 盲肠前动脉 anterior cecal artery；3. 阑尾动脉 appendicular artery

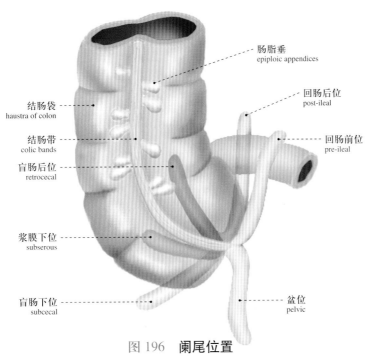

肠脂垂
epiploic appendices

结肠袋
haustra of colon

结肠带
colic bands

盲肠后位
retrocecal

浆膜下位
subserous

盲肠下位
subcecal

回肠后位
post-ileal

回肠前位
pre-ileal

盆位
pelvic

图 196　**阑尾位置**
Positions of the vermiform appendix

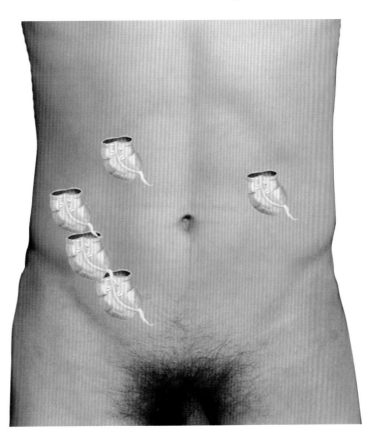

图 197　**阑尾位置的变异**
Variations of the vermiform appendicular position

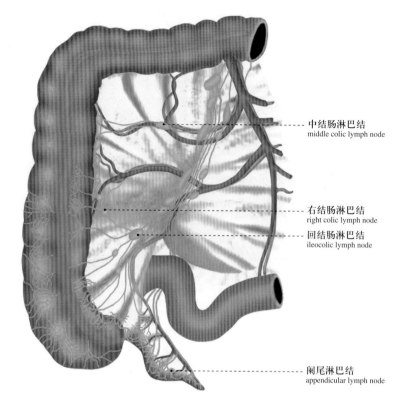

中结肠淋巴结
middle colic lymph node

右结肠淋巴结
right colic lymph node

回结肠淋巴结
ileocolic lymph node

阑尾淋巴结
appendicular lymph node

图 198　大肠的淋巴管和淋巴结（前面观）
Lymph vessels and lymph nodes of the large intestine (anterior aspect)

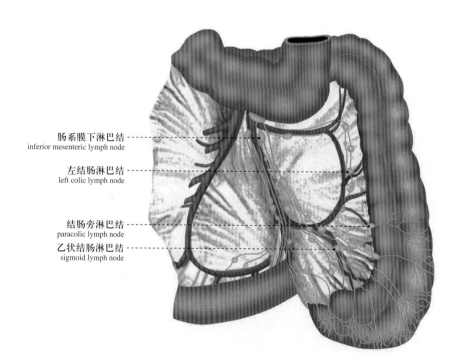

肠系膜下淋巴结
inferior mesenteric lymph node

左结肠淋巴结
left colic lymph node

结肠旁淋巴结
paracolic lymph node

乙状结肠淋巴结
sigmoid lymph node

图 199　大肠的淋巴管和淋巴结（后面观）
Lymph vessels and the lymph nodes of the large intestine (posterior aspect)

第五节

腹膜后隙

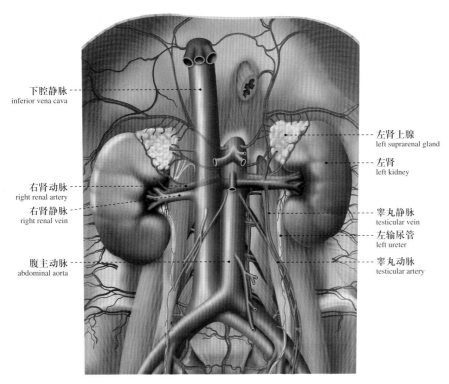

下腔静脉
inferior vena cava

左肾上腺
left suprarenal gland

左肾
left kidney

右肾动脉
right renal artery

右肾静脉
right renal vein

睾丸静脉
testicular vein

左输尿管
left ureter

腹主动脉
abdominal aorta

睾丸动脉
testicular artery

图 200　肾
Kidney

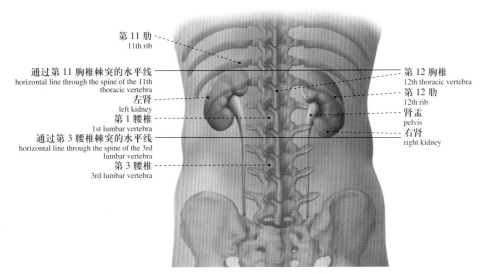

第 11 肋
11th rib

通过第 11 胸椎棘突的水平线
horizontal line through the spine of the 11th thoracic vertebra

左肾
left kidney

第 1 腰椎
1st lumbar vertebra

通过第 3 腰椎棘突的水平线
horizontal line through the spine of the 3rd lumbar vertebra

第 3 腰椎
3rd lumbar vertebra

第 12 胸椎
12th thoracic vertebra

第 12 肋
12th rib

肾盂
pelvis

右肾
right kidney

图 201　肾和输尿管的体表投影
Surface projection of kidney and ureter

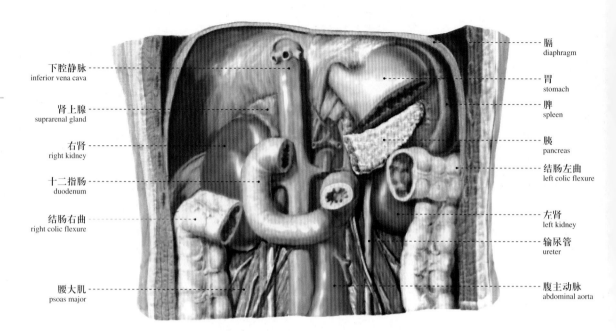

下腔静脉
inferior vena cava

肾上腺
suprarenal gland

右肾
right kidney

十二指肠
duodenum

结肠右曲
right colic flexure

腰大肌
psoas major

膈
diaphragm

胃
stomach

脾
spleen

胰
pancreas

结肠左曲
left colic flexure

左肾
left kidney

输尿管
ureter

腹主动脉
abdominal aorta

图 202　肾的位置和毗邻（前面观）
Position and neighbourhood of the kidneys (anterior aspect)

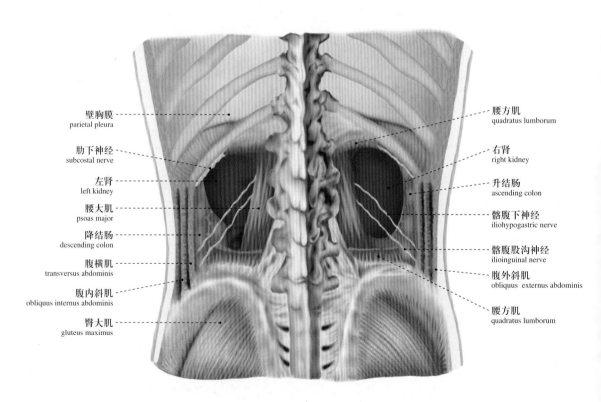

壁胸膜
parietal pleura

肋下神经
subcostal nerve

左肾
left kidney

腰大肌
psoas major

降结肠
descending colon

腹横肌
transversus abdominis

腹内斜肌
obliquus internus abdominis

臀大肌
gluteus maximus

腰方肌
quadratus lumborum

右肾
right kidney

升结肠
ascending colon

髂腹下神经
iliohypogastric nerve

髂腹股沟神经
ilioinguinal nerve

腹外斜肌
obliquus externus abdominis

腰方肌
quadratus lumborum

图 203　肾的位置和毗邻（后面观）
Position and neighbourhood of the kidneys (posterior aspect)

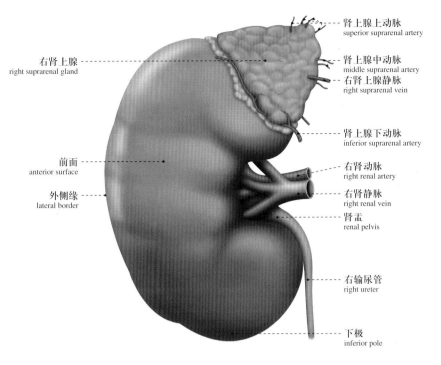

右肾上腺
right suprarenal gland

前面
anterior surface

外侧缘
lateral border

肾上腺上动脉
superior suprarenal artery

肾上腺中动脉
middle suprarenal artery

右肾上腺静脉
right suprarenal vein

肾上腺下动脉
inferior suprarenal artery

右肾动脉
right renal artery

右肾静脉
right renal vein

肾盂
renal pelvis

右输尿管
right ureter

下极
inferior pole

图 204 肾的形状（前面观）
Shape of the kidney (anterior aspect)

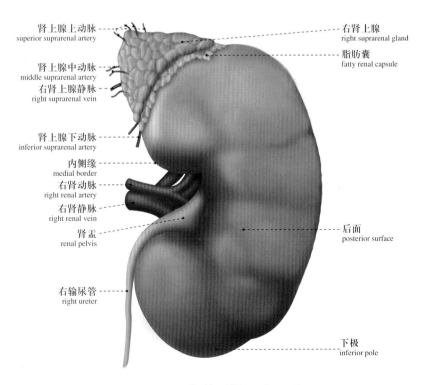

肾上腺上动脉
superior suprarenal artery

肾上腺中动脉
middle suprarenal artery

右肾上腺静脉
right suprarenal vein

肾上腺下动脉
inferior suprarenal artery

内侧缘
medial border

右肾动脉
right renal artery

右肾静脉
right renal vein

肾盂
renal pelvis

右输尿管
right ureter

右肾上腺
right suprarenal gland

脂肪囊
fatty renal capsule

后面
posterior surface

下极
inferior pole

图 205 肾的形状（后面观）
Shape of the kidney (posterior aspect)

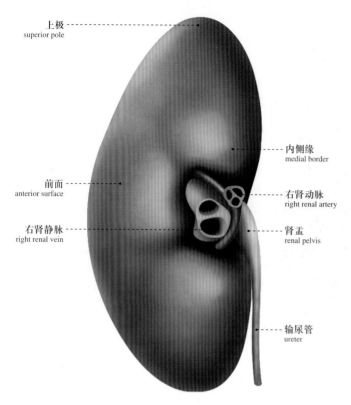

上极
superior pole

内侧缘
medial border

前面
anterior surface

右肾动脉
right renal artery

右肾静脉
right renal vein

肾盂
renal pelvis

输尿管
ureter

图 206　肾的形状（内面观）
Shape of the kidney (medial aspect)

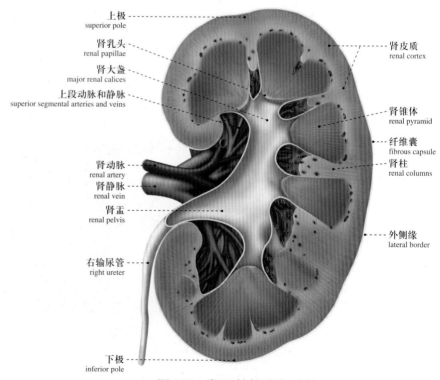

上极
superior pole

肾乳头
renal papillae

肾大盏
major renal calices

上段动脉和静脉
superior segmental arteries and veins

肾皮质
renal cortex

肾锥体
renal pyramid

纤维囊
fibrous capsule

肾动脉
renal artery

肾静脉
renal vein

肾盂
renal pelvis

肾柱
renal columns

右输尿管
right ureter

外侧缘
lateral border

下极
inferior pole

图 207　肾盂的构造和形状
Structure and shape of the renal pelvis

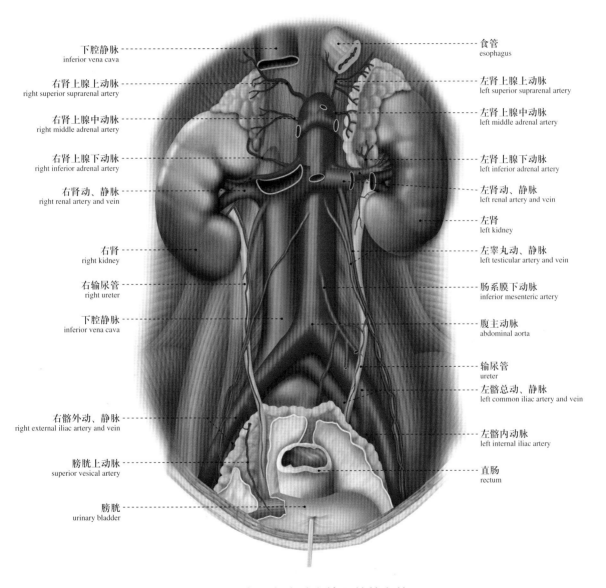

下腔静脉
inferior vena cava

右肾上腺上动脉
right superior suprarenal artery

右肾上腺中动脉
right middle adrenal artery

右肾上腺下动脉
right inferior adrenal artery

右肾动、静脉
right renal artery and vein

右肾
right kidney

右输尿管
right ureter

下腔静脉
inferior vena cava

右髂外动、静脉
right external iliac artery and vein

膀胱上动脉
superior vesical artery

膀胱
urinary bladder

食管
esophagus

左肾上腺上动脉
left superior suprarenal artery

左肾上腺中动脉
left middle adrenal artery

左肾上腺下动脉
left inferior adrenal artery

左肾动、静脉
left renal artery and vein

左肾
left kidney

左睾丸动、静脉
left testicular artery and vein

肠系膜下动脉
inferior mesenteric artery

腹主动脉
abdominal aorta

输尿管
ureter

左髂总动、静脉
left common iliac artery and vein

左髂内动脉
left internal iliac artery

直肠
rectum

图 208 肾、肾上腺和输尿管的血管
Blood vessels of the kidney, adrenal gland and ureter

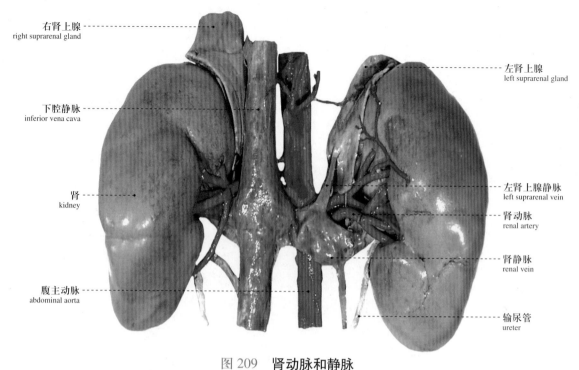

右肾上腺
right suprarenal gland

下腔静脉
inferior vena cava

肾
kidney

腹主动脉
abdominal aorta

左肾上腺
left suprarenal gland

左肾上腺静脉
left suprarenal vein

肾动脉
renal artery

肾静脉
renal vein

输尿管
ureter

图 209　肾动脉和静脉
Arteries and veins of the kidney

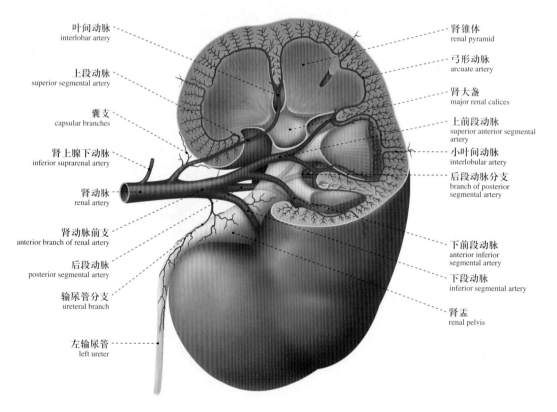

叶间动脉
interlobar artery

上段动脉
superior segmental artery

囊支
capsular branches

肾上腺下动脉
inferior suprarenal artery

肾动脉
renal artery

肾动脉前支
anterior branch of renal artery

后段动脉
posterior segmental artery

输尿管分支
ureteral branch

左输尿管
left ureter

肾锥体
renal pyramid

弓形动脉
arcuate artery

肾大盏
major renal calices

上前段动脉
superior anterior segmental artery

小叶间动脉
interlobular artery

后段动脉分支
branch of posterior segmental artery

下前段动脉
anterior inferior segmental artery

下段动脉
inferior segmental artery

肾盂
renal pelvis

图 210　肾动脉的分支
Branches of renal artery

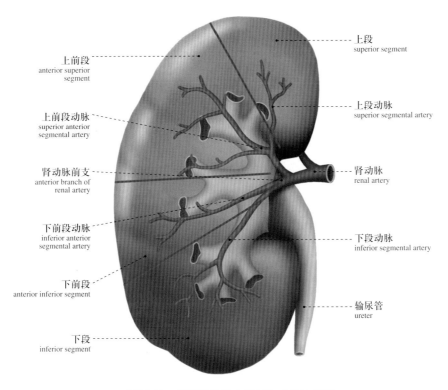

上前段
anterior superior
segment

上前段动脉
superior anterior
segmental artery

肾动脉前支
anterior branch of
renal artery

下前段动脉
inferior anterior
segmental artery

下前段
anterior inferior segment

下段
inferior segment

上段
superior segment

上段动脉
superior segmental artery

肾动脉
renal artery

下段动脉
inferior segmental artery

输尿管
ureter

图 211　肾段动脉与肾段（前面观）
Renal segment artery and renal segment (anterior aspect)

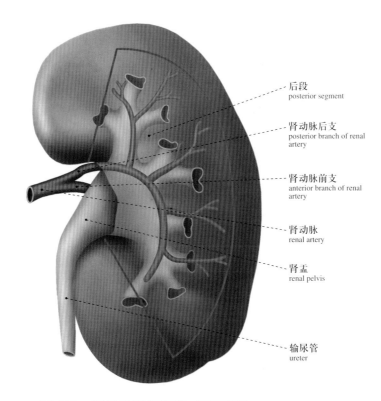

后段
posterior segment

肾动脉后支
posterior branch of renal
artery

肾动脉前支
anterior branch of renal
artery

肾动脉
renal artery

肾盂
renal pelvis

输尿管
ureter

图 212　肾段动脉与肾段（后面观）
Renal segment artery and renal segment (posterior aspect)

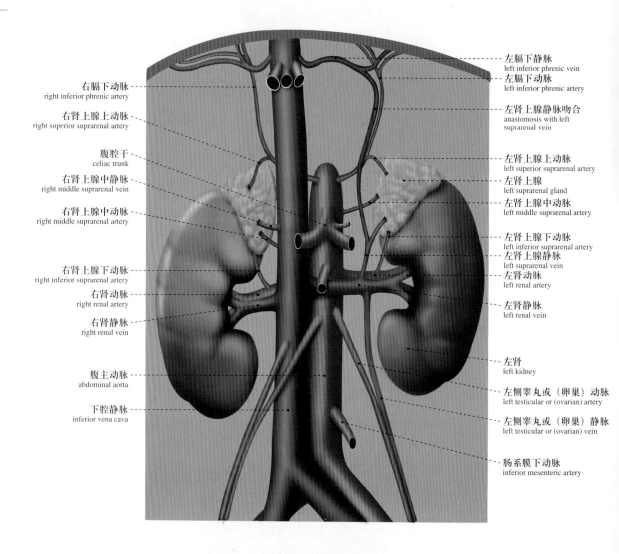

右膈下动脉
right inferior phrenic artery

右肾上腺上动脉
right superior suprarenal artery

腹腔干
celiac trunk

右肾上腺中静脉
right middle suprarenal vein

右肾上腺中动脉
right middle suprarenal artery

右肾上腺下动脉
right inferior suprarenal artery

右肾动脉
right renal artery

右肾静脉
right renal vein

腹主动脉
abdominal aorta

下腔静脉
inferior vena cava

左膈下静脉
left inferior phrenic vein

左膈下动脉
left inferior phrenic artery

左肾上腺静脉吻合
anastomosis with left
suprarenal vein

左肾上腺上动脉
left superior suprarenal artery

左肾上腺
left suprarenal gland

左肾上腺中动脉
left middle suprarenal artery

左肾上腺下动脉
left inferior suprarenal artery

左肾上腺静脉
left suprarenal vein

左肾动脉
left renal artery

左肾静脉
left renal vein

左肾
left kidney

左侧睾丸或（卵巢）动脉
left testicular or (ovarian) artery

左侧睾丸或（卵巢）静脉
left testicular or (ovarian) vein

肠系膜下动脉
inferior mesenteric artery

图 213 肾的动脉和静脉及肾上腺
Arteries and veins of the kidneys and suprarenal glands

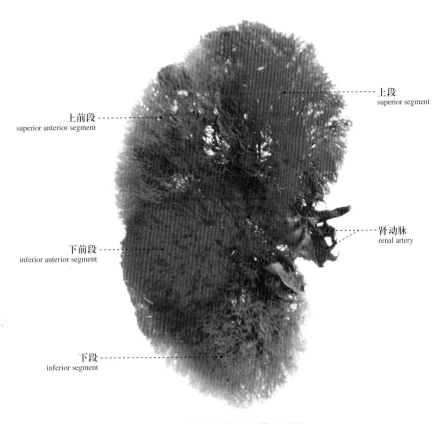

上前段
superior anterior segment

上段
superior segment

肾动脉
renal artery

下前段
inferior anterior segment

下段
inferior segment

图 214　肾段铸型（前面观）
Cast of the renal segments (anterior aspect)

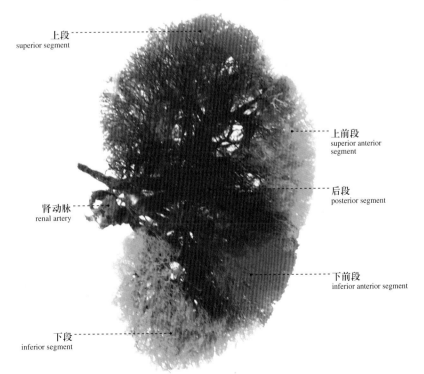

上段
superior segment

上前段
superior anterior segment

后段
posterior segment

肾动脉
renal artery

下前段
inferior anterior segment

下段
inferior segment

图 215　肾段铸型（后面观）
Cast of the renal segments (posterior aspect)

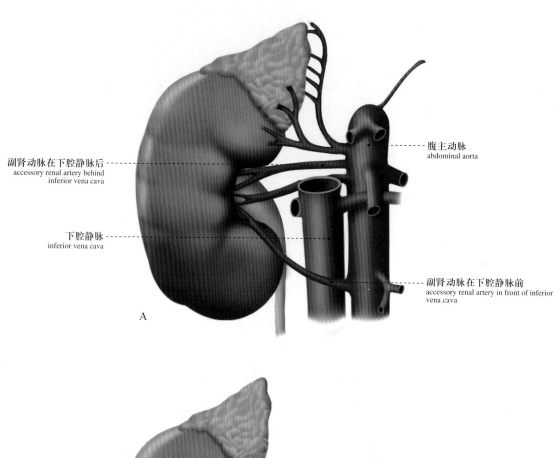

副肾动脉在下腔静脉后
accessory renal artery behind
inferior vena cava

腹主动脉
abdominal aorta

下腔静脉
inferior vena cava

副肾动脉在下腔静脉前
accessory renal artery in front of inferior
vena cava

A

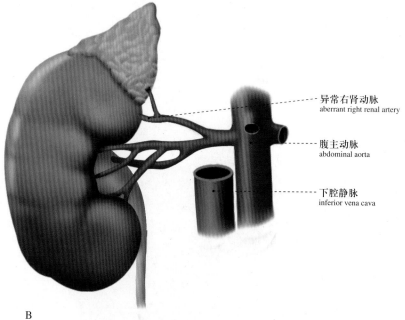

异常右肾动脉
aberrant right renal artery

腹主动脉
abdominal aorta

下腔静脉
inferior vena cava

B

图 216　肾动脉的变异

Variations in the renal artery

A. 低位右肾动脉通过下腔静脉前方；B. 肾动脉多分支

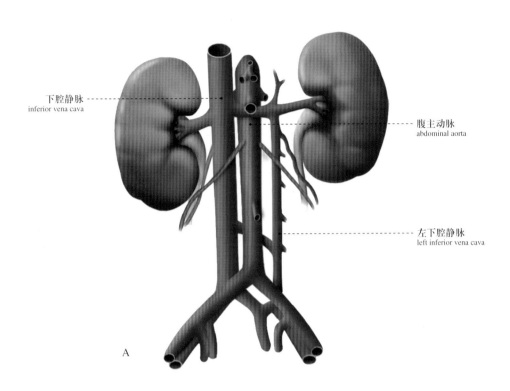

下腔静脉
inferior vena cava

腹主动脉
abdominal aorta

左下腔静脉
left inferior vena cava

A

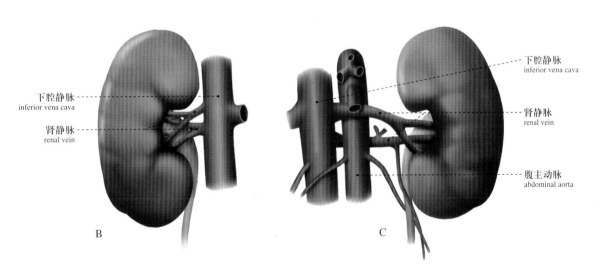

下腔静脉
inferior vena cava

肾静脉
renal vein

B

下腔静脉
inferior vena cava

肾静脉
renal vein

腹主动脉
abdominal aorta

C

图 217　肾静脉的变异
Variations in the renal vein

A. 左下腔静脉加入到左肾静脉；B. 多根肾静脉；C. 双左肾静脉围绕腹主动脉

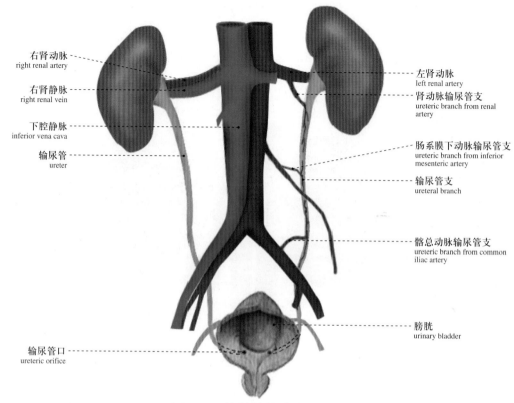

右肾动脉
right renal artery

右肾静脉
right renal vein

下腔静脉
inferior vena cava

输尿管
ureter

输尿管口
ureteric orifice

左肾动脉
left renal artery

肾动脉输尿管支
ureteric branch from renal artery

肠系膜下动脉输尿管支
ureteric branch from inferior mesenteric artery

输尿管支
ureteral branch

髂总动脉输尿管支
ureteric branch from common iliac artery

膀胱
urinary bladder

图 218　输尿管的动脉
Ureteral arteries

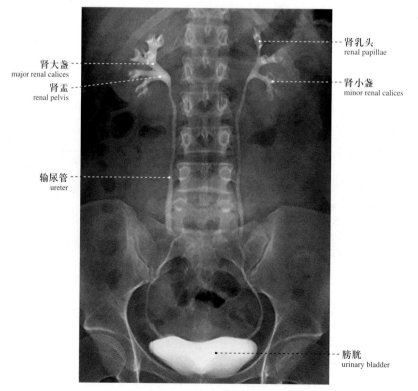

肾大盏
major renal calices

肾盂
renal pelvis

输尿管
ureter

肾乳头
renal papillae

肾小盏
minor renal calices

膀胱
urinary bladder

图 219　泌尿系造影
Ureteropyelography

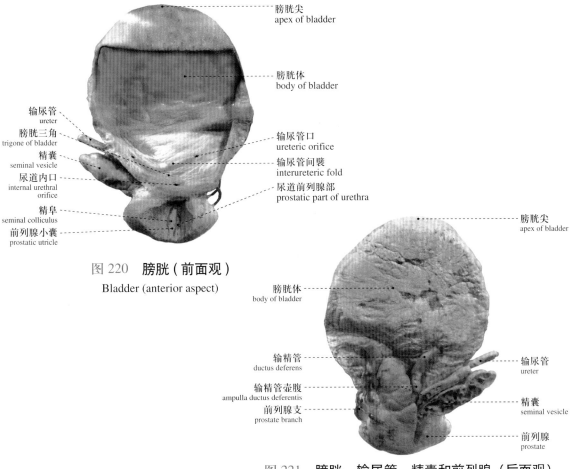

膀胱尖
apex of bladder

膀胱体
body of bladder

输尿管
ureter

膀胱三角
trigone of bladder

精囊
seminal vesicle

尿道内口
internal urethral orifice

精阜
seminal colliculus

前列腺小囊
prostatic utricle

输尿管口
ureteric orifice

输尿管间襞
interureteric fold

尿道前列腺部
prostatic part of urethra

图 220　膀胱（前面观）
Bladder (anterior aspect)

膀胱尖
apex of bladder

膀胱体
body of bladder

输精管
ductus deferens

输精管壶腹
ampulla ductus deferentis

前列腺支
prostate branch

输尿管
ureter

精囊
seminal vesicle

前列腺
prostate

图 221　膀胱、输尿管、精囊和前列腺（后面观）
Bladder, ureter, seminal vesicle and prostate (posterior aspect)

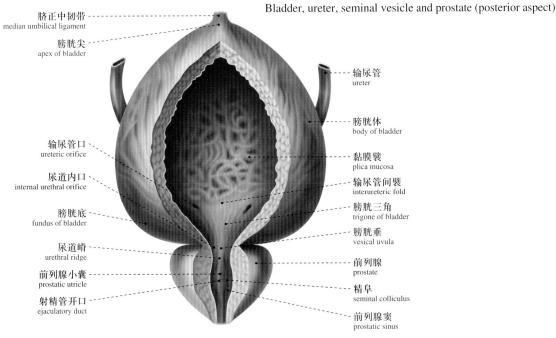

脐正中韧带
median umbilical ligament

膀胱尖
apex of bladder

输尿管口
ureteric orifice

尿道内口
internal urethral orifice

膀胱底
fundus of bladder

尿道嵴
urethral ridge

前列腺小囊
prostatic utricle

射精管开口
ejaculatory duct

输尿管
ureter

膀胱体
body of bladder

黏膜襞
plica mucosa

输尿管间襞
interureteric fold

膀胱三角
trigone of bladder

膀胱垂
vesical uvula

前列腺
prostate

精阜
seminal colliculus

前列腺窦
prostatic sinus

图 222　膀胱及男性尿道前列腺部（前面观）
Bladder and the prostatic part of the male urethra (anterior aspect)

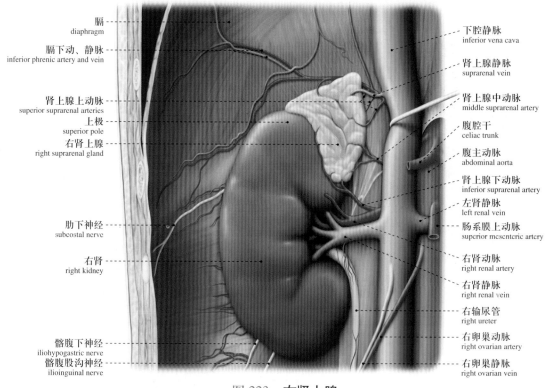

膈
diaphragm

膈下动、静脉
inferior phrenic artery and vein

肾上腺上动脉
superior suprarenal arteries

上极
superior pole

右肾上腺
right suprarenal gland

肋下神经
subcostal nerve

右肾
right kidney

髂腹下神经
iliohypogastric nerve

髂腹股沟神经
ilioinguinal nerve

下腔静脉
inferior vena cava

肾上腺静脉
suprarenal vein

肾上腺中动脉
middle suprarenal artery

腹腔干
celiac trunk

腹主动脉
abdominal aorta

肾上腺下动脉
inferior suprarenal artery

左肾静脉
left renal vein

肠系膜上动脉
superior mesenteric artery

右肾动脉
right renal artery

右肾静脉
right renal vein

右输尿管
right ureter

右卵巢动脉
right ovarian artery

右卵巢静脉
right ovarian vein

图 223　右肾上腺
Right suprarenal gland

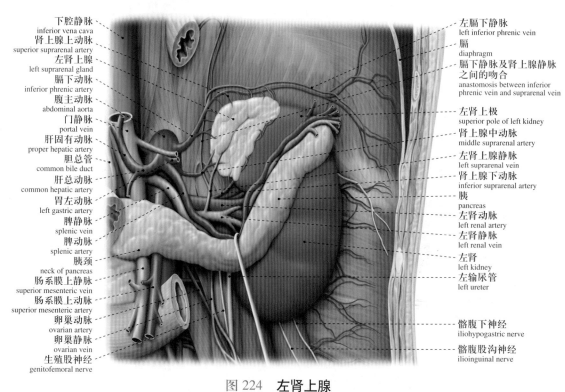

下腔静脉
inferior vena cava

肾上腺上动脉
superior suprarenal artery

左肾上腺
left suprarenal gland

膈下动脉
inferior phrenic artery

腹主动脉
abdominal aorta

门静脉
portal vein

肝固有动脉
proper hepatic artery

胆总管
common bile duct

肝总动脉
common hepatic artery

胃左动脉
left gastric artery

脾静脉
splenic vein

脾动脉
splenic artery

胰颈
neck of pancreas

肠系膜上静脉
superior mesenteric vein

肠系膜上动脉
superior mesenteric artery

卵巢动脉
ovarian artery

卵巢静脉
ovarian vein

生殖股神经
genitofemoral nerve

左膈下静脉
left inferior phrenic vein

膈
diaphragm

膈下静脉及肾上腺静脉
之间的吻合
anastomosis between inferior
phrenic vein and suprarenal vein

左肾上极
superior pole of left kidney

肾上腺中动脉
middle suprarenal artery

左肾上腺静脉
left suprarenal vein

肾上腺下动脉
inferior suprarenal artery

胰
pancreas

左肾动脉
left renal artery

左肾静脉
left renal vein

左肾
left kidney

左输尿管
left ureter

髂腹下神经
iliohypogastric nerve

髂腹股沟神经
ilioinguinal nerve

图 224　左肾上腺
Left suprarenal gland

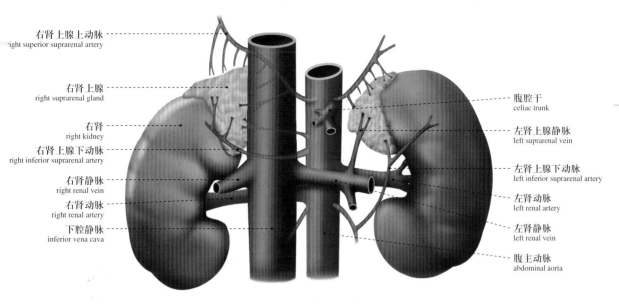

右肾上腺上动脉
right superior suprarenal artery

右肾上腺
right suprarenal gland

右肾
right kidney

右肾上腺下动脉
right inferior suprarenal artery

右肾静脉
right renal vein

右肾动脉
right renal artery

下腔静脉
inferior vena cava

腹腔干
celiac trunk

左肾上腺静脉
left suprarenal vein

左肾上腺下动脉
left inferior suprarenal artery

左肾动脉
left renal artery

左肾静脉
left renal vein

腹主动脉
abdominal aorta

图 225　肾上腺的血管 1

Blood vessels of the suprarenal gland 1

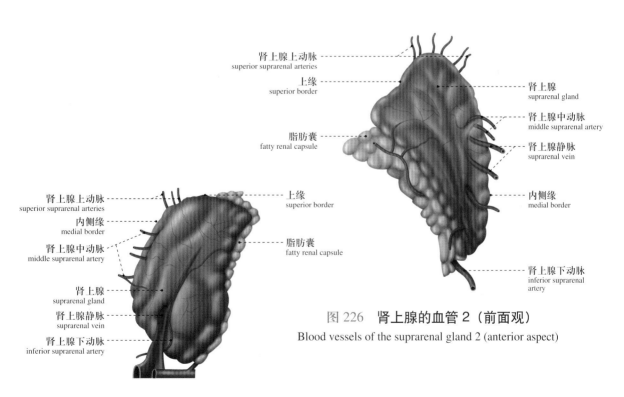

肾上腺上动脉
superior suprarenal arteries

上缘
superior border

脂肪囊
fatty renal capsule

肾上腺
suprarenal gland

肾上腺中动脉
middle suprarenal artery

肾上腺静脉
suprarenal vein

内侧缘
medial border

肾上腺下动脉
inferior suprarenal artery

图 226　肾上腺的血管 2（前面观）

Blood vessels of the suprarenal gland 2 (anterior aspect)

肾上腺上动脉
superior suprarenal arteries

内侧缘
medial border

肾上腺中动脉
middle suprarenal artery

肾上腺
suprarenal gland

肾上腺静脉
suprarenal vein

肾上腺下动脉
inferior suprarenal artery

上缘
superior border

脂肪囊
fatty renal capsule

图 227　肾上腺的血管 3（后面观）

Blood vessels of the suprarenal gland 3 (posterior aspect)

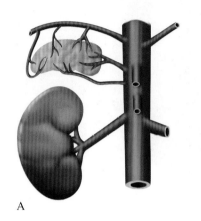

A

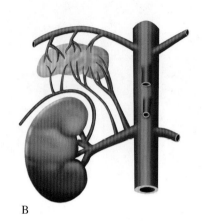

B

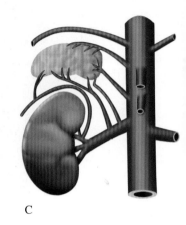

C

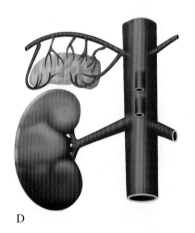

D

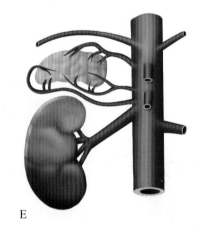

E

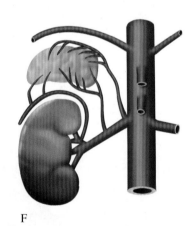

F

图 228　肾上腺动脉的变异

Variations of suprarenal gland artery

A. 起自膈下动脉和腹主动脉；B. 起自膈下动脉和肾动脉；C. 起自腹主动脉和肾动脉；
D. 起自膈下动脉；E. 起自腹主动脉；F. 起自肾动脉

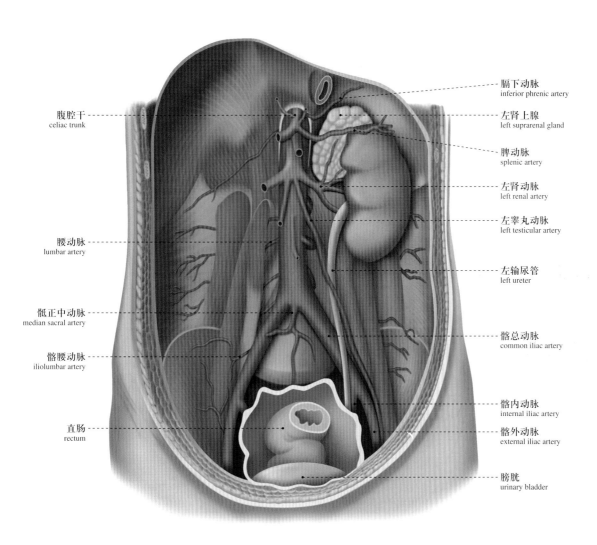

膈下动脉
inferior phrenic artery

左肾上腺
left suprarenal gland

脾动脉
splenic artery

左肾动脉
left renal artery

左睾丸动脉
left testicular artery

左输尿管
left ureter

髂总动脉
common iliac artery

髂内动脉
internal iliac artery

髂外动脉
external iliac artery

膀胱
urinary bladder

腹腔干
celiac trunk

腰动脉
lumbar artery

骶正中动脉
median sacral artery

髂腰动脉
iliolumbar artery

直肠
rectum

图 229　腹主动脉及其分支
Abdominal aorta and its branches

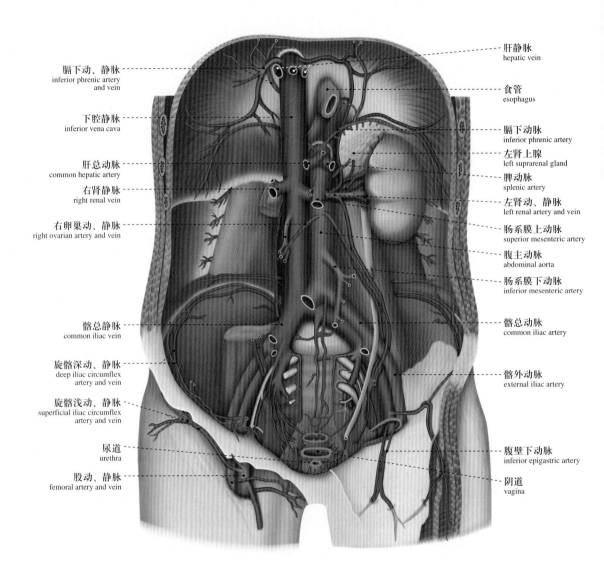

膈下动、静脉
inferior phrenic artery
and vein

下腔静脉
inferior vena cava

肝总动脉
common hepatic artery

右肾静脉
right renal vein

右卵巢动、静脉
right ovarian artery and vein

髂总静脉
common iliac vein

旋髂深动、静脉
deep iliac circumflex
artery and vein

旋髂浅动、静脉
superficial iliac circumflex
artery and vein

尿道
urethra

股动、静脉
femoral artery and vein

肝静脉
hepatic vein

食管
esophagus

膈下动脉
inferior phrenic artery

左肾上腺
left suprarenal gland

脾动脉
splenic artery

左肾动、静脉
left renal artery and vein

肠系膜上动脉
superior mesenteric artery

腹主动脉
abdominal aorta

肠系膜下动脉
inferior mesenteric artery

髂总动脉
common iliac artery

髂外动脉
external iliac artery

腹壁下动脉
inferior epigastric artery

阴道
vagina

图 230　腹膜后隙的大血管
Large vessels of the retroperitoneal space

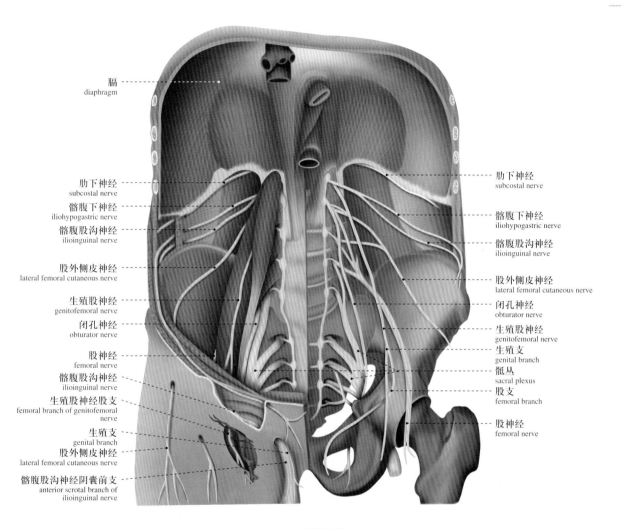

膈
diaphragm

肋下神经
subcostal nerve

髂腹下神经
iliohypogastric nerve

髂腹股沟神经
ilioinguinal nerve

股外侧皮神经
lateral femoral cutaneous nerve

生殖股神经
genitofemoral nerve

闭孔神经
obturator nerve

股神经
femoral nerve

髂腹股沟神经
ilioinguinal nerve

生殖股神经股支
femoral branch of genitofemoral nerve

生殖支
genital branch

股外侧皮神经
lateral femoral cutaneous nerve

髂腹股沟神经阴囊前支
anterior scrotal branch of ilioinguinal nerve

肋下神经
subcostal nerve

髂腹下神经
iliohypogastric nerve

髂腹股沟神经
ilioinguinal nerve

股外侧皮神经
lateral femoral cutaneous nerve

闭孔神经
obturator nerve

生殖股神经
genitofemoral nerve

生殖支
genital branch

骶丛
sacral plexus

股支
femoral branch

股神经
femoral nerve

图 231　腰骶丛
Plexus lumbosacralis

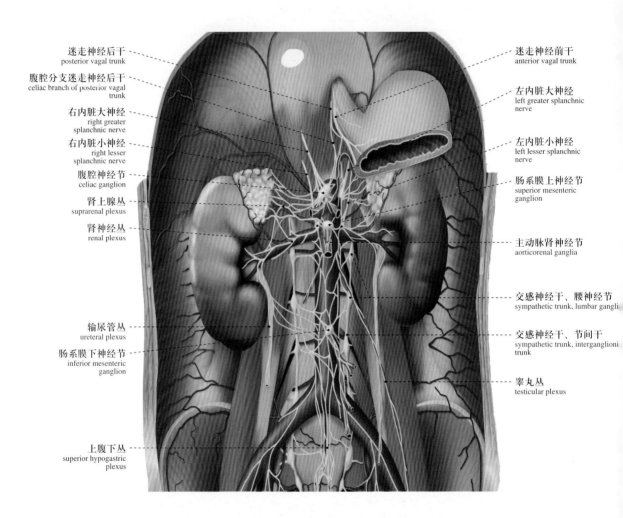

迷走神经后干
posterior vagal trunk

腹腔分支迷走神经后干
celiac branch of posterior vagal
trunk

右内脏大神经
right greater
splanchnic nerve

右内脏小神经
right lesser
splanchnic nerve

腹腔神经节
celiac ganglion

肾上腺丛
suprarenal plexus

肾神经丛
renal plexus

输尿管丛
ureteral plexus

肠系膜下神经节
inferior mesenteric
ganglion

上腹下丛
superior hypogastric
plexus

迷走神经前干
anterior vagal trunk

左内脏大神经
left greater splanchnic
nerve

左内脏小神经
left lesser splanchnic
nerve

肠系膜上神经节
superior mesenteric
ganglion

主动脉肾神经节
aorticorenal ganglia

交感神经干、腰神经节
sympathetic trunk, lumbar gangli

交感神经干、节间干
sympathetic trunk, interganglioni
trunk

睾丸丛
testicular plexus

图 232　腹膜后隙的自主神经节和神经丛
Autonomic ganglia and plexuses of the retroperitoneal space

第六节

腹部断面

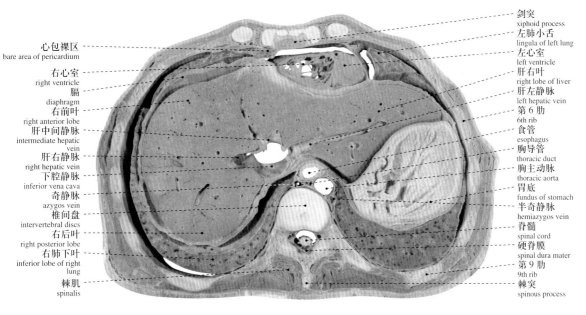

心包裸区
bare area of pericardium

右心室
right ventricle

膈
diaphragm

右前叶
right anterior lobe

肝中间静脉
intermediate hepatic vein

肝右静脉
right hepatic vein

下腔静脉
inferior vena cava

奇静脉
azygos vein

椎间盘
intervertebral discs

右后叶
right posterior lobe

右肺下叶
inferior lobe of right lung

棘肌
spinalis

剑突
xiphoid process

左肺小舌
lingula of left lung

左心室
left ventricle

肝右叶
right lobe of liver

肝左静脉
left hepatic vein

第 6 肋
6th rib

食管
esophagus

胸导管
thoracic duct

胸主动脉
thoracic aorta

胃底
fundus of stomach

半奇静脉
hemiazygos vein

脊髓
spinal cord

硬脊膜
spinal dura mater

第 9 肋
9th rib

棘突
spinous process

图 233　腹部水平断面 1

Horizontal section of the abdomen 1

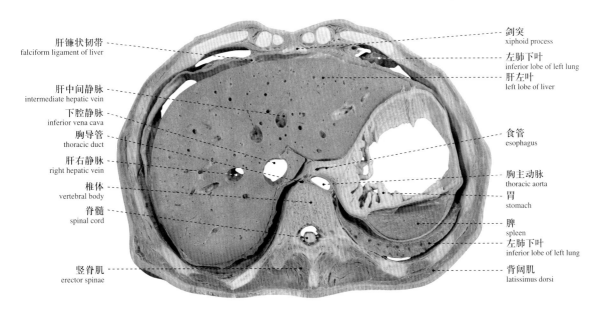

肝镰状韧带
falciform ligament of liver

肝中间静脉
intermediate hepatic vein

下腔静脉
inferior vena cava

胸导管
thoracic duct

肝右静脉
right hepatic vein

椎体
vertebral body

脊髓
spinal cord

竖脊肌
erector spinae

剑突
xiphoid process

左肺下叶
inferior lobe of left lung

肝左叶
left lobe of liver

食管
esophagus

胸主动脉
thoracic aorta

胃
stomach

脾
spleen

左肺下叶
inferior lobe of left lung

背阔肌
latissimus dorsi

图 234　腹部水平断面 2

Horizontal section of the abdomen 2

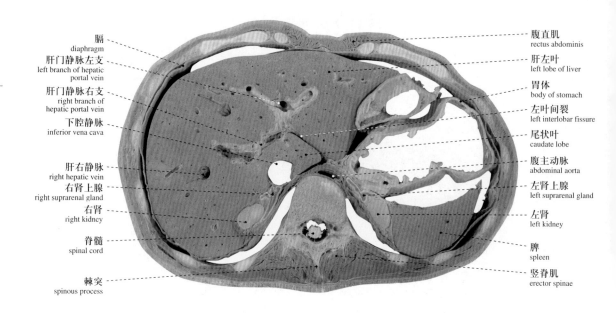

膈
diaphragm

肝门静脉左支
left branch of hepatic portal vein

肝门静脉右支
right branch of hepatic portal vein

下腔静脉
inferior vena cava

肝右静脉
right hepatic vein

右肾上腺
right suprarenal gland

右肾
right kidney

脊髓
spinal cord

棘突
spinous process

腹直肌
rectus abdominis

肝左叶
left lobe of liver

胃体
body of stomach

左叶间裂
left interlobar fissure

尾状叶
caudate lobe

腹主动脉
abdominal aorta

左肾上腺
left suprarenal gland

左肾
left kidney

脾
spleen

竖脊肌
erector spinae

图 235　腹部水平断面 3

Horizontal section of the abdomen 3

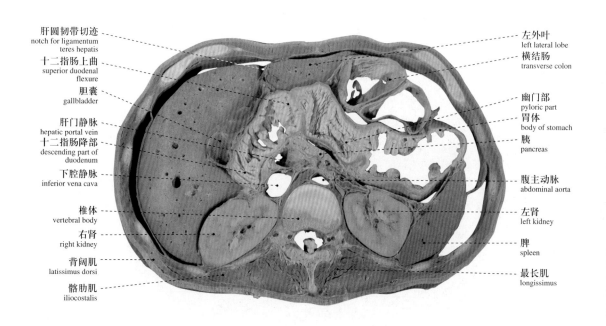

肝圆韧带切迹
notch for ligamentum teres hepatis

十二指肠上曲
superior duodenal flexure

胆囊
gallbladder

肝门静脉
hepatic portal vein

十二指肠降部
descending part of duodenum

下腔静脉
inferior vena cava

椎体
vertebral body

右肾
right kidney

背阔肌
latissimus dorsi

髂肋肌
iliocostalis

左外叶
left lateral lobe

横结肠
transverse colon

幽门部
pyloric part

胃体
body of stomach

胰
pancreas

腹主动脉
abdominal aorta

左肾
left kidney

脾
spleen

最长肌
longissimus

图 236　腹部水平断面 4

Horizontal section of the abdomen 4

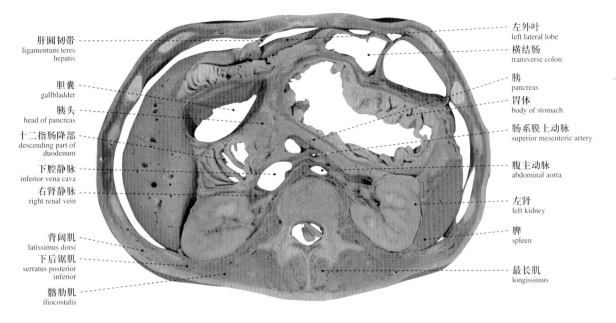

肝圆韧带
ligamentum teres
hepatis

胆囊
gallbladder

胰头
head of pancreas

十二指肠降部
descending part of
duodenum

下腔静脉
inferior vena cava

右肾静脉
right renal vein

背阔肌
latissimus dorsi

下后锯肌
serratus posterior
inferior

髂肋肌
iliocostalis

左外叶
left lateral lobe

横结肠
transverse colon

胰
pancreas

胃体
body of stomach

肠系膜上动脉
superior mesenteric artery

腹主动脉
abdominal aorta

左肾
left kidney

脾
spleen

最长肌
longissimus

图 237 腹部水平断面 5
Horizontal section of the abdomen 5

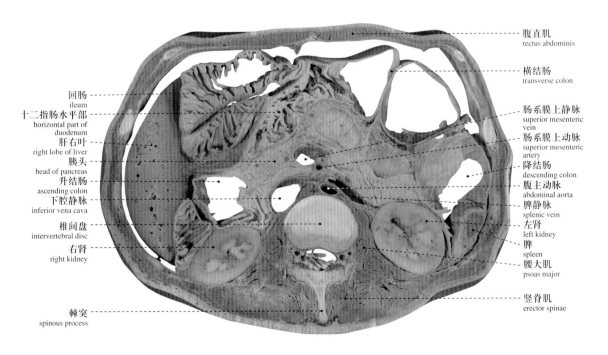

回肠
ileum

十二指肠水平部
horizontal part of
duodenum

肝右叶
right lobe of liver

胰头
head of pancreas

升结肠
ascending colon

下腔静脉
inferior vena cava

椎间盘
intervertebral disc

右肾
right kidney

棘突
spinous process

腹直肌
rectus abdominis

横结肠
transverse colon

肠系膜上静脉
superior mesenteric
vein

肠系膜上动脉
superior mesenteric
artery

降结肠
descending colon

腹主动脉
abdominal aorta

脾静脉
splenic vein

左肾
left kidney

脾
spleen

腰大肌
psoas major

竖脊肌
erector spinae

图 238 腹部水平断面 6
Horizontal section of the abdomen 6

盆部分区

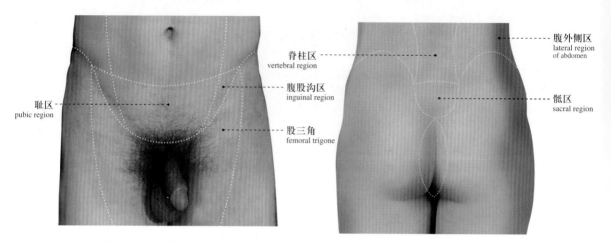

脊柱区
vertebral region

腹股沟区
inguinal region

股三角
femoral trigone

耻区
pubic region

腹外侧区
lateral region
of abdomen

骶区
sacral region

图 239　男性盆部分区
Regions of the male pelvis

图 240　骶部分区
Regions of the sacral

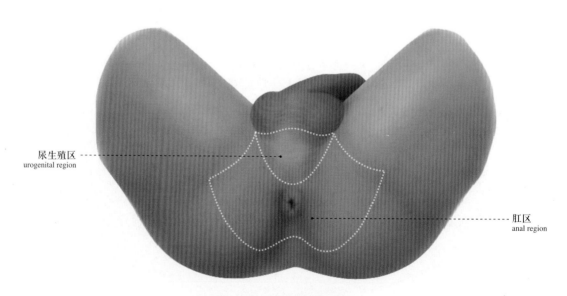

尿生殖区
urogenital region

肛区
anal region

图 241　男性会阴分区
Regions of the male perineum

第二节

骨 盆

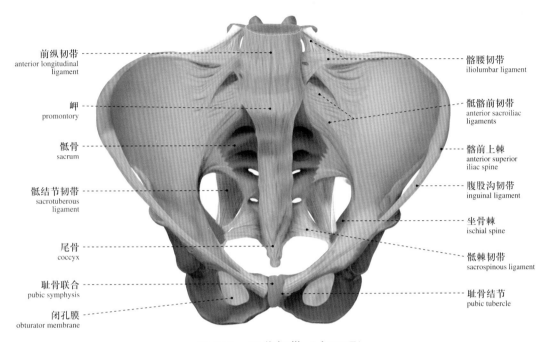

前纵韧带
anterior longitudinal ligament

岬
promontory

骶骨
sacrum

骶结节韧带
sacrotuberous ligament

尾骨
coccyx

耻骨联合
pubic symphysis

闭孔膜
obturator membrane

髂腰韧带
iliolumbar ligament

骶髂前韧带
anterior sacroiliac ligaments

髂前上棘
anterior superior iliac spine

腹股沟韧带
inguinal ligament

坐骨棘
ischial spine

骶棘韧带
sacrospinous ligament

耻骨结节
pubic tubercle

图 242　骨盆韧带（上面观）
Ligaments of the pelvic (superior aspect)

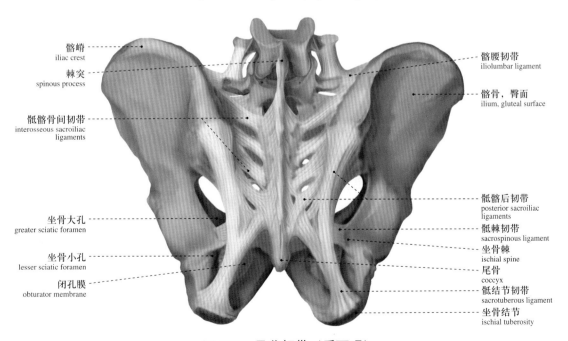

髂嵴
iliac crest

棘突
spinous process

骶髂骨间韧带
interosseous sacroiliac ligaments

坐骨大孔
greater sciatic foramen

坐骨小孔
lesser sciatic foramen

闭孔膜
obturator membrane

髂腰韧带
iliolumbar ligament

髂骨，臀面
ilium, gluteal surface

骶髂后韧带
posterior sacroiliac ligaments

骶棘韧带
sacrospinous ligament

坐骨棘
ischial spine

尾骨
coccyx

骶结节韧带
sacrotuberous ligament

坐骨结节
ischial tuberosity

图 243　骨盆韧带（后面观）
Ligaments of the pelvic (posterior aspect)

137

第三节

盆 部

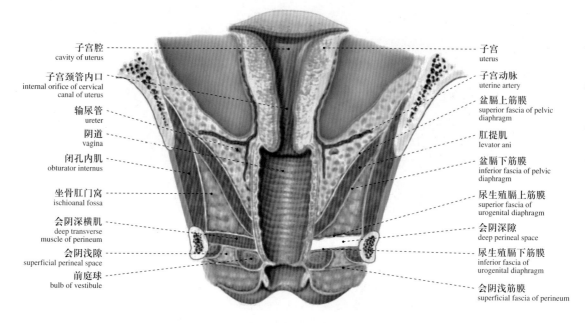

子宫腔 cavity of uterus	子宫 uterus
子宫颈管内口 internal orifice of cervical canal of uterus	子宫动脉 uterine artery
输尿管 ureter	盆膈上筋膜 superior fascia of pelvic diaphragm
阴道 vagina	肛提肌 levator ani
闭孔内肌 obturator internus	盆膈下筋膜 inferior fascia of pelvic diaphragm
坐骨肛门窝 ischioanal fossa	尿生殖膈上筋膜 superior fascia of urogenital diaphragm
会阴深横肌 deep transverse muscle of perineum	会阴深隙 deep perineal space
会阴浅隙 superficial perineal space	尿生殖膈下筋膜 inferior fascia of urogenital diaphragm
前庭球 bulb of vestibule	会阴浅筋膜 superficial fascia of perineum

图 244　女性盆腔冠状切面（模式图）
Coronal section of the female pelvic cavity (diagram)

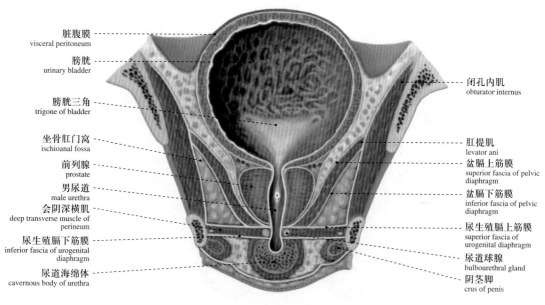

脏腹膜 visceral peritoneum	
膀胱 urinary bladder	
膀胱三角 trigone of bladder	闭孔内肌 obturator internus
坐骨肛门窝 ischioanal fossa	肛提肌 levator ani
前列腺 prostate	盆膈上筋膜 superior fascia of pelvic diaphragm
男尿道 male urethra	盆膈下筋膜 inferior fascia of pelvic diaphragm
会阴深横肌 deep transverse muscle of perineum	尿生殖膈上筋膜 superior fascia of urogenital diaphragm
尿生殖膈下筋膜 inferior fascia of urogenital diaphragm	尿道球腺 bulbourethral gland
尿道海绵体 cavernous body of urethra	阴茎脚 crus of penis

图 245　男性盆腔冠状切面（模式图）
Coronal section of the male pelvic cavity (diagram)

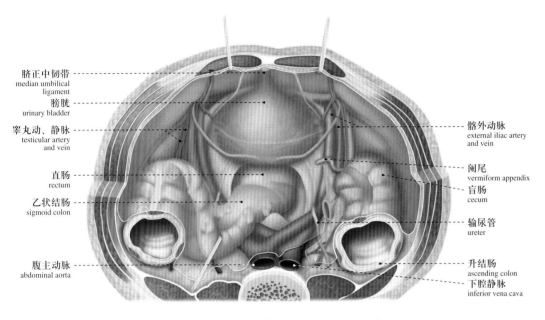

图 246　男性盆腔内容（上面观）

Male pelvic contents (superior aspect)

脐正中韧带 median umbilical ligament

膀胱 urinary bladder

睾丸动、静脉 testicular artery and vein

直肠 rectum

乙状结肠 sigmoid colon

腹主动脉 abdominal aorta

髂外动脉 external iliac artery and vein

阑尾 vermiform appendix

盲肠 cecum

输尿管 ureter

升结肠 ascending colon

下腔静脉 inferior vena cava

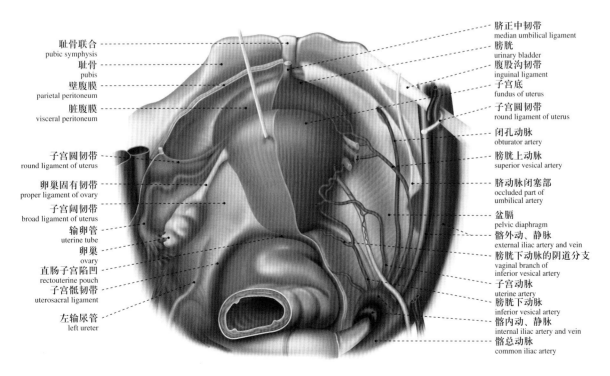

图 247　女性子宫和膀胱（上面观）

Ureters and bladder in the female（superior aspect）

耻骨联合 pubic symphysis

耻骨 pubis

壁腹膜 parietal peritoneum

脏腹膜 visceral peritoneum

子宫圆韧带 round ligament of uterus

卵巢固有韧带 proper ligament of ovary

子宫阔韧带 broad ligament of uterus

输卵管 uterine tube

卵巢 ovary

直肠子宫陷凹 rectouterine pouch

子宫骶韧带 uterosacral ligament

左输尿管 left ureter

脐正中韧带 median umbilical ligament

膀胱 urinary bladder

腹股沟韧带 inguinal ligament

子宫底 fundus of uterus

子宫圆韧带 round ligament of uterus

闭孔动脉 obturator artery

膀胱上动脉 superior vesical artery

脐动脉闭塞部 occluded part of umbilical artery

盆膈 pelvic diaphragm

髂外动、静脉 external iliac artery and vein

膀胱下动脉的阴道分支 vaginal branch of inferior vesical artery

子宫动脉 uterine artery

膀胱下动脉 inferior vesical artery

髂内动、静脉 internal iliac artery and vein

髂总动脉 common iliac artery

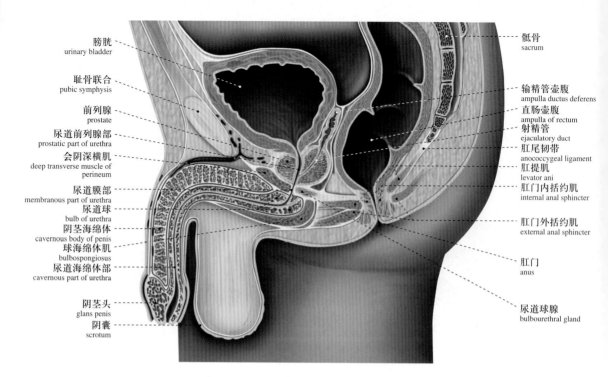

膀胱
urinary bladder

耻骨联合
pubic symphysis

前列腺
prostate

尿道前列腺部
prostatic part of urethra

会阴深横肌
deep transverse muscle of perineum

尿道膜部
membranous part of urethra

尿道球
bulb of urethra

阴茎海绵体
cavernous body of penis

球海绵体肌
bulbospongiosus

尿道海绵体部
cavernous part of urethra

阴茎头
glans penis

阴囊
scrotum

骶骨
sacrum

输精管壶腹
ampulla ductus deferens

直肠壶腹
ampulla of rectum

射精管
ejaculatory duct

肛尾韧带
anococcygeal ligament

肛提肌
levator ani

肛门内括约肌
internal anal sphincter

肛门外括约肌
external anal sphincter

肛门
anus

尿道球腺
bulbourethral gland

图 248　男性盆腔（正中矢状断）
Male pelvic cavity (median sagittal section)

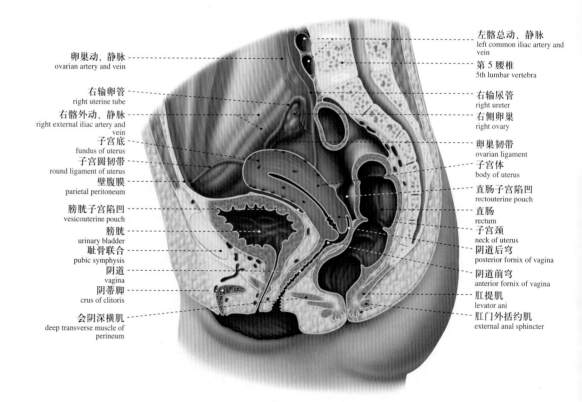

卵巢动、静脉
ovarian artery and vein

右输卵管
right uterine tube

右髂外动、静脉
right external iliac artery and vein

子宫底
fundus of uterus

子宫圆韧带
round ligament of uterus

壁腹膜
parietal peritoneum

膀胱子宫陷凹
vesicouterine pouch

膀胱
urinary bladder

耻骨联合
pubic symphysis

阴道
vagina

阴蒂脚
crus of clitoris

会阴深横肌
deep transverse muscle of perineum

左髂总动、静脉
left common iliac artery and vein

第 5 腰椎
5th lumbar vertebra

右输尿管
right ureter

右侧卵巢
right ovary

卵巢韧带
ovarian ligament

子宫体
body of uterus

直肠子宫陷凹
rectouterine pouch

直肠
rectum

子宫颈
neck of uterus

阴道后穹
posterior fornix of vagina

阴道前穹
anterior fornix of vagina

肛提肌
levator ani

肛门外括约肌
external anal sphincter

图 249　女性盆腔（正中矢状断）
Female pelvic cavity (median sagittal section)

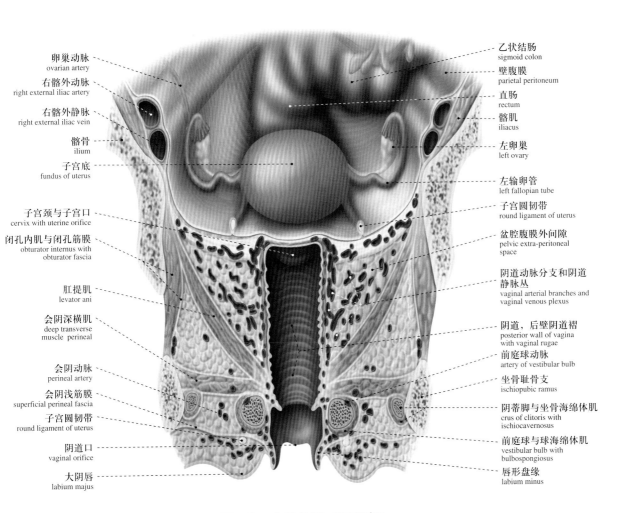

卵巢动脉
ovarian artery

右髂外动脉
right external iliac artery

右髂外静脉
right external iliac vein

髂骨
ilium

子宫底
fundus of uterus

子宫颈与子宫口
cervix with uterine orifice

闭孔内肌与闭孔筋膜
obturator internus with obturator fascia

肛提肌
levator ani

会阴深横肌
deep transverse muscle perineal

会阴动脉
perineal artery

会阴浅筋膜
superficial perineal fascia

子宫圆韧带
round ligament of uterus

阴道口
vaginal orifice

大阴唇
labium majus

乙状结肠
sigmoid colon

壁腹膜
parietal peritoneum

直肠
rectum

髂肌
iliacus

左卵巢
left ovary

左输卵管
left fallopian tube

子宫圆韧带
round ligament of uterus

盆腔腹膜外间隙
pelvic extra-peritoneal space

阴道动脉分支和阴道静脉丛
vaginal arterial branches and vaginal venous plexus

阴道，后壁阴道褶
posterior wall of vagina with vaginal rugae

前庭球动脉
artery of vestibular bulb

坐骨耻骨支
ischiopubic ramus

阴蒂脚与坐骨海绵体肌
crus of clitoris with ischiocavernosus

前庭球与球海绵体肌
vestibular bulb with bulbospongiosus

唇形盘缘
labium minus

图 250　女性盆腔（冠状断）

Female pelvic cavity (coronal section)

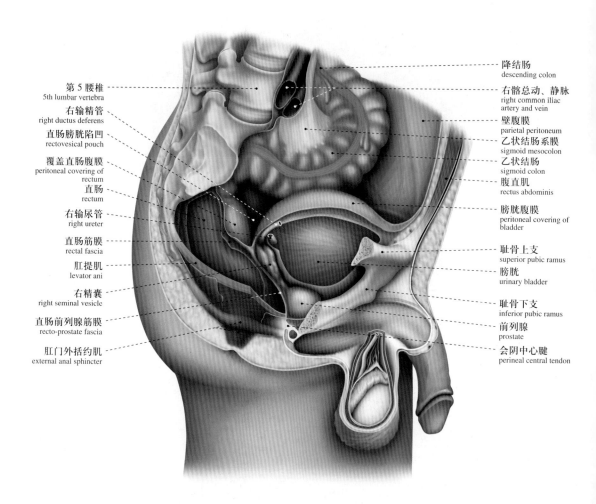

第 5 腰椎
5th lumbar vertebra

右输精管
right ductus deferens

直肠膀胱陷凹
rectovesical pouch

覆盖直肠腹膜
peritoneal covering of rectum

直肠
rectum

右输尿管
right ureter

直肠筋膜
rectal fascia

肛提肌
levator ani

右精囊
right seminal vesicle

直肠前列腺筋膜
recto-prostate fascia

肛门外括约肌
external anal sphincter

降结肠
descending colon

右髂总动、静脉
right common iliac artery and vein

壁腹膜
parietal peritoneum

乙状结肠系膜
sigmoid mesocolon

乙状结肠
sigmoid colon

腹直肌
rectus abdominis

膀胱腹膜
peritoneal covering of bladder

耻骨上支
superior pubic ramus

膀胱
urinary bladder

耻骨下支
inferior pubic ramus

前列腺
prostate

会阴中心腱
perineal central tendon

图 251 男性盆腔脏器与腹膜的关系
Relationship between male pelvic organs and peritoneum

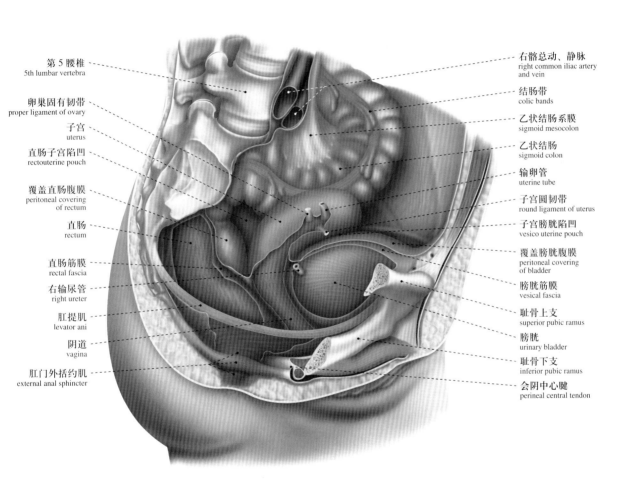

第 5 腰椎
5th lumbar vertebra

卵巢固有韧带
proper ligament of ovary

子宫
uterus

直肠子宫陷凹
rectouterine pouch

覆盖直肠腹膜
peritoneal covering
of rectum

直肠
rectum

直肠筋膜
rectal fascia

右输尿管
right ureter

肛提肌
levator ani

阴道
vagina

肛门外括约肌
external anal sphincter

右髂总动、静脉
right common iliac artery
and vein

结肠带
colic bands

乙状结肠系膜
sigmoid mesocolon

乙状结肠
sigmoid colon

输卵管
uterine tube

子宫圆韧带
round ligament of uterus

子宫膀胱陷凹
vesico uterine pouch

覆盖膀胱腹膜
peritoneal covering
of bladder

膀胱筋膜
vesical fascia

耻骨上支
superior pubic ramus

膀胱
urinary bladder

耻骨下支
inferior pubic ramus

会阴中心腱
perineal central tendon

图 252　女性盆腔脏器与腹膜的关系
Relationship between female pelvic organs and peritoneum

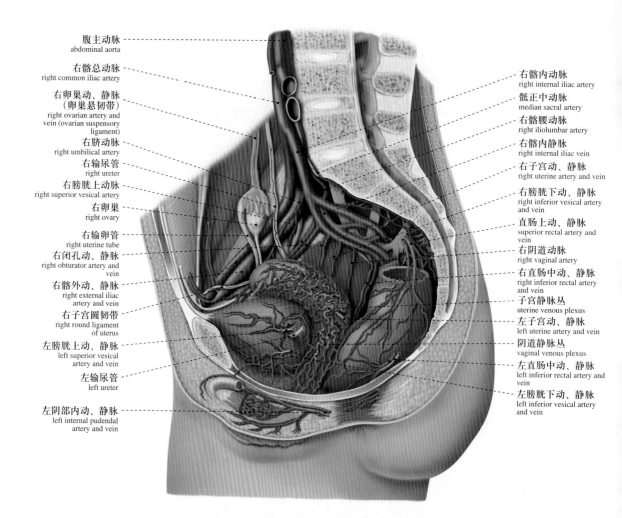

腹主动脉
abdominal aorta

右髂总动脉
right common iliac artery

右卵巢动、静脉
（卵巢悬韧带）
right ovarian artery and
vein (ovarian suspensory
ligament)

右脐动脉
right umbilical artery

右输尿管
right ureter

右膀胱上动脉
right superior vesical artery

右卵巢
right ovary

右输卵管
right uterine tube

右闭孔动、静脉
right obturator artery and
vein

右髂外动、静脉
right external iliac
artery and vein

右子宫圆韧带
right round ligament
of uterus

左膀胱上动、静脉
left superior vesical
artery and vein

左输尿管
left ureter

左阴部内动、静脉
left internal pudendal
artery and vein

右髂内动脉
right internal iliac artery

骶正中动脉
median sacral artery

右髂腰动脉
right iliolumbar artery

右髂内静脉
right internal iliac vein

右子宫动、静脉
right uterine artery and vein

右膀胱下动、静脉
right inferior vesical artery
and vein

直肠上动、静脉
superior rectal artery and
vein

右阴道动脉
right vaginal artery

右直肠中动、静脉
right inferior rectal artery
and vein

子宫静脉丛
uterine venous plexus

左子宫动、静脉
left uterine artery and vein

阴道静脉丛
vaginal venous plexus

左直肠中动、静脉
left inferior rectal artery and
vein

左膀胱下动、静脉
left inferior vesical artery
and vein

图 253　女性盆腔器官的动脉和静脉
Arteries and veins of the pelvic organs in the female

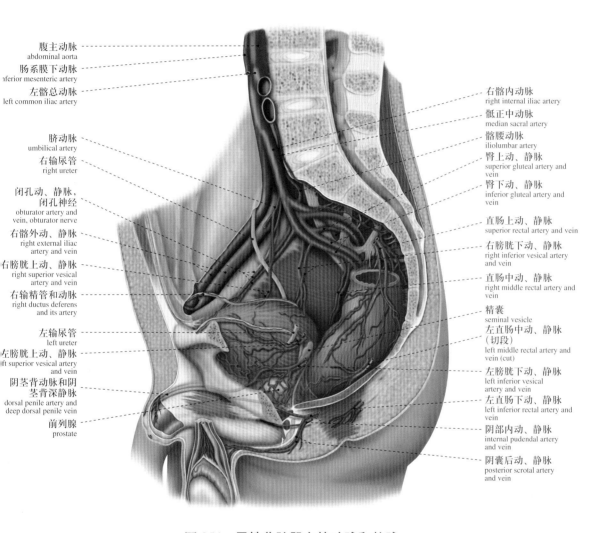

腹主动脉
abdominal aorta

肠系膜下动脉
inferior mesenteric artery

左髂总动脉
left common iliac artery

脐动脉
umbilical artery

右输尿管
right ureter

闭孔动、静脉，闭孔神经
obturator artery and vein, obturator nerve

右髂外动、静脉
right external iliac artery and vein

右膀胱上动、静脉
right superior vesical artery and vein

右输精管和动脉
right ductus deferens and its artery

左输尿管
left ureter

左膀胱上动、静脉
left superior vesical artery and vein

阴茎背动脉和阴茎背深静脉
dorsal penile artery and deep dorsal penile vein

前列腺
prostate

右髂内动脉
right internal iliac artery

骶正中动脉
median sacral artery

髂腰动脉
iliolumbar artery

臀上动、静脉
superior gluteal artery and vein

臀下动、静脉
inferior gluteal artery and vein

直肠上动、静脉
superior rectal artery and vein

右膀胱下动、静脉
right inferior vesical artery and vein

直肠中动、静脉
right middle rectal artery and vein

精囊
seminal vesicle

左直肠中动、静脉（切段）
left middle rectal artery and vein (cut)

左膀胱下动、静脉
left inferior vesical artery and vein

左直肠下动、静脉
left inferior rectal artery and vein

阴部内动、静脉
internal pudendal artery and vein

阴囊后动、静脉
posterior scrotal artery and vein

图 254 男性盆腔器官的动脉和静脉
Arteries and veins of the pelvic organs in the male

145

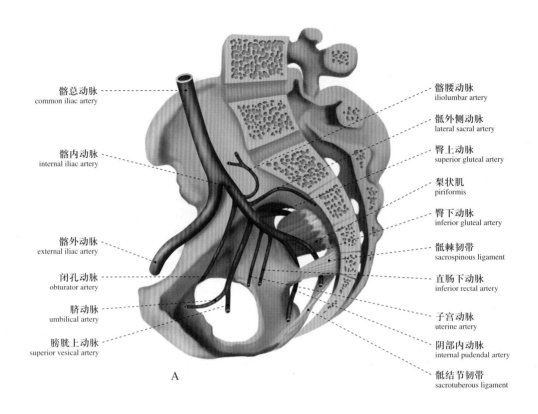

髂总动脉 common iliac artery	髂腰动脉 iliolumbar artery
	骶外侧动脉 lateral sacral artery
髂内动脉 internal iliac artery	臀上动脉 superior gluteal artery
	梨状肌 piriformis
	臀下动脉 inferior gluteal artery
髂外动脉 external iliac artery	骶棘韧带 sacrospinous ligament
闭孔动脉 obturator artery	直肠下动脉 inferior rectal artery
脐动脉 umbilical artery	子宫动脉 uterine artery
膀胱上动脉 superior vesical artery	阴部内动脉 internal pudendal artery
	骶结节韧带 sacrotuberous ligament

A

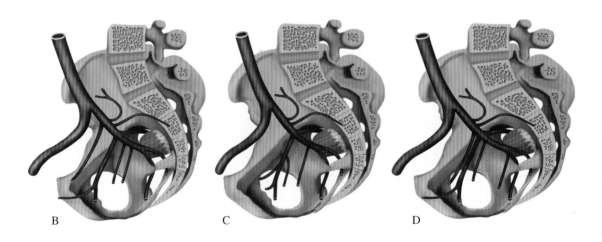

B   C   D

图 255 髂内动脉分支的变异
Branch variations of the internal iliac artery

A. 所有分支都起自髂内动脉本干；B. 髂内动脉分为两条主要分支；C. 髂内动脉分成三条主要分支；
D. 髂内动脉分出三条以上主要分支

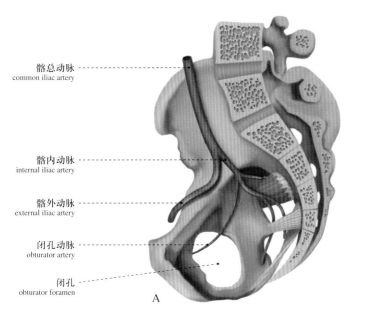
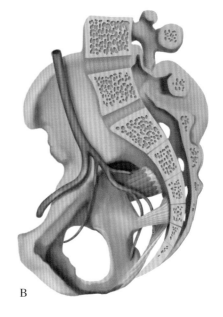

髂总动脉
common iliac artery

髂内动脉
internal iliac artery

髂外动脉
external iliac artery

闭孔动脉
obturator artery

闭孔
obturator foramen

A

B

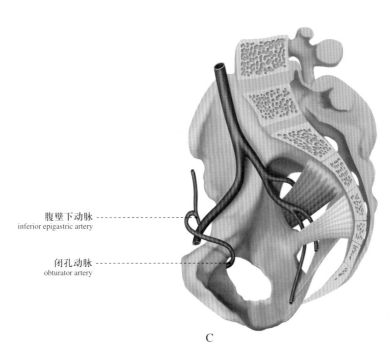

腹壁下动脉
inferior epigastric artery

闭孔动脉
obturator artery

C

图 256　闭孔动脉的变异
Variations of the obturator artery

A. 起自髂内动脉前支；B. 单独起自髂内动脉；C. 起自髂外动脉仅 75% 的闭孔动脉是髂内动脉干的分支

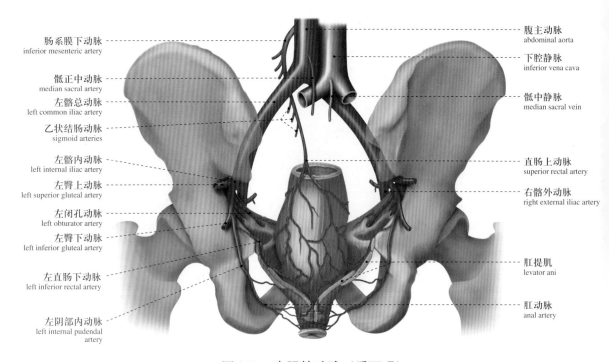

肠系膜下动脉
inferior mesenteric artery

骶正中动脉
median sacral artery

左髂总动脉
left common iliac artery

乙状结肠动脉
sigmoid arteries

左髂内动脉
left internal iliac artery

左臀上动脉
left superior gluteal artery

左闭孔动脉
left obturator artery

左臀下动脉
left inferior gluteal artery

左直肠下动脉
left inferior rectal artery

左阴部内动脉
left internal pudendal
artery

腹主动脉
abdominal aorta

下腔静脉
inferior vena cava

骶中静脉
median sacral vein

直肠上动脉
superior rectal artery

右髂外动脉
right external iliac artery

肛提肌
levator ani

肛动脉
anal artery

图 257　直肠的动脉（后面观）
Arteries of the rectum (posterior aspect)

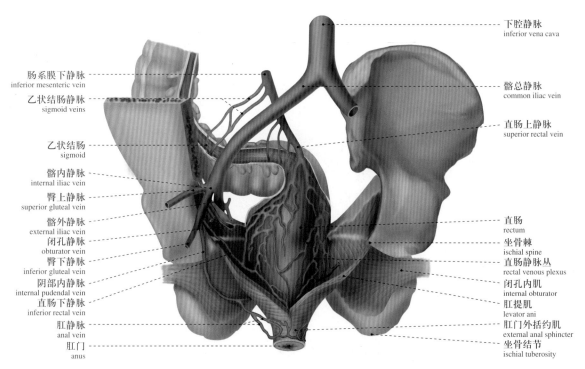

肠系膜下静脉
inferior mesenteric vein

乙状结肠静脉
sigmoid veins

乙状结肠
sigmoid

髂内静脉
internal iliac vein

臀上静脉
superior gluteal vein

髂外静脉
external iliac vein

闭孔静脉
obturator vein

臀下静脉
inferior gluteal vein

阴部内静脉
internal pudendal vein

直肠下静脉
inferior rectal vein

肛静脉
anal vein

肛门
anus

下腔静脉
inferior vena cava

髂总静脉
common iliac vein

直肠上静脉
superior rectal vein

直肠
rectum

坐骨棘
ischial spine

直肠静脉丛
rectal venous plexus

闭孔内肌
internal obturator

肛提肌
levator ani

肛门外括约肌
external anal sphincter

坐骨结节
ischial tuberosity

图 258　直肠的静脉（后面观）
Veins of the rectum (posterior aspect)

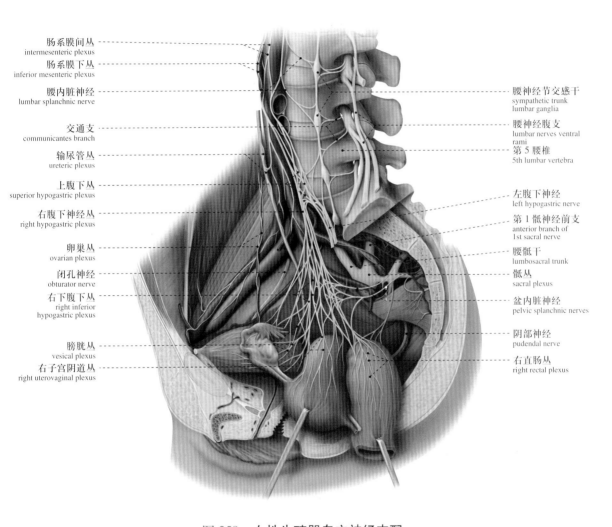

肠系膜间丛
intermesenteric plexus

肠系膜下丛
inferior mesenteric plexus

腰内脏神经
lumbar splanchnic nerve

交通支
communicantes branch

输尿管丛
ureteric plexus

上腹下丛
superior hypogastric plexus

右腹下神经丛
right hypogastric plexus

卵巢丛
ovarian plexus

闭孔神经
obturator nerve

右下腹下丛
right inferior
hypogastric plexus

膀胱丛
vesical plexus

右子宫阴道丛
right uterovaginal plexus

腰神经节交感干
sympathetic trunk
lumbar ganglia

腰神经腹支
lumbar nerves ventral
rami

第 5 腰椎
5th lumbar vertebra

左腹下神经
left hypogastric nerve

第 1 骶神经前支
anterior branch of
1st sacral nerve

腰骶干
lumbosacral trunk

骶丛
sacral plexus

盆内脏神经
pelvic splanchnic nerves

阴部神经
pudendal nerve

右直肠丛
right rectal plexus

图 259　女性生殖器自主神经支配
Autonomic innervation of the female genitalia

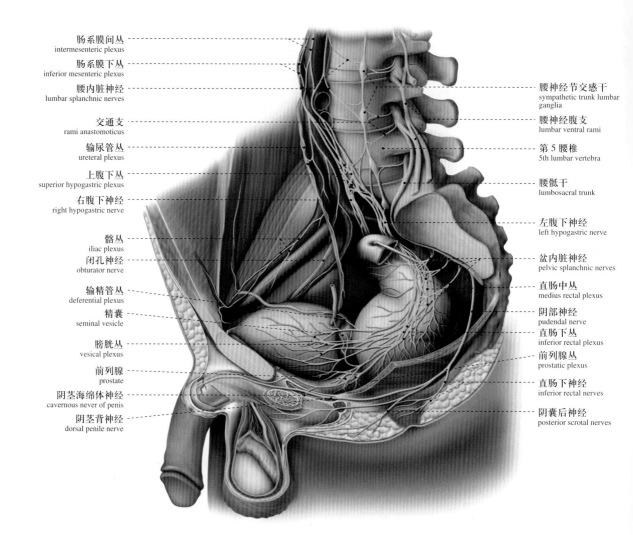

肠系膜间丛
intermesenteric plexus

肠系膜下丛
inferior mesenteric plexus

腰内脏神经
lumbar splanchnic nerves

交通支
rami anastomoticus

输尿管丛
ureteral plexus

上腹下丛
superior hypogastric plexus

右腹下神经
right hypogastric nerve

髂丛
iliac plexus

闭孔神经
obturator nerve

输精管丛
deferential plexus

精囊
seminal vesicle

膀胱丛
vesical plexus

前列腺
prostate

阴茎海绵体神经
cavernous never of penis

阴茎背神经
dorsal penile nerve

腰神经节交感干
sympathetic trunk lumbar ganglia

腰神经腹支
lumbar ventral rami

第 5 腰椎
5th lumbar vertebra

腰骶干
lumbosacral trunk

左腹下神经
left hypogastric nerve

盆内脏神经
pelvic splanchnic nerves

直肠中丛
medius rectal plexus

阴部神经
pudendal nerve

直肠下丛
inferior rectal plexus

前列腺丛
prostatic plexus

直肠下神经
inferior rectal nerves

阴囊后神经
posterior scrotal nerves

图 260　男性生殖器自主神经支配
Autonomic innervation of the male genitalia

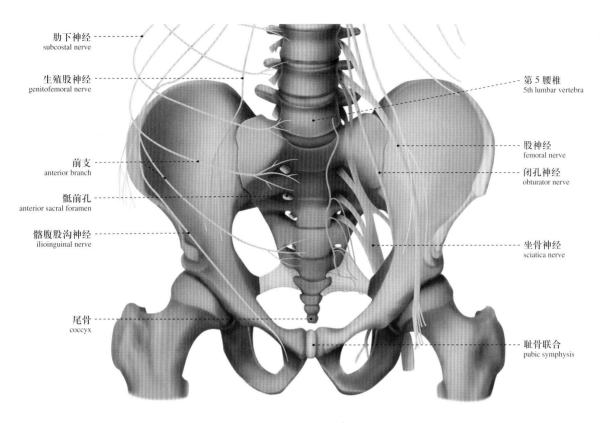

肋下神经
subcostal nerve

生殖股神经
genitofemoral nerve

前支
anterior branch

骶前孔
anterior sacral foramen

髂腹股沟神经
ilioinguinal nerve

尾骨
coccyx

第 5 腰椎
5th lumbar vertebra

股神经
femoral nerve

闭孔神经
obturator nerve

坐骨神经
sciatica nerve

耻骨联合
pubic symphysis

图 261　盆腔的神经
Pelvic nerves

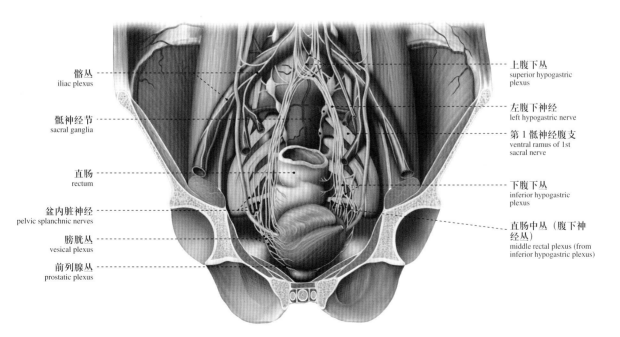

髂丛
iliac plexus

骶神经节
sacral ganglia

直肠
rectum

盆内脏神经
pelvic splanchnic nerves

膀胱丛
vesical plexus

前列腺丛
prostatic plexus

上腹下丛
superior hypogastric plexus

左腹下神经
left hypogastric nerve

第 1 骶神经腹支
ventral ramus of 1st sacral nerve

下腹下丛
inferior hypogastric plexus

直肠中丛（腹下神经丛）
middle rectal plexus (from inferior hypogastric plexus)

图 262　膀胱和直肠的自主神经支配
Autonomic innervation of the bladder and rectum

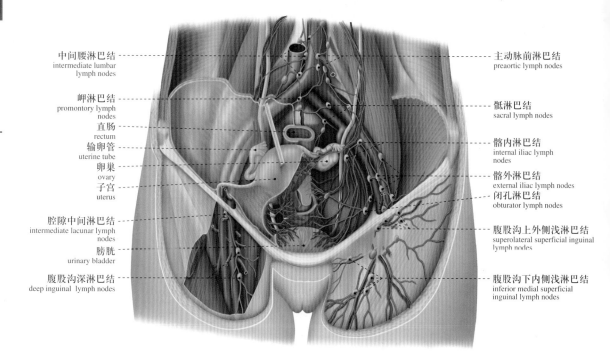

中间腰淋巴结
intermediate lumbar
lymph nodes

岬淋巴结
promontory lymph
nodes

直肠
rectum

输卵管
uterine tube

卵巢
ovary

子宫
uterus

腔隙中间淋巴结
intermediate lacunar lymph
nodes

膀胱
urinary bladder

腹股沟深淋巴结
deep inguinal lymph nodes

主动脉前淋巴结
preaortic lymph nodes

骶淋巴结
sacral lymph nodes

髂内淋巴结
internal iliac lymph
nodes

髂外淋巴结
external iliac lymph nodes

闭孔淋巴结
obturator lymph nodes

腹股沟上外侧浅淋巴结
superolateral superficial inguinal
lymph nodes

腹股沟下内侧浅淋巴结
inferior medial superficial
inguinal lymph nodes

图 263　女性生殖器的淋巴
Lymph of the female genitalis

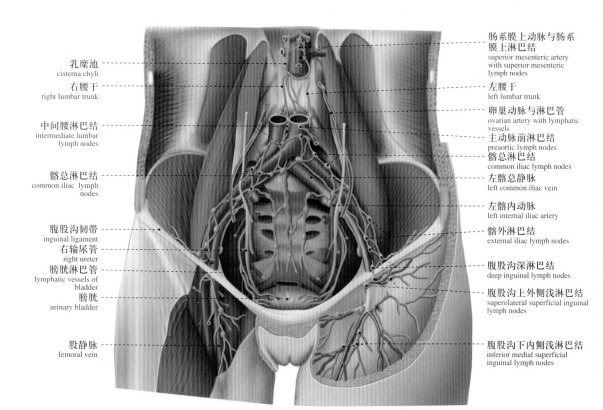

乳糜池
cisterna chyli

右腰干
right lumbar trunk

中间腰淋巴结
intermediate lumbar
lymph nodes

髂总淋巴结
common iliac lymph
nodes

腹股沟韧带
inguinal ligament

右输尿管
right ureter

膀胱淋巴管
lymphatic vessels of
bladder

膀胱
urinary bladder

股静脉
femoral vein

肠系膜上动脉与肠系
膜上淋巴结
superior mesenteric artery
with superior mesenteric
lymph nodes

左腰干
left lumbar trunk

卵巢动脉与淋巴管
ovarian artery with lymphatic
vessels

主动脉前淋巴结
preaortic lymph nodes

髂总淋巴结
common iliac lymph nodes

左髂总静脉
left common iliac vein

左髂内动脉
left internal iliac artery

髂外淋巴结
external iliac lymph nodes

腹股沟深淋巴结
deep inguinal lymph nodes

腹股沟上外侧浅淋巴结
superolateral superficial inguinal
lymph nodes

腹股沟下内侧浅淋巴结
inferior medial superficial
inguinal lymph nodes

图 264　膀胱的盆腔淋巴结和淋巴回流（女性）
Pelvic lymph nodes and the lymphatic drainage of the bladder (female)

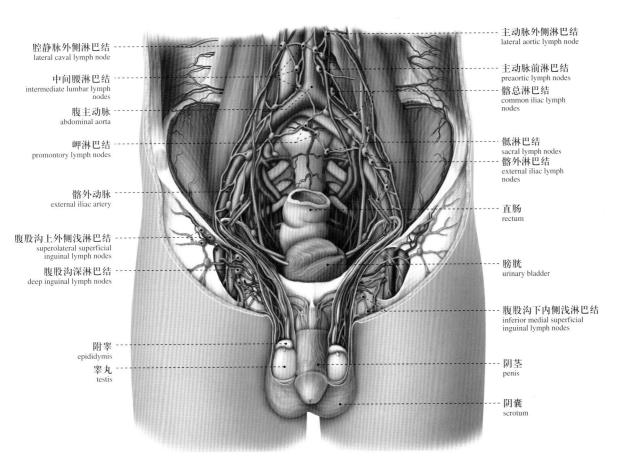

腔静脉外侧淋巴结
lateral caval lymph node

中间腰淋巴结
intermediate lumbar lymph
nodes

腹主动脉
abdominal aorta

岬淋巴结
promontory lymph nodes

髂外动脉
external iliac artery

腹股沟上外侧浅淋巴结
superolateral superficial
inguinal lymph nodes

腹股沟深淋巴结
deep inguinal lymph nodes

附睾
epididymis

睾丸
testis

主动脉外侧淋巴结
lateral aortic lymph node

主动脉前淋巴结
preaortic lymph nodes

髂总淋巴结
common iliac lymph
nodes

骶淋巴结
sacral lymph nodes

髂外淋巴结
external iliac lymph
nodes

直肠
rectum

膀胱
urinary bladder

腹股沟下内侧浅淋巴结
inferior medial superficial
inguinal lymph nodes

阴茎
penis

阴囊
scrotum

图 265　男性生殖器的淋巴
Lymph of the male genitalis

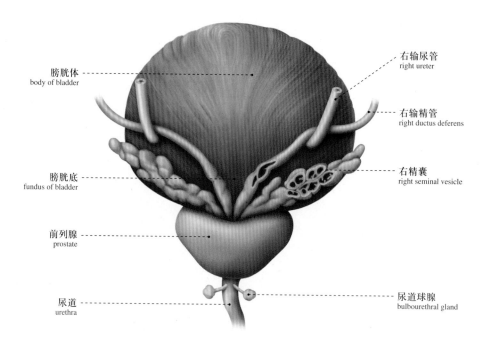

膀胱体
body of bladder

右输尿管
right ureter

右输精管
right ductus deferens

膀胱底
fundus of bladder

右精囊
right seminal vesicle

前列腺
prostate

尿道
urethra

尿道球腺
bulbourethral gland

图 266　膀胱、前列腺及精囊腺（后面观）
Urinary bladder, prostate and seminal vesicles (posterior aspect)

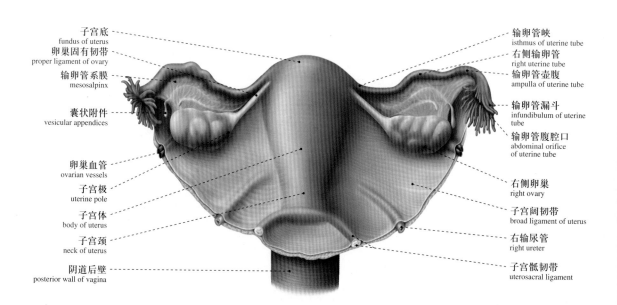

子宫底
fundus of uterus

卵巢固有韧带
proper ligament of ovary

输卵管系膜
mesosalpinx

囊状附件
vesicular appendices

卵巢血管
ovarian vessels

子宫极
uterine pole

子宫体
body of uterus

子宫颈
neck of uterus

阴道后壁
posterior wall of vagina

输卵管峡
isthmus of uterine tube

右侧输卵管
right uterine tube

输卵管壶腹
ampulla of uterine tube

输卵管漏斗
infundibulum of uterine tube

输卵管腹腔口
abdominal orifice of uterine tube

右侧卵巢
right ovary

子宫阔韧带
broad ligament of uterus

右输尿管
right ureter

子宫骶韧带
uterosacral ligament

图 267　子宫及附件（后上面观）
Uterus and the adnexa (posterosuperior aspect)

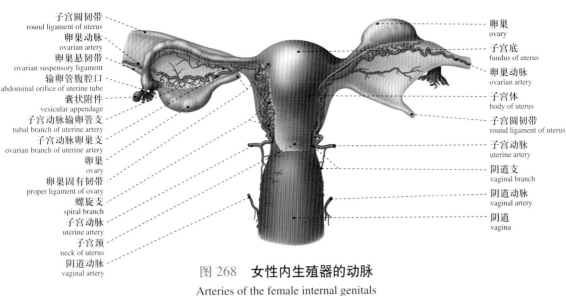

子宫圆韧带
round ligament of uterus

卵巢动脉
ovarian artery

卵巢悬韧带
ovarian suspensory ligament

输卵管腹腔口
abdominal orifice of uterine tube

囊状附件
vesicular appendage

子宫动脉输卵管支
tubal branch of uterine artery

子宫动脉卵巢支
ovarian branch of uterine artery

卵巢
ovary

卵巢固有韧带
proper ligament of ovary

螺旋支
spiral branch

子宫动脉
uterine artery

子宫颈
neck of uterus

阴道动脉
vaginal artery

卵巢
ovary

子宫底
fundus of uterus

卵巢动脉
ovarian artery

子宫体
body of uterus

子宫圆韧带
round ligament of uterus

子宫动脉
uterine artery

阴道支
vaginal branch

阴道动脉
vaginal artery

阴道
vagina

图 268 女性内生殖器的动脉
Arteries of the female internal genitals

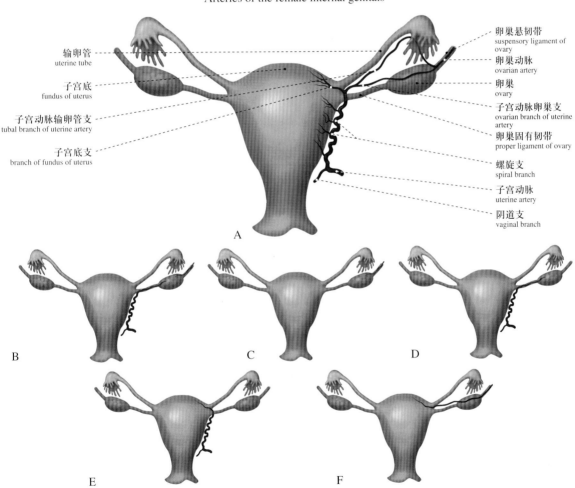

输卵管
uterine tube

子宫底
fundus of uterus

子宫动脉输卵管支
tubal branch of uterine artery

子宫底支
branch of fundus of uterus

卵巢悬韧带
suspensory ligament of ovary

卵巢动脉
ovarian artery

卵巢
ovary

子宫动脉卵巢支
ovarian branch of uterine artery

卵巢固有韧带
proper ligament of ovary

螺旋支
spiral branch

子宫动脉
uterine artery

阴道支
vaginal branch

A

B   C   D

E   F

图 269 女性内生殖器的动脉变异
Arterial variations of the female internal genitals

A. 营养子宫的血管；B. 营养卵巢的血管；C. 营养卵巢的血管；D. 营养卵巢的血管；
E. 营养子宫底的血管；F. 营养子宫底的血管

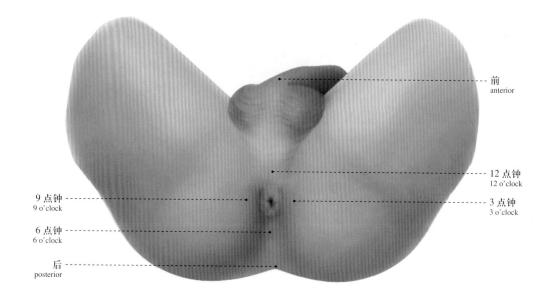

前
anterior

12 点钟
12 o'clock

9 点钟
9 o'clock

3 点钟
3 o'clock

6 点钟
6 o'clock

后
posterior

图 270　男性会阴体表
Surface of the male perineum

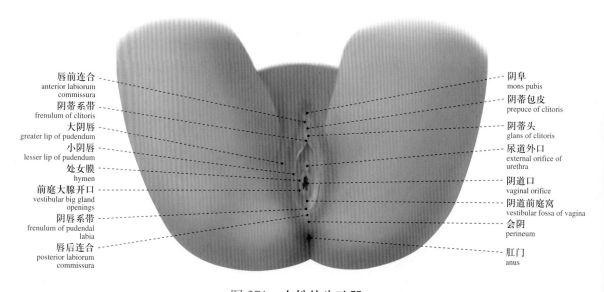

唇前连合
anterior labiorum
commissura

阴蒂系带
frenulum of clitoris

大阴唇
greater lip of pudendum

小阴唇
lesser lip of pudendum

处女膜
hymen

前庭大腺开口
vestibular big gland
openings

阴唇系带
frenulum of pudendal
labia

唇后连合
posterior labiorum
commissura

阴阜
mons pubis

阴蒂包皮
prepuce of clitoris

阴蒂头
glans of clitoris

尿道外口
external orifice of
urethra

阴道口
vaginal orifice

阴道前庭窝
vestibular fossa of vagina

会阴
perineum

肛门
anus

图 271　女性外生殖器
External genital organs of the female

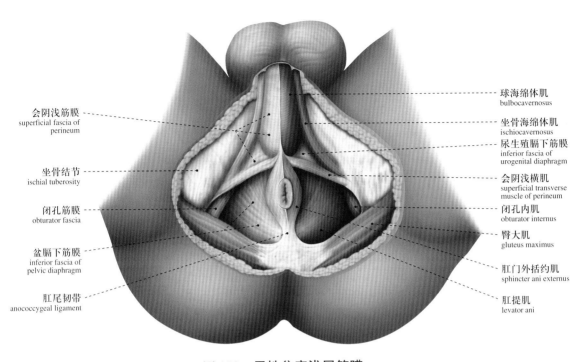

会阴浅筋膜
superficial fascia of
perineum

坐骨结节
ischial tuberosity

闭孔筋膜
obturator fascia

盆膈下筋膜
inferior fascia of
pelvic diaphragm

肛尾韧带
anococcygeal ligament

球海绵体肌
bulbocavernosus

坐骨海绵体肌
ischiocavernosus

尿生殖膈下筋膜
inferior fascia of
urogenital diaphragm

会阴浅横肌
superficial transverse
muscle of perineum

闭孔内肌
obturator internus

臀大肌
gluteus maximus

肛门外括约肌
sphincter ani externus

肛提肌
levator ani

图 272　男性盆底浅层筋膜
Superficial fasciae of the male pelvic floor

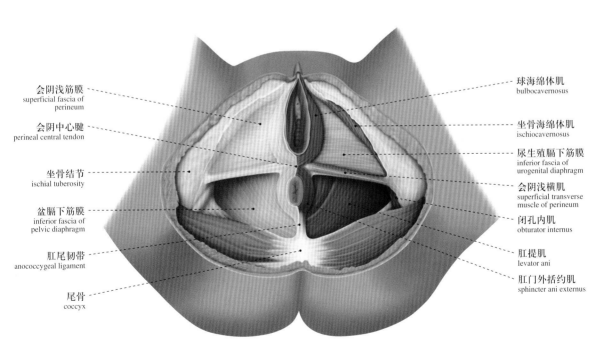

会阴浅筋膜
superficial fascia of
perineum

会阴中心腱
perineal central tendon

坐骨结节
ischial tuberosity

盆膈下筋膜
inferior fascia of
pelvic diaphragm

肛尾韧带
anococcygeal ligament

尾骨
coccyx

球海绵体肌
bulbocavernosus

坐骨海绵体肌
ischiocavernosus

尿生殖膈下筋膜
inferior fascia of
urogenital diaphragm

会阴浅横肌
superficial transverse
muscle of perineum

闭孔内肌
obturator internus

肛提肌
levator ani

肛门外括约肌
sphincter ani externus

图 273　女性盆底浅层筋膜
Superficial fasciae of the female pelvic floor

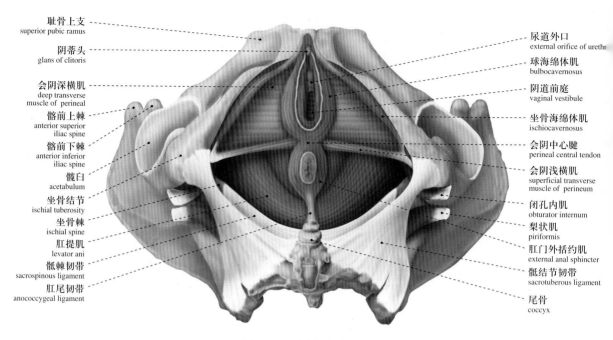

耻骨上支
superior pubic ramus

阴蒂头
glans of clitoris

会阴深横肌
deep transverse
muscle of perineal

髂前上棘
anterior superior
iliac spine

髂前下棘
anterior inferior
iliac spine

髋臼
acetabulum

坐骨结节
ischial tuberosity

坐骨棘
ischial spine

肛提肌
levator ani

骶棘韧带
sacrospinous ligament

肛尾韧带
anococcygeal ligament

尿道外口
external orifice of urethra

球海绵体肌
bulbocavernosus

阴道前庭
vaginal vestibule

坐骨海绵体肌
ischiocavernosus

会阴中心腱
perineal central tendon

会阴浅横肌
superficial transverse
muscle of perineum

闭孔内肌
obturator internus

梨状肌
piriformis

肛门外括约肌
external anal sphincter

骶结节韧带
sacrotuberous ligament

尾骨
coccyx

图 274　女性盆底肌 1
Muscles of the female pelvic floor 1

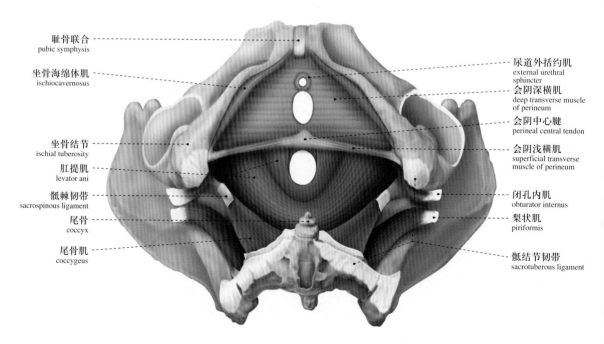

耻骨联合
pubic symphysis

坐骨海绵体肌
ischiocavernosus

坐骨结节
ischial tuberosity

肛提肌
levator ani

骶棘韧带
sacrospinous ligament

尾骨
coccyx

尾骨肌
coccygeus

尿道外括约肌
external urethral
sphincter

会阴深横肌
deep transverse muscle
of perineum

会阴中心腱
perineal central tendon

会阴浅横肌
superficial transverse
muscle of perineum

闭孔内肌
obturator internus

梨状肌
piriformis

骶结节韧带
sacrotuberous ligament

图 275　女性盆底肌 2
Muscles of the female pelvic floor 2

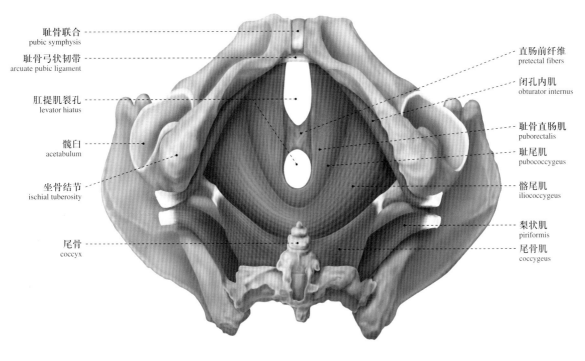

图 276　女性盆底肌 3
Muscles of the female pelvic floor 3

耻骨联合　pubic symphysis
耻骨弓状韧带　arcuate pubic ligament
肛提肌裂孔　levator hiatus
髋臼　acetabulum
坐骨结节　ischial tuberosity
尾骨　coccyx

直肠前纤维　pretectal fibers
闭孔内肌　obturator internus
耻骨直肠肌　puborectalis
耻尾肌　pubococcygeus
髂尾肌　iliococcygeus
梨状肌　piriformis
尾骨肌　coccygeus

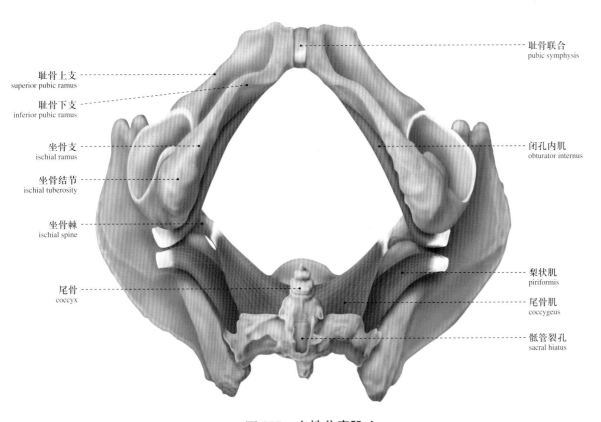

图 277　女性盆底肌 4
Muscles of the female pelvic floor 4

耻骨上支　superior pubic ramus
耻骨下支　inferior pubic ramus
坐骨支　ischial ramus
坐骨结节　ischial tuberosity
坐骨棘　ischial spine
尾骨　coccyx

耻骨联合　pubic symphysis
闭孔内肌　obturator internus
梨状肌　piriformis
尾骨肌　coccygeus
骶管裂孔　sacral hiatus

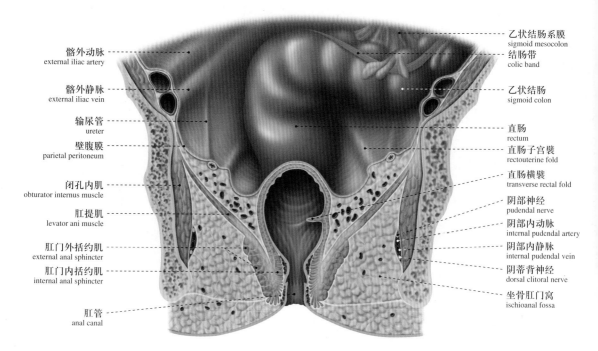

髂外动脉
external iliac artery

髂外静脉
external iliac vein

输尿管
ureter

壁腹膜
parietal peritoneum

闭孔内肌
obturator internus muscle

肛提肌
levator ani muscle

肛门外括约肌
external anal sphincter

肛门内括约肌
internal anal sphincter

肛管
anal canal

乙状结肠系膜
sigmoid mesocolon

结肠带
colic band

乙状结肠
sigmoid colon

直肠
rectum

直肠子宫襞
rectouterine fold

直肠横襞
transverse rectal fold

阴部神经
pudendal nerve

阴部内动脉
internal pudendal artery

阴部内静脉
internal pudendal vein

阴蒂背神经
dorsal clitoral nerve

坐骨肛门窝
ischioanal fossa

图 278　坐骨直肠窝（冠状断）
Ischioanal fossa (coronary section)

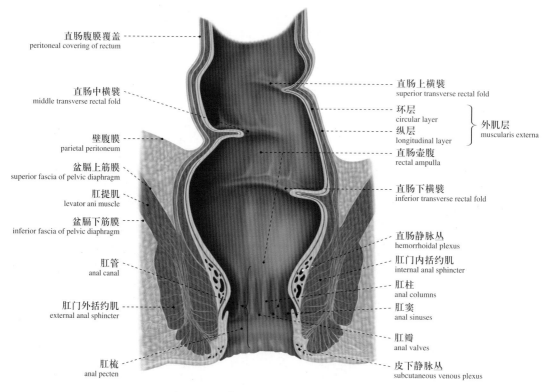

直肠腹膜覆盖
peritoneal covering of rectum

直肠中横襞
middle transverse rectal fold

壁腹膜
parietal peritoneum

盆膈上筋膜
superior fascia of pelvic diaphragm

肛提肌
levator ani muscle

盆膈下筋膜
inferior fascia of pelvic diaphragm

肛管
anal canal

肛门外括约肌
external anal sphincter

肛梳
anal pecten

直肠上横襞
superior transverse rectal fold

环层
circular layer

纵层
longitudinal layer

外肌层
muscularis externa

直肠壶腹
rectal ampulla

直肠下横襞
inferior transverse rectal fold

直肠静脉丛
hemorrhoidal plexus

肛门内括约肌
internal anal sphincter

肛柱
anal columns

肛窦
anal sinuses

肛瓣
anal valves

皮下静脉丛
subcutaneous venous plexus

图 279　直肠及肛门（冠状断）
Rectum and anus (coronary section)

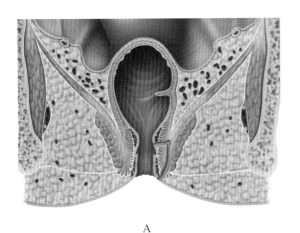

A

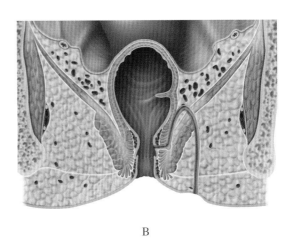

B

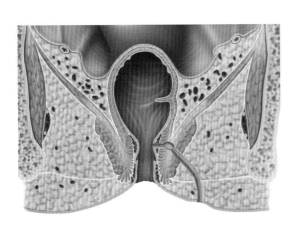

C

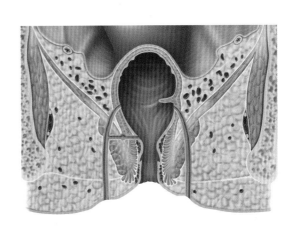

D

图 280　肛瘘的解剖学类型
Anatomy types of anal fistula

A. 肛管括约肌间型；B. 肛管括约肌间上型；C. 经肛管括约肌型；D. 经肛管括约肌外型

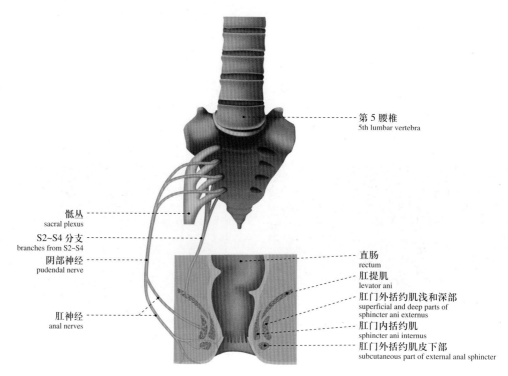

第 5 腰椎
5th lumbar vertebra

骶丛
sacral plexus

S2~S4 分支
branches from S2~S4

阴部神经
pudendal nerve

肛神经
anal nerves

直肠
rectum

肛提肌
levator ani

肛门外括约肌浅和深部
superficial and deep parts of
sphincter ani externus

肛门内括约肌
sphincter ani internus

肛门外括约肌皮下部
subcutaneous part of external anal sphincter

图 281 肛门的躯体运动和躯体神经支配
Somatomotor and somatosensory innervation of the anus

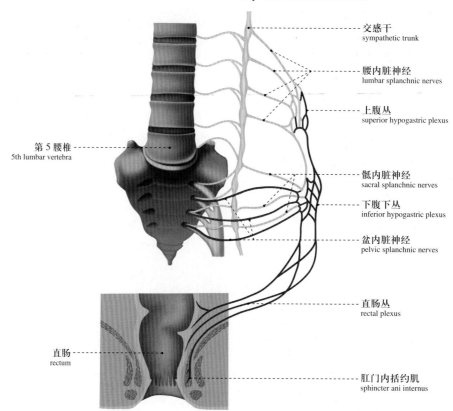

交感干
sympathetic trunk

腰内脏神经
lumbar splanchnic nerves

上腹丛
superior hypogastric plexus

骶内脏神经
sacral splanchnic nerves

下腹下丛
inferior hypogastric plexus

盆内脏神经
pelvic splanchnic nerves

第 5 腰椎
5th lumbar vertebra

直肠丛
rectal plexus

直肠
rectum

肛门内括约肌
sphincter ani internus

图 282 肛门的内脏运动和内脏感觉神经支配
Visceromotor and viscerosensory innervation of the anus

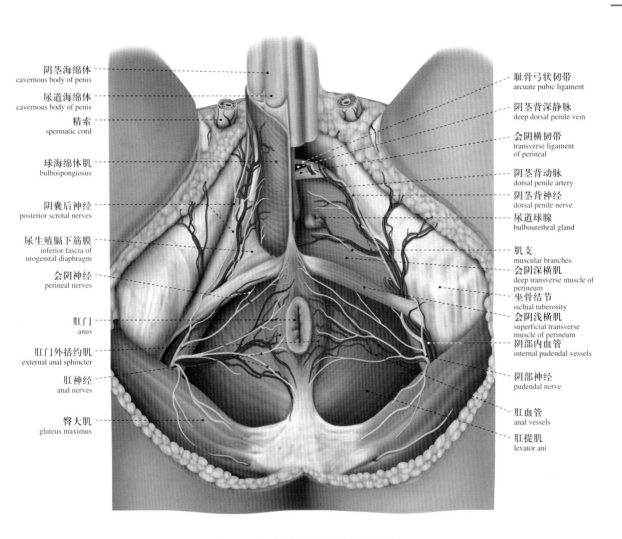

阴茎海绵体
cavernous body of penis

尿道海绵体
cavernous body of penis

精索
spermatic cord

球海绵体肌
bulbospongiosus

阴囊后神经
posterior scrotal nerves

尿生殖膈下筋膜
inferior fascia of
urogenital diaphragm

会阴神经
perineal nerves

肛门
anus

肛门外括约肌
external anal sphincter

肛神经
anal nerves

臀大肌
gluteus maximus

耻骨弓状韧带
arcuate pubic ligament

阴茎背深静脉
deep dorsal penile vein

会阴横韧带
transverse ligament
of perineal

阴茎背动脉
dorsal penile artery

阴茎背神经
dorsal penile nerve

尿道球腺
bulbourethral gland

肌支
muscular branches

会阴深横肌
deep transverse muscle of
perineum

坐骨结节
ischial tuberosity

会阴浅横肌
superficial transverse
muscle of perineum

阴部内血管
internal pudendal vessels

阴部神经
pudendal nerve

肛血管
anal vessels

肛提肌
levator ani

图 283 男性会阴部血管和神经
Blood vessels and nerves of the male perineum

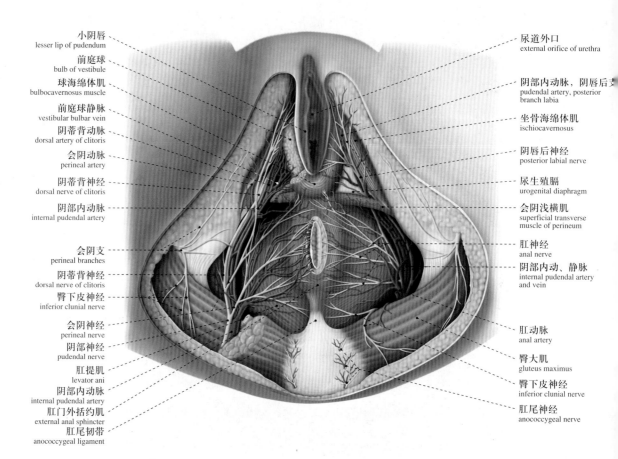

小阴唇
lesser lip of pudendum

前庭球
bulb of vestibule

球海绵体肌
bulbocavernosus muscle

前庭球静脉
vestibular bulbar vein

阴蒂背动脉
dorsal artery of clitoris

会阴动脉
perineal artery

阴蒂背神经
dorsal nerve of clitoris

阴部内动脉
internal pudendal artery

会阴支
perineal branches

阴蒂背神经
dorsal nerve of clitoris

臀下皮神经
inferior clunial nerve

会阴神经
perineal nerve

阴部神经
pudendal nerve

肛提肌
levator ani

阴部内动脉
internal pudendal artery

肛门外括约肌
external anal sphincter

肛尾韧带
anococcygeal ligament

尿道外口
external orifice of urethra

阴部内动脉，阴唇后支
pudendal artery, posterior branch labia

坐骨海绵体肌
ischiocavernosus

阴唇后神经
posterior labial nerve

尿生殖膈
urogenital diaphragm

会阴浅横肌
superficial transverse muscle of perineum

肛神经
anal nerve

阴部内动、静脉
internal pudendal artery and vein

肛动脉
anal artery

臀大肌
gluteus maximus

臀下皮神经
inferior clunial nerve

肛尾神经
anococcygeal nerve

图 284 女性会阴区和外生殖器的血管、神经
Female perineal region and blood vessels, nerves

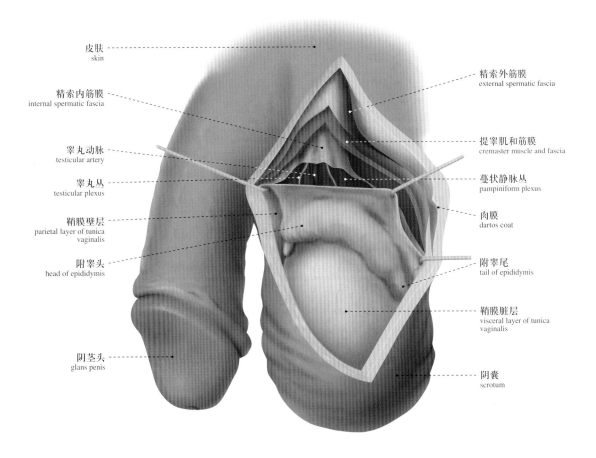

皮肤
skin

精索外筋膜
external spermatic fascia

精索内筋膜
internal spermatic fascia

提睾肌和筋膜
cremaster muscle and fascia

睾丸动脉
testicular artery

蔓状静脉丛
pampiniform plexus

睾丸丛
testicular plexus

肉膜
dartos coat

鞘膜壁层
parietal layer of tunica vaginalis

附睾头
head of epididymis

附睾尾
tail of epididymis

鞘膜脏层
visceral layer of tunica vaginalis

阴茎头
glans penis

阴囊
scrotum

图 285　阴囊结构
Structure of the scrotum

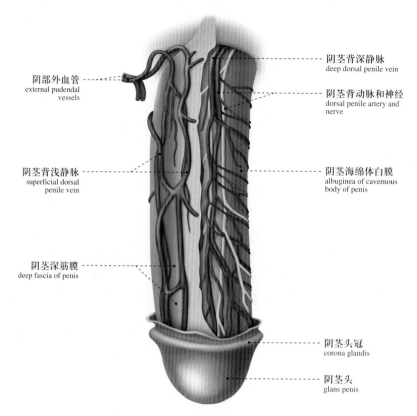

阴部外血管
external pudendal
vessels

阴茎背浅静脉
superficial dorsal
penile vein

阴茎深筋膜
deep fascia of penis

阴茎背深静脉
deep dorsal penile vein

阴茎背动脉和神经
dorsal penile artery and
nerve

阴茎海绵体白膜
albuginea of cavernous
body of penis

阴茎头冠
corona glandis

阴茎头
glans penis

图 286　阴茎背部血管和神经
Dorsal blood vessels and nerves of the penis

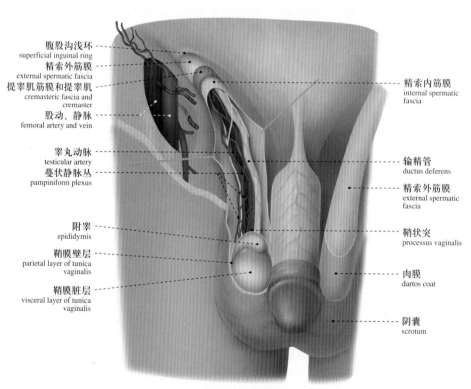

腹股沟浅环
superficial inguinal ring

精索外筋膜
external spermatic fascia

提睾肌筋膜和提睾肌
cremasteric fascia and
cremaster

股动、静脉
femoral artery and vein

睾丸动脉
testicular artery

蔓状静脉丛
pampiniform plexus

附睾
epididymis

鞘膜壁层
parietal layer of tunica
vaginalis

鞘膜脏层
visceral layer of tunica
vaginalis

精索内筋膜
internal spermatic
fascia

输精管
ductus deferens

精索外筋膜
external spermatic
fascia

鞘状突
processus vaginalis

肉膜
dartos coat

阴囊
scrotum

图 287　阴茎、阴囊和精索
Penis, scrotum and spermatic cord

第四节

盆部断面

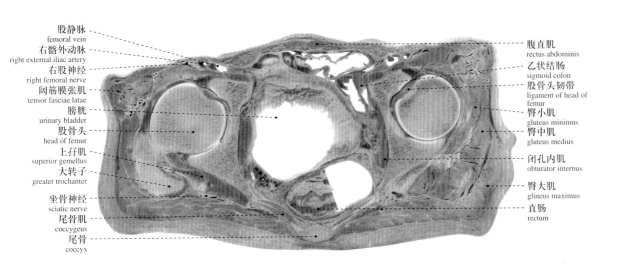

股静脉
femoral vein

右髂外动脉
right external iliac artery

右股神经
right femoral nerve

阔筋膜张肌
tensor fasciae latae

膀胱
urinary bladder

股骨头
head of femur

上孖肌
superior gemellus

大转子
greater trochanter

坐骨神经
sciatic nerve

尾骨肌
coccygeus

尾骨
coccyx

腹直肌
rectus abdominis

乙状结肠
sigmoid colon

股骨头韧带
ligament of head of femur

臀小肌
gluteus minimus

臀中肌
gluteus medius

闭孔内肌
obturator internus

臀大肌
gluteus maximus

直肠
rectum

图 288　盆部水平断面 1（男）

Horizontal section of the pelvis 1 (male)

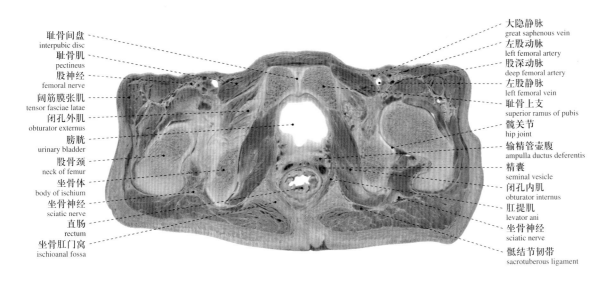

耻骨间盘
interpubic disc

耻骨肌
pectineus

股神经
femoral nerve

阔筋膜张肌
tensor fasciae latae

闭孔外肌
obturator externus

膀胱
urinary bladder

股骨颈
neck of femur

坐骨体
body of ischium

坐骨神经
sciatic nerve

直肠
rectum

坐骨肛门窝
ischioanal fossa

大隐静脉
great saphenous vein

左股动脉
left femoral artery

股深动脉
deep femoral artery

左股静脉
left femoral vein

耻骨上支
superior ramus of pubis

髋关节
hip joint

输精管壶腹
ampulla ductus deferentis

精囊
seminal vesicle

闭孔内肌
obturator internus

肛提肌
levator ani

坐骨神经
sciatic nerve

骶结节韧带
sacrotuberous ligament

图 289　盆部水平断面 2（男）

Horizontal section of the pelvis 2 (male)

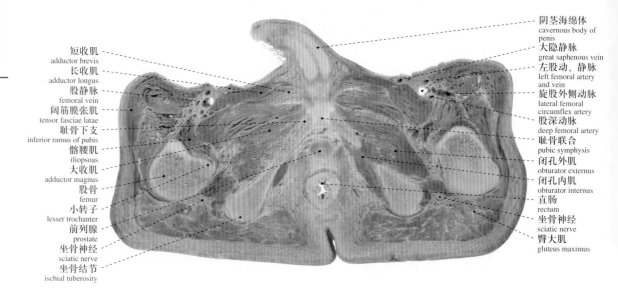

短收肌
adductor brevis
长收肌
adductor longus
股静脉
femoral vein
阔筋膜张肌
tensor fasciae latae
耻骨下支
inferior ramus of pubis
髂腰肌
iliopsoas
大收肌
adductor magnus
股骨
femur
小转子
lesser trochanter
前列腺
prostate
坐骨神经
sciatic nerve
坐骨结节
ischial tuberosity

阴茎海绵体
cavernous body of penis
大隐静脉
great saphenous vein
左股动、静脉
left femoral artery and vein
旋股外侧动脉
lateral femoral circumflex artery
股深动脉
deep femoral artery
耻骨联合
pubic symphysis
闭孔外肌
obturator externus
闭孔内肌
obturator internus
直肠
rectum
坐骨神经
sciatic nerve
臀大肌
gluteus maximus

图 290　盆部水平断面 3（男）

Horizontal section of the pelvis 3 (male)

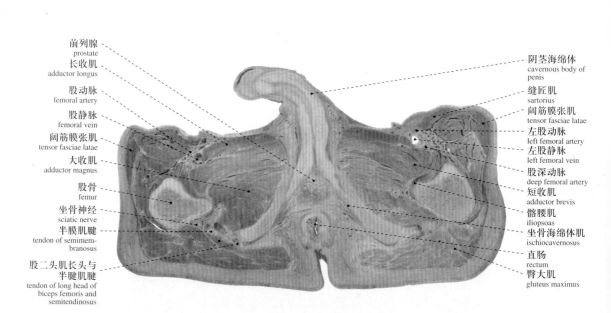

前列腺
prostate
长收肌
adductor longus
股动脉
femoral artery
股静脉
femoral vein
阔筋膜张肌
tensor fasciae latae
大收肌
adductor magnus
股骨
femur
坐骨神经
sciatic nerve
半膜肌腱
tendon of semimembranosus
股二头肌长头与
半腱肌腱
tendon of long head of biceps femoris and semitendinosus

阴茎海绵体
cavernous body of penis
缝匠肌
sartorius
阔筋膜张肌
tensor fasciae latae
左股动脉
left femoral artery
左股静脉
left femoral vein
股深动脉
deep femoral artery
短收肌
adductor brevis
髂腰肌
iliopsoas
坐骨海绵体肌
ischiocavernosus
直肠
rectum
臀大肌
gluteus maximus

图 291　盆部水平断面 4（男）

Horizontal section of the pelvis 4 (male)

脊　柱

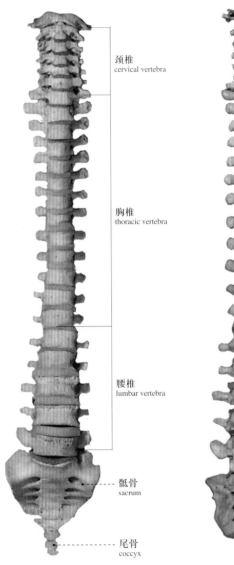

图 292　脊柱（前面观）
Vertebral column (norma anterior)

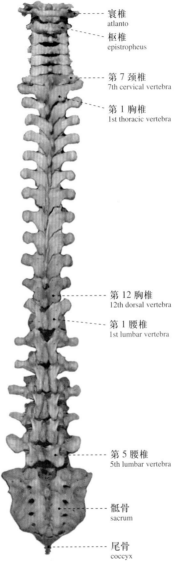

图 293　脊柱（后面观）
Vertebral column (norma occipitalis)

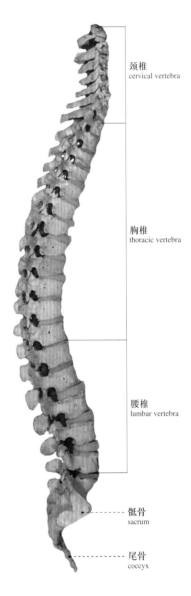

图 294　脊柱（侧面观）
Vertebral column (lateral aspect)

颈椎
cervical vertebra

胸椎
thoracic vertebra

腰椎
lumbar vertebra

骶骨
sacrum

尾骨
coccyx

寰椎
atlanto

枢椎
epistropheus

第 7 颈椎
7th cervical vertebra

第 1 胸椎
1st thoracic vertebra

第 12 胸椎
12th dorsal vertebra

第 1 腰椎
1st lumbar vertebra

第 5 腰椎
5th lumbar vertebra

骶骨
sacrum

尾骨
coccyx

颈椎
cervical vertebra

胸椎
thoracic vertebra

腰椎
lumbar vertebra

骶骨
sacrum

尾骨
coccyx

第二节

椎骨连接及椎管

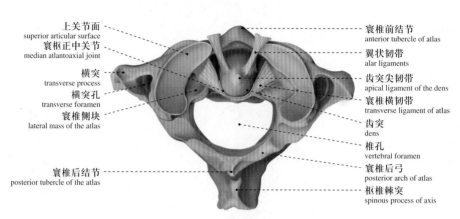

上关节面
superior articular surface
寰枢正中关节
median atlantoaxial joint
横突
transverse process
横突孔
transverse foramen
寰椎侧块
lateral mass of the atlas

寰椎后结节
posterior tubercle of the atlas

寰椎前结节
anterior tubercle of atlas
翼状韧带
alar ligaments
齿突尖韧带
apical ligament of the dens
寰椎横韧带
transverse ligament of atlas
齿突
dens
椎孔
vertebral foramen
寰椎后弓
posterior arch of atlas
枢椎棘突
spinous process of axis

图 295　寰枢正中关节韧带
Ligaments of the median atlanto-axial joint

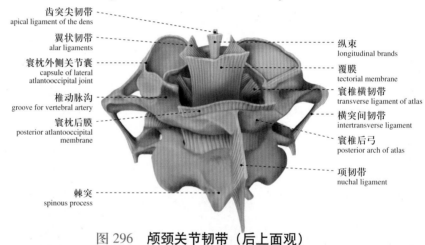

齿突尖韧带
apical ligament of the dens
翼状韧带
alar ligaments
寰枕外侧关节囊
capsule of lateral
atlantooccipital joint
椎动脉沟
groove for vertebral artery
寰枕后膜
posterior atlantooccipital
membrane

棘突
spinous process

纵束
longitudinal brands
覆膜
tectorial membrane
寰椎横韧带
transverse ligament of atlas
横突间韧带
intertransverse ligament
寰椎后弓
posterior arch of atlas
项韧带
nuchal ligament

图 296　颅颈关节韧带（后上面观）
Ligaments of the craniovertebral joints (posterosuperior aspect)

翼状韧带
alar ligament
上关节面
superior articular surface
寰椎前弓
anterior arch of atlas
寰枢外侧关节
lateral atlantoaxial joint
横突
transverse process
横突孔
transverse foramen

寰枕后膜
posterior atlantooccipital
membrane
纵束
longitudinal brands
齿突尖韧带
apical ligament of the dens
覆膜
tectorial membrane
齿突
dens
寰枢正中关节
median atlantaxial joint
寰椎前结节
anterior tubercle of atlas

图 297　颅颈关节韧带（前上面观）
Ligaments of the craniovertebral joints (anterosuperior aspect)

170

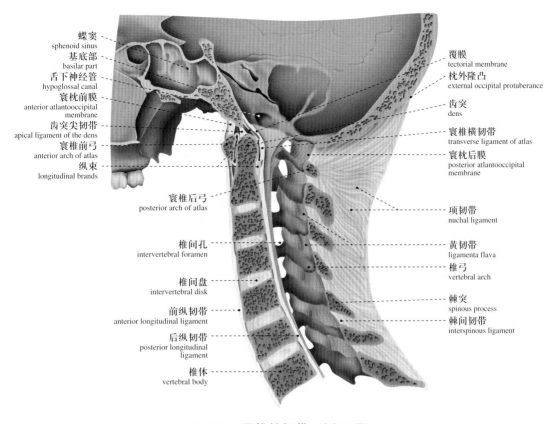

蝶窦
sphenoid sinus

基底部
basilar part

舌下神经管
hypoglossal canal

寰枕前膜
anterior atlantooccipital membrane

齿突尖韧带
apical ligament of the dens

寰椎前弓
anterior arch of atlas

纵束
longitudinal brands

寰椎后弓
posterior arch of atlas

椎间孔
intervertebral foramen

椎间盘
intervertebral disk

前纵韧带
anterior longitudinal ligament

后纵韧带
posterior longitudinal ligament

椎体
vertebral body

覆膜
tectorial membrane

枕外隆凸
external occipital protuberance

齿突
dens

寰椎横韧带
transverse ligament of atlas

寰枕后膜
posterior atlantooccipital membrane

项韧带
nuchal ligament

黄韧带
ligamenta flava

椎弓
vertebral arch

棘突
spinous process

棘间韧带
interspinous ligament

图 298 颈椎的韧带（侧面观）
Ligaments of the cervical vertebrae (lateral aspect)

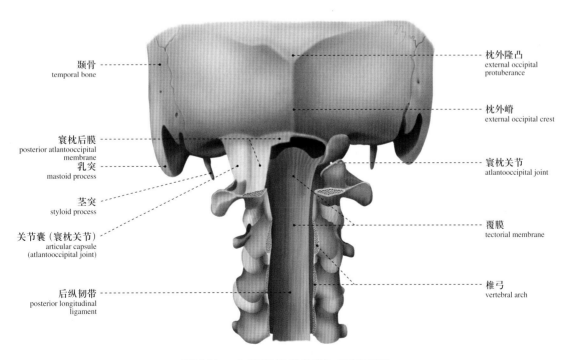

颞骨
temporal bone

寰枕后膜
posterior atlantooccipital membrane

乳突
mastoid process

茎突
styloid process

关节囊（寰枕关节）
articular capsule (atlantooccipital joint)

后纵韧带
posterior longitudinal ligament

枕外隆凸
external occipital protuberance

枕外嵴
external occipital crest

寰枕关节
atlantooccipital joint

覆膜
tectorial membrane

椎弓
vertebral arch

图 299 上部颈椎的韧带（后面观）
Ligaments of the upper cervical spine (posterior aspect)

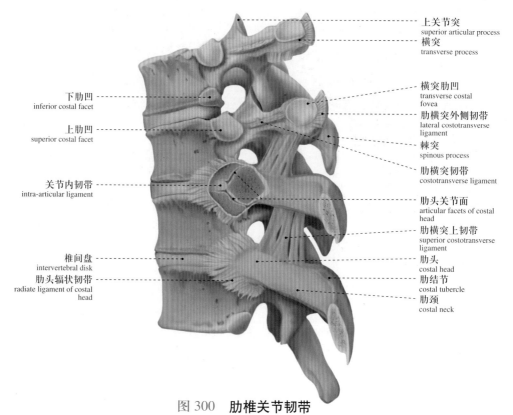

上关节突
superior articular process

横突
transverse process

下肋凹
inferior costal facet

横突肋凹
transverse costal
fovea

上肋凹
superior costal facet

肋横突外侧韧带
lateral costotransverse
ligament

棘突
spinous process

肋横突韧带
costotransverse ligament

关节内韧带
intra-articular ligament

肋头关节面
articular facets of costal
head

肋横突上韧带
superior costotransverse
ligament

椎间盘
intervertebral disk

肋头辐状韧带
radiate ligament of costal
head

肋头
costal head

肋结节
costal tubercle

肋颈
costal neck

图 300　肋椎关节韧带
Ligaments of the costovertebral joints

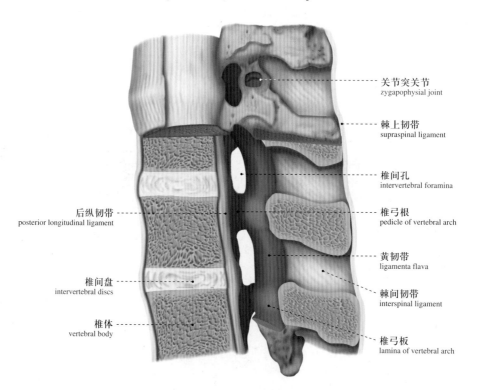

关节突关节
zygapophysial joint

棘上韧带
supraspinal ligament

椎间孔
intervertebral foramina

后纵韧带
posterior longitudinal ligament

椎弓根
pedicle of vertebral arch

黄韧带
ligamenta flava

椎间盘
intervertebral discs

棘间韧带
interspinal ligament

椎体
vertebral body

椎弓板
lamina of vertebral arch

图 301　椎管
Vertebral canal

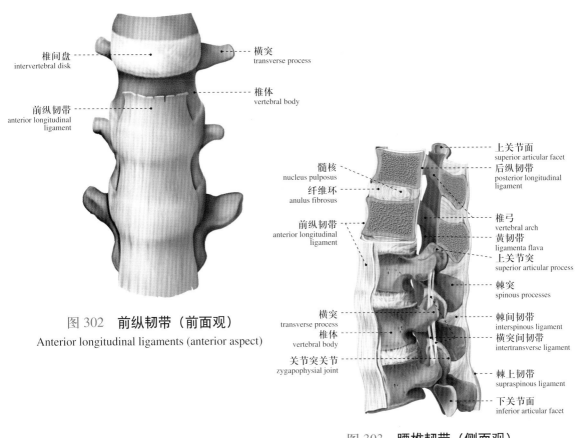

椎间盘
intervertebral disk

横突
transverse process

椎体
vertebral body

前纵韧带
anterior longitudinal
ligament

图 302　前纵韧带（前面观）

Anterior longitudinal ligaments (anterior aspect)

髓核
nucleus pulposus

纤维环
anulus fibrosus

前纵韧带
anterior longitudinal
ligament

横突
transverse process
椎体
vertebral body
关节突关节
zygapophysial joint

上关节面
superior articular facet

后纵韧带
posterior longitudinal
ligament

椎弓
vertebral arch
黄韧带
ligamenta flava
上关节突
superior articular process

棘突
spinous processes

棘间韧带
interspinous ligament
横突间韧带
intertransverse ligament

棘上韧带
supraspinous ligament

下关节面
inferior articular facet

图 303　腰椎韧带（侧面观）

Ligaments of the lumbar vertebras (lateral aspect)

椎弓根
pedicle of vertebral
arch

椎间盘
intervertebral discs

后纵韧带
posterior
longitudinal
ligament

椎体
vertebral body

图 304　后纵韧带（后面观）

Posterior longitudinal ligaments (posterior aspect)

横突间韧带
intertransverse
ligament

横突
transverse process

后纵韧带
posterior longitudinal
ligament
前纵韧带
anterior longitudinal
ligament
棘突
spinous process

上关节突
superior articular
process

椎弓板
lamina of vertebral
arch

黄韧带
ligamenta flava

上关节突
superior articular
process

下关节面
inferior articular
surface

图 305　黄韧带和横突间韧带（前面观）

Ligamenta flava and intertransverse ligaments (anterior aspect)

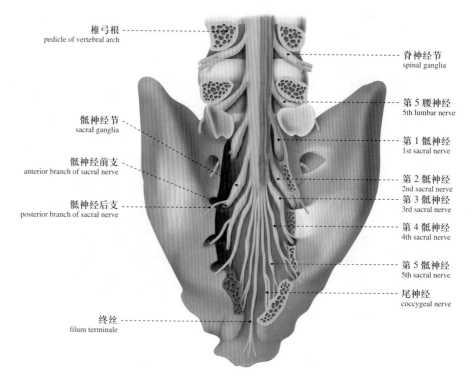

椎弓根
pedicle of vertebral arch

脊神经节
spinal ganglia

第 5 腰神经
5th lumbar nerve

骶神经节
sacral ganglia

第 1 骶神经
1st sacral nerve

骶神经前支
anterior branch of sacral nerve

第 2 骶神经
2nd sacral nerve

第 3 骶神经
3rd sacral nerve

骶神经后支
posterior branch of sacral nerve

第 4 骶神经
4th sacral nerve

第 5 骶神经
5th sacral nerve

尾神经
coccygeal nerve

终丝
filum terminale

图 306　骶管及其内容物
Sacral canal and its contents

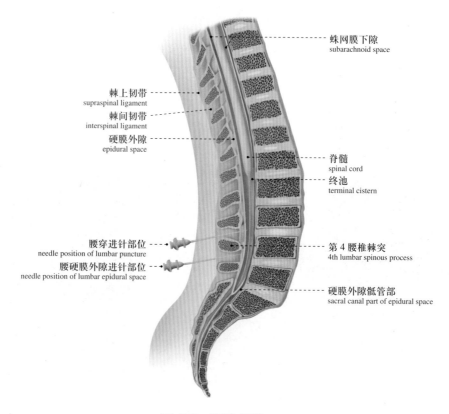

蛛网膜下隙
subarachnoid space

棘上韧带
supraspinal ligament

棘间韧带
interspinal ligament

硬膜外隙
epidural space

脊髓
spinal cord

终池
terminal cistern

腰穿进针部位
needle position of lumbar puncture

腰硬膜外隙进针部位
needle position of lumbar epidural space

第 4 腰椎棘突
4th lumbar spinous process

硬膜外隙骶管部
sacral canal part of epidural space

图 307　腰穿部位
Lumbar puncture site

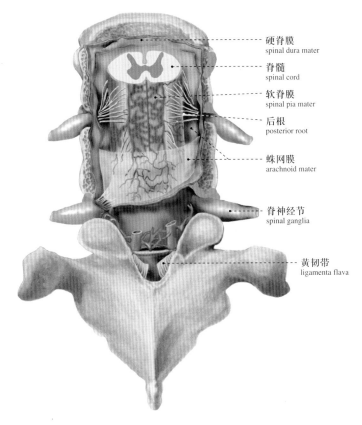

硬脊膜
spinal dura mater

脊髓
spinal cord

软脊膜
spinal pia mater

后根
posterior root

蛛网膜
arachnoid mater

脊神经节
spinal ganglia

黄韧带
ligamenta flava

图 308　脊髓的被膜
Meninges of the spinal cord

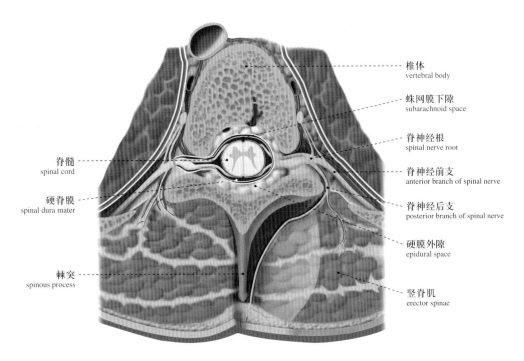

脊髓
spinal cord

硬脊膜
spinal dura mater

棘突
spinous process

椎体
vertebral body

蛛网膜下隙
subarachnoid space

脊神经根
spinal nerve root

脊神经前支
anterior branch of spinal nerve

脊神经后支
posterior branch of spinal nerve

硬膜外隙
epidural space

竖脊肌
erector spinae

图 309　椎管及其内容（水平断）
Spinal canal and its contents (horizontal section)

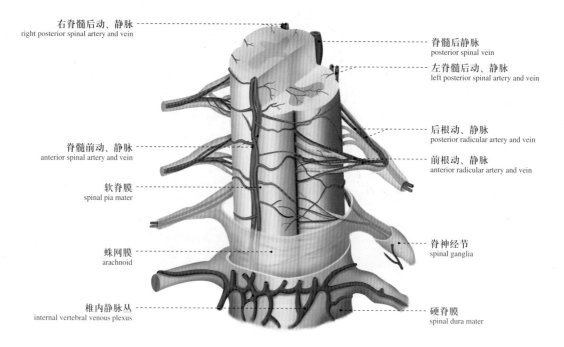

右脊髓后动、静脉
right posterior spinal artery and vein

脊髓后静脉
posterior spinal vein

左脊髓后动、静脉
left posterior spinal artery and vein

后根动、静脉
posterior radicular artery and vein

脊髓前动、静脉
anterior spinal artery and vein

前根动、静脉
anterior radicular artery and vein

软脊膜
spinal pia mater

蛛网膜
arachnoid

脊神经节
spinal ganglia

椎内静脉丛
internal vertebral venous plexus

硬脊膜
spinal dura mater

图 310　脊髓的血管（模式图）
Blood vessels of Spinal cord (diagram)

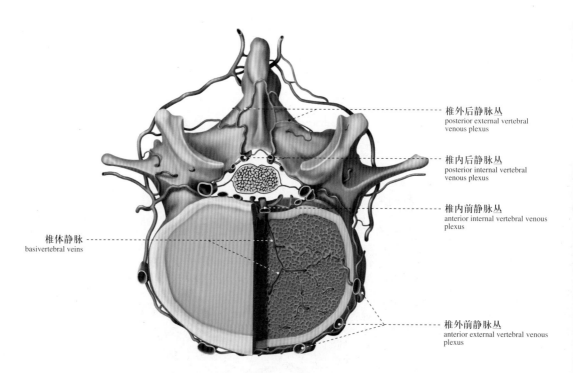

椎外后静脉丛
posterior external vertebral venous plexus

椎内后静脉丛
posterior internal vertebral venous plexus

椎内前静脉丛
anterior internal vertebral venous plexus

椎体静脉
basivertebral veins

椎外前静脉丛
anterior external vertebral venous plexus

图 311　胸椎周围静脉
Veins around thoracic vertebrae

第三节

层次结构

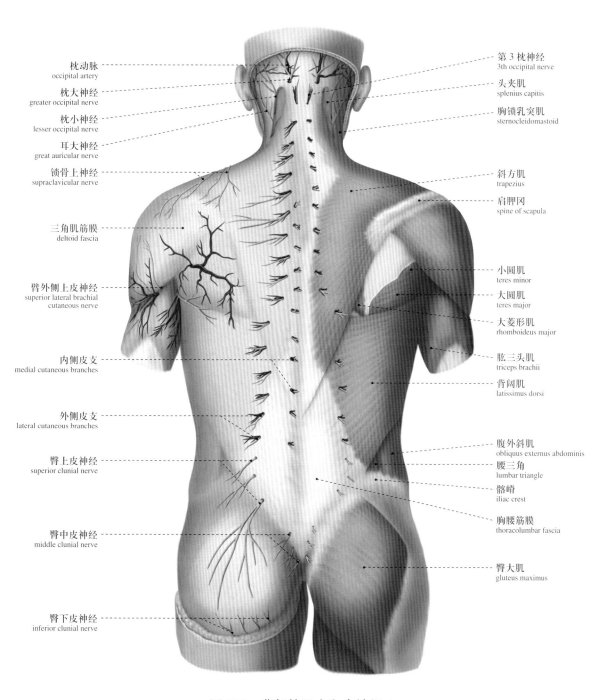

枕动脉
occipital artery

枕大神经
greater occipital nerve

枕小神经
lesser occipital nerve

耳大神经
great auricular nerve

锁骨上神经
supraclavicular nerve

三角肌筋膜
deltoid fascia

臂外侧上皮神经
superior lateral brachial cutaneous nerve

内侧皮支
medial cutaneous branches

外侧皮支
lateral cutaneous branches

臀上皮神经
superior clunial nerve

臀中皮神经
middle clunial nerve

臀下皮神经
inferior clunial nerve

第 3 枕神经
3th occipital nerve

头夹肌
splenius capitis

胸锁乳突肌
sternocleidomastoid

斜方肌
trapezius

肩胛冈
spine of scapula

小圆肌
teres minor

大圆肌
teres major

大菱形肌
rhomboideus major

肱三头肌
triceps brachii

背阔肌
latissimus dorsi

腹外斜肌
obliquus externus abdominis

腰三角
lumbar triangle

髂嵴
iliac crest

胸腰筋膜
thoracolumbar fascia

臀大肌
gluteus maximus

图 312　背部的肌肉和皮神经 1
Muscles and cutaneous nerves of the back 1

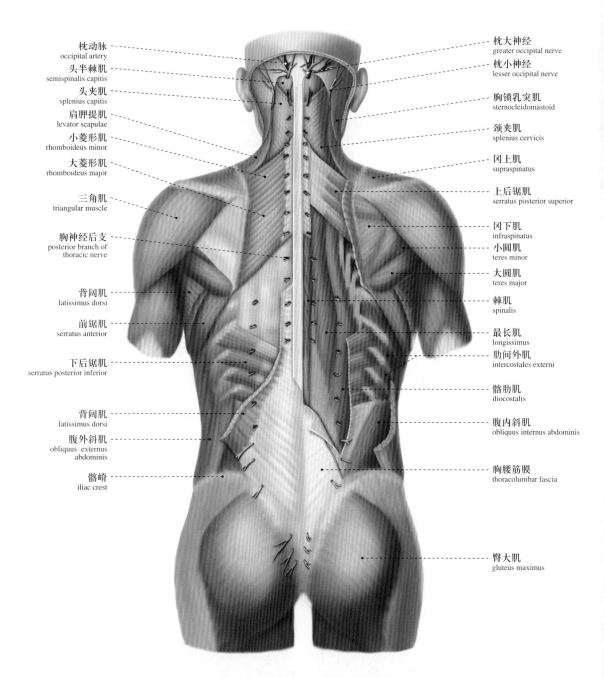

枕动脉
occipital artery

头半棘肌
semispinalis capitis

头夹肌
splenius capitis

肩胛提肌
levator scapulae

小菱形肌
rhomboideus minor

大菱形肌
rhomboideus major

三角肌
triangular muscle

胸神经后支
posterior branch of
thoracic nerve

背阔肌
latissimus dorsi

前锯肌
serratus anterior

下后锯肌
serratus posterior inferior

背阔肌
latissimus dorsi

腹外斜肌
obliquus externus
abdominis

髂嵴
iliac crest

枕大神经
greater occipital nerve

枕小神经
lesser occipital nerve

胸锁乳突肌
sternocleidomastoid

颈夹肌
splenius cervicis

冈上肌
supraspinatus

上后锯肌
serratus posterior superior

冈下肌
infraspinatus

小圆肌
teres minor

大圆肌
teres major

棘肌
spinalis

最长肌
longissimus

肋间外肌
intercostales externi

髂肋肌
iliocostalis

腹内斜肌
obliquus internus abdominis

胸腰筋膜
thoracolumbar fascia

臀大肌
gluteus maximus

图 313 背部的肌肉和皮神经 2
Muscles and cutaneous nerves of the back 2

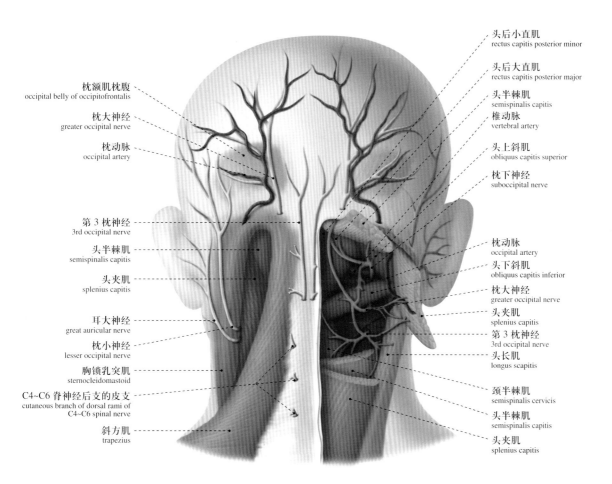

枕额肌枕腹
occipital belly of occipitofrontalis

枕大神经
greater occipital nerve

枕动脉
occipital artery

第 3 枕神经
3rd occipital nerve

头半棘肌
semispinalis capitis

头夹肌
splenius capitis

耳大神经
great auricular nerve

枕小神经
lesser occipital nerve

胸锁乳突肌
sternocleidomastoid

C4~C6 脊神经后支的皮支
cutaneous branch of dorsal rami of
C4~C6 spinal nerve

斜方肌
trapezius

头后小直肌
rectus capitis posterior minor

头后大直肌
rectus capitis posterior major

头半棘肌
semispinalis capitis

椎动脉
vertebral artery

头上斜肌
obliquus capitis superior

枕下神经
suboccipital nerve

枕动脉
occipital artery

头下斜肌
obliquus capitis inferior

枕大神经
greater occipital nerve

头夹肌
splenius capitis

第 3 枕神经
3rd occipital nerve

头长肌
longus scapitis

颈半棘肌
semispinalis cervicis

头半棘肌
semispinalis capitis

头夹肌
splenius capitis

图 314　枕下三角
Suboccipital triangle

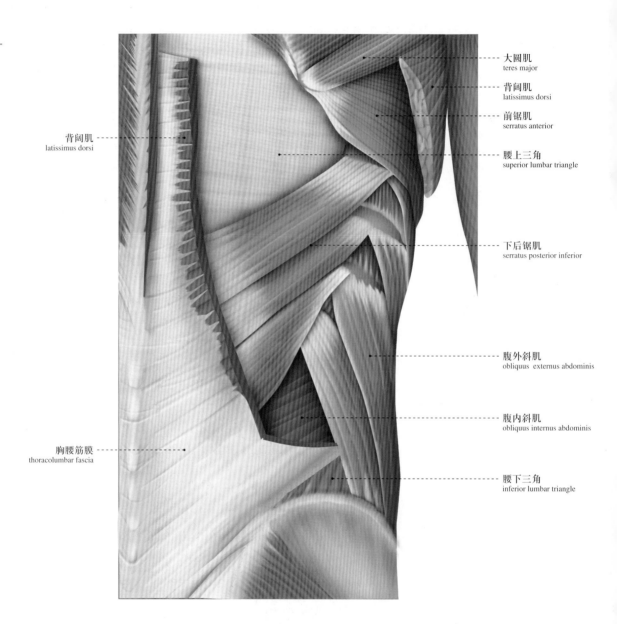

大圆肌
teres major

背阔肌
latissimus dorsi

前锯肌
serratus anterior

腰上三角
superior lumbar triangle

下后锯肌
serratus posterior inferior

腹外斜肌
obliquus externus abdominis

腹内斜肌
obliquus internus abdominis

腰下三角
inferior lumbar triangle

背阔肌
latissimus dorsi

胸腰筋膜
thoracolumbar fascia

图 315　腰上三角和腰下三角
Superior lumbar triangle and inferior lumbar triangle

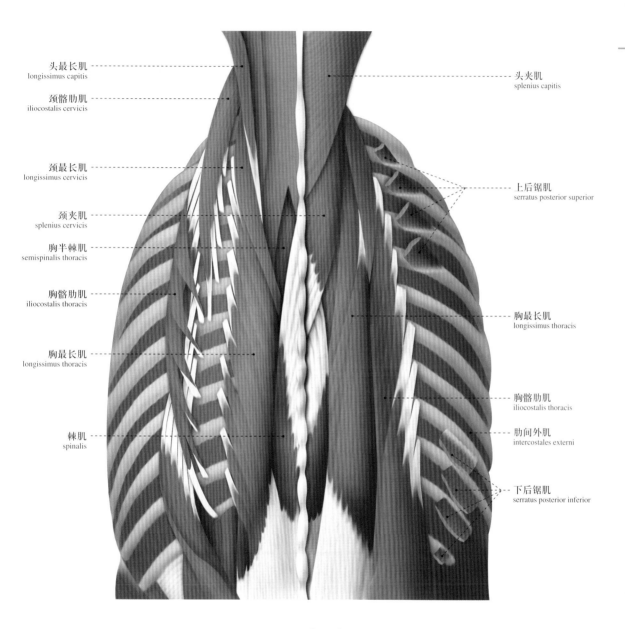

头最长肌
longissimus capitis

颈髂肋肌
iliocostalis cervicis

颈最长肌
longissimus cervicis

颈夹肌
splenius cervicis

胸半棘肌
semispinalis thoracis

胸髂肋肌
iliocostalis thoracis

胸最长肌
longissimus thoracis

棘肌
spinalis

头夹肌
splenius capitis

上后锯肌
serratus posterior superior

胸最长肌
longissimus thoracis

胸髂肋肌
iliocostalis thoracis

肋间外肌
intercostales externi

下后锯肌
serratus posterior inferior

图 316 背固有肌
Intrinsic back muscles

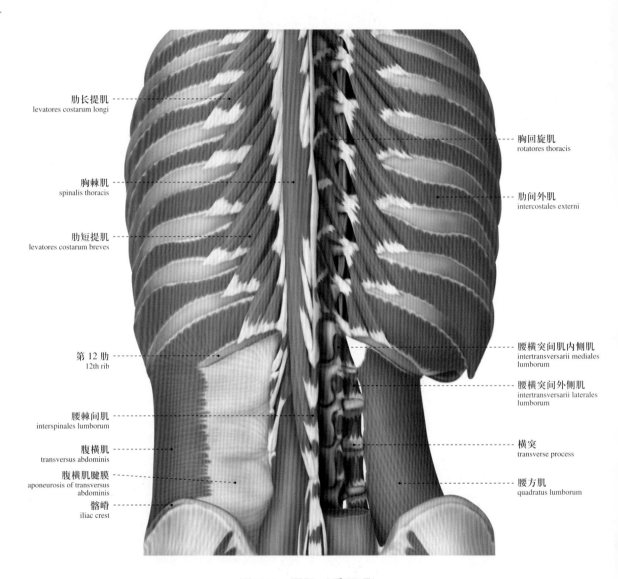

肋长提肌
levatores costarum longi

胸棘肌
spinalis thoracis

肋短提肌
levatores costarum breves

第 12 肋
12th rib

腰棘间肌
interspinales lumborum

腹横肌
transversus abdominis

腹横肌腱膜
aponeurosis of transversus abdominis

髂嵴
iliac crest

胸回旋肌
rotatores thoracis

肋间外肌
intercostales externi

腰横突间肌内侧肌
intertransversarii mediales lumborum

腰横突间外侧肌
intertransversarii laterales lumborum

横突
transverse process

腰方肌
quadratus lumborum

图 317　腰肌（后面观）
Lumbar muscles (posterior aspect)

第一节

肩 部

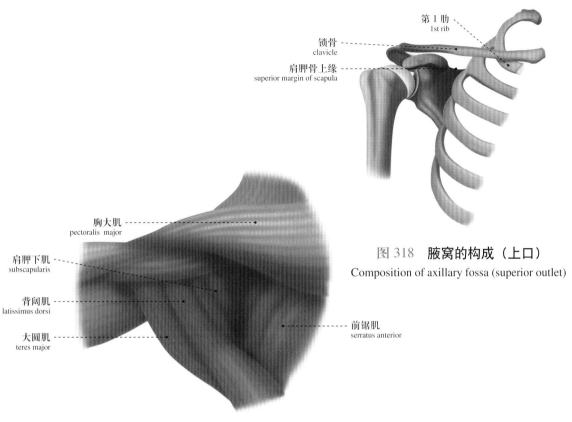

第 1 肋
1st rib

锁骨
clavicle

肩胛骨上缘
superior margin of scapula

图 318　腋窝的构成（上口）
Composition of axillary fossa (superior outlet)

胸大肌
pectoralis major

肩胛下肌
subscapularis

背阔肌
latissimus dorsi

大圆肌
teres major

前锯肌
serratus anterior

图 319　腋窝的后壁（前面观）
Posterior wall of the axilla (anterior aspect)

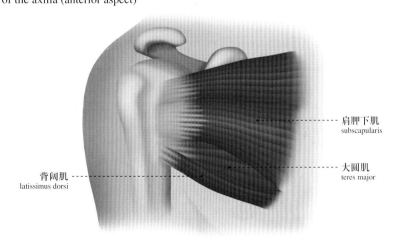

肩胛下肌
subscapularis

大圆肌
teres major

背阔肌
latissimus dorsi

图 320　腋窝的后壁（后面观）
Posterior wall of the axilla (posterior aspect)

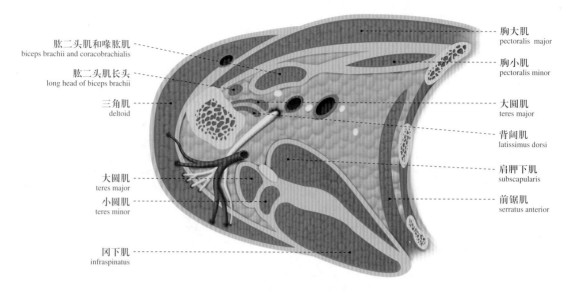

肱二头肌和喙肱肌
biceps brachii and coracobrachialis

肱二头肌长头
long head of biceps brachii

三角肌
deltoid

大圆肌
teres major

小圆肌
teres minor

冈下肌
infraspinatus

胸大肌
pectoralis major

胸小肌
pectoralis minor

大圆肌
teres major

背阔肌
latissimus dorsi

肩胛下肌
subscapularis

前锯肌
serratus anterior

图 321　腋窝的构成（水平断）
Composition of axillary fossa (horizontal section)

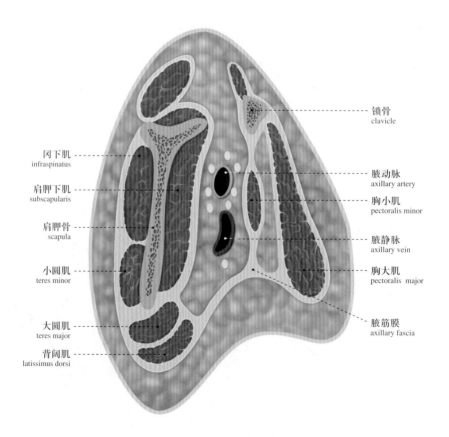

冈下肌
infraspinatus

肩胛下肌
subscapularis

肩胛骨
scapula

小圆肌
teres minor

大圆肌
teres major

背阔肌
latissimus dorsi

锁骨
clavicle

腋动脉
axillary artery

胸小肌
pectoralis minor

腋静脉
axillary vein

胸大肌
pectoralis major

腋筋膜
axillary fascia

图 322　腋窝的构成（矢状断）
Composition of axillary fossa (sagittal section)

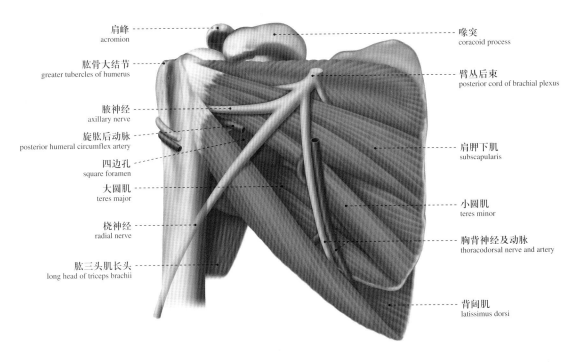

图 323　腋窝后壁及三边孔和四边孔（前面观）

Axillary posterior wall and trilateral foramen, square foramen (anterior aspect)

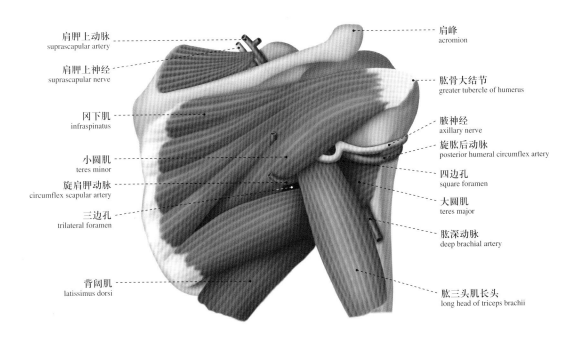

图 324　腋窝后壁及三边孔和四边孔（后面观）

Axillary posterior wall and trilateral foramen, square foramen (posterior aspect)

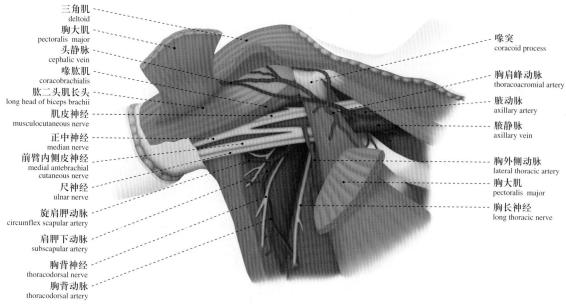

三角肌
deltoid

胸大肌
pectoralis major

头静脉
cephalic vein

喙肱肌
coracobrachialis

肱二头肌长头
long head of biceps brachii

肌皮神经
musculocutaneous nerve

正中神经
median nerve

前臂内侧皮神经
medial antebrachial cutaneous nerve

尺神经
ulnar nerve

旋肩胛动脉
circumflex scapular artery

肩胛下动脉
subscapular artery

胸背神经
thoracodorsal nerve

胸背动脉
thoracodorsal artery

喙突
coracoid process

胸肩峰动脉
thoracoacromial artery

腋动脉
axillary artery

腋静脉
axillary vein

胸外侧动脉
lateral thoracic artery

胸大肌
pectoralis major

胸长神经
long thoracic nerve

图 325 腋窝的内容
Axillary contents

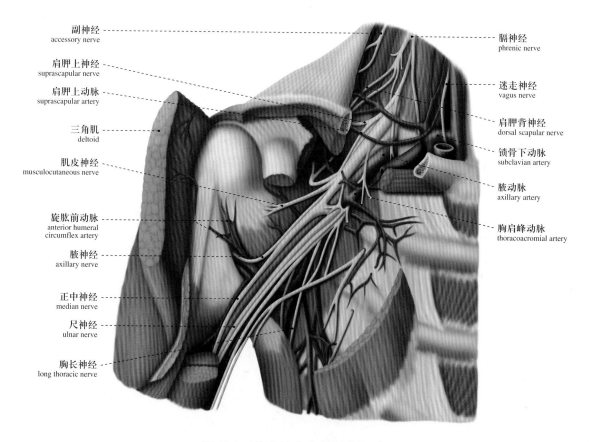

副神经
accessory nerve

肩胛上神经
suprascapular nerve

肩胛上动脉
suprascapular artery

三角肌
deltoid

肌皮神经
musculocutaneous nerve

旋肱前动脉
anterior humeral circumflex artery

腋神经
axillary nerve

正中神经
median nerve

尺神经
ulnar nerve

胸长神经
long thoracic nerve

膈神经
phrenic nerve

迷走神经
vagus nerve

肩胛背神经
dorsal scapular nerve

锁骨下动脉
subclavian artery

腋动脉
axillary artery

胸肩峰动脉
thoracoacromial artery

图 326 腋窝的内容与臂丛组成
Axillary contents and brachial composition

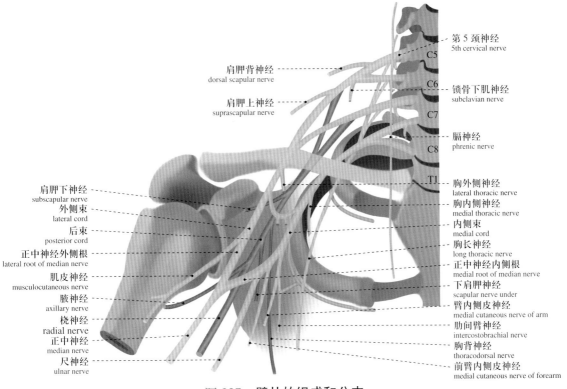

图 327　臂丛的组成和分支
Constitution and branches of the brachial plexus

第 5 颈神经
5th cervical nerve
肩胛背神经
dorsal scapular nerve
锁骨下肌神经
subclavian nerve
肩胛上神经
suprascapular nerve
膈神经
phrenic nerve
肩胛下神经
subscapular nerve
外侧束
lateral cord
后束
posterior cord
正中神经外侧根
lateral root of median nerve
肌皮神经
musculocutaneous nerve
腋神经
axillary nerve
桡神经
radial nerve
正中神经
median nerve
尺神经
ulnar nerve
胸外侧神经
lateral thoracic nerve
胸内侧神经
medial thoracic nerve
内侧束
medial cord
胸长神经
long thoracic nerve
正中神经内侧根
medial root of median nerve
下肩胛神经
scapular nerve under
臂内侧皮神经
medial cutaneous nerve of arm
肋间臂神经
intercostobrachial nerve
胸背神经
thoracodorsal nerve
前臂内侧皮神经
medial cutaneous nerve of forearm

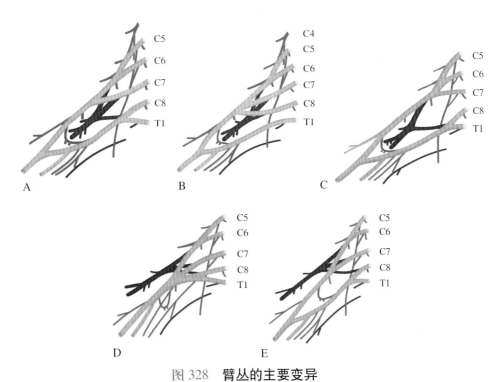

图 328　臂丛的主要变异
Principle variations of the brachial plexus

A. 根异位:C5、C6 居前斜角肌前方；B. 根变异：前置型，有 C4 参加；干变异：四干型；C. 干变异：双干型，C5 ~ C7 成上干，
C8、T1 成下干；D. 股、束变异：二束型，内外侧束合成前束，三后股合成后束；E. 束异位：后束向外移位

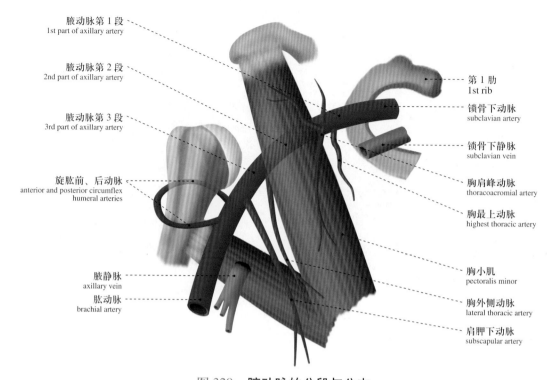

腋动脉第 1 段
1st part of axillary artery

腋动脉第 2 段
2nd part of axillary artery

腋动脉第 3 段
3rd part of axillary artery

旋肱前、后动脉
anterior and posterior circumflex
humeral arteries

腋静脉
axillary vein

肱动脉
brachial artery

第 1 肋
1st rib

锁骨下动脉
subclavian artery

锁骨下静脉
subclavian vein

胸肩峰动脉
thoracoacromial artery

胸最上动脉
highest thoracic artery

胸小肌
pectoralis minor

胸外侧动脉
lateral thoracic artery

肩胛下动脉
subscapular artery

图 329　腋动脉的分段与分支
Segments and branches of the axillary artery

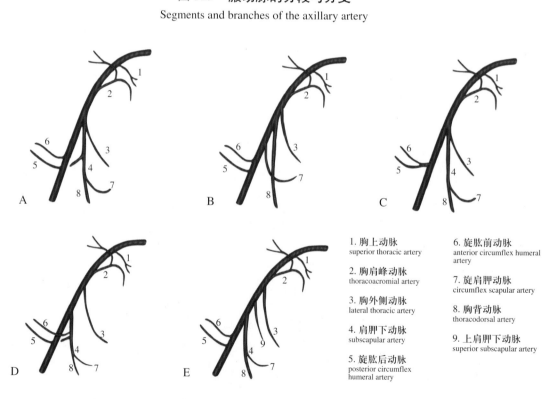

1. 胸上动脉
superior thoracic artery

2. 胸肩峰动脉
thoracoacromial artery

3. 胸外侧动脉
lateral thoracic artery

4. 肩胛下动脉
subscapular artery

5. 旋肱后动脉
posterior circumflex
humeral artery

6. 旋肱前动脉
anterior circumflex humeral
artery

7. 旋肩胛动脉
circumflex scapular artery

8. 胸背动脉
thoracodorsal artery

9. 上肩胛下动脉
superior subscapular artery

图 330　腋动脉的分支类型
Forms of the branches of the axillary artery

A.胸外侧动脉、肩胛下动脉、旋肱后动脉共干；B.胸背动脉和旋肩胛动脉单独起始，无肩胛下动脉；C.胸外侧动脉与肩胛下
动脉共干，旋肱前、后动脉共干；D.肩胛下动脉和旋肱前、后动脉共干；E.存在上肩胛下动脉

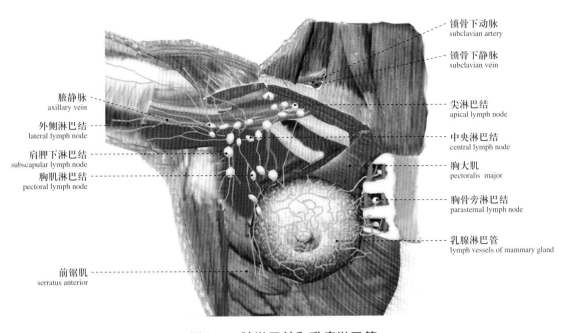

锁骨下动脉
subclavian artery

锁骨下静脉
subclavian vein

尖淋巴结
apical lymph node

中央淋巴结
central lymph node

胸大肌
pectoralis major

胸骨旁淋巴结
parasternal lymph node

乳腺淋巴管
lymph vessels of mammary gland

腋静脉
axillary vein

外侧淋巴结
lateral lymph node

肩胛下淋巴结
subscapular lymph node

胸肌淋巴结
pectoral lymph node

前锯肌
serratus anterior

图 331　腋淋巴结和乳房淋巴管
Axillary lymph nodes and mamma lymph vessels

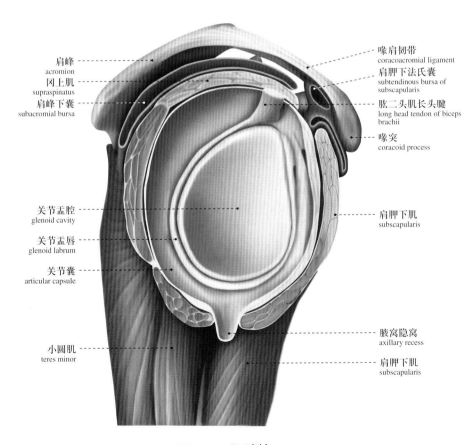

肩峰
acromion

冈上肌
supraspinatus

肩峰下囊
subacromial bursa

喙肩韧带
coracoacromial ligament

肩胛下法氏囊
subtendinous bursa of subscapularis

肱二头肌长头腱
long head tendon of biceps brachii

喙突
coracoid process

关节盂腔
glenoid cavity

关节盂唇
glenoid labrum

关节囊
articular capsule

肩胛下肌
subscapularis

小圆肌
teres minor

腋窝隐窝
axillary recess

肩胛下肌
subscapularis

图 332　肌腱袖
Tendon sleeves

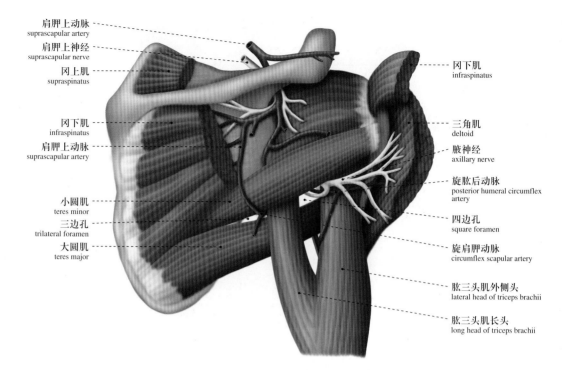

肩胛上动脉
suprascapular artery

肩胛上神经
suprascapular nerve

冈上肌
supraspinatus

冈下肌
infraspinatus

肩胛上动脉
suprascapular artery

小圆肌
teres minor

三边孔
trilateral foramen

大圆肌
teres major

冈下肌
infraspinatus

三角肌
deltoid

腋神经
axillary nerve

旋肱后动脉
posterior humeral circumflex
artery

四边孔
square foramen

旋肩胛动脉
circumflex scapular artery

肱三头肌外侧头
lateral head of triceps brachii

肱三头肌长头
long head of triceps brachii

图 333　三角肌区及肩胛区的结构
Structure of deltoid region and scapular region

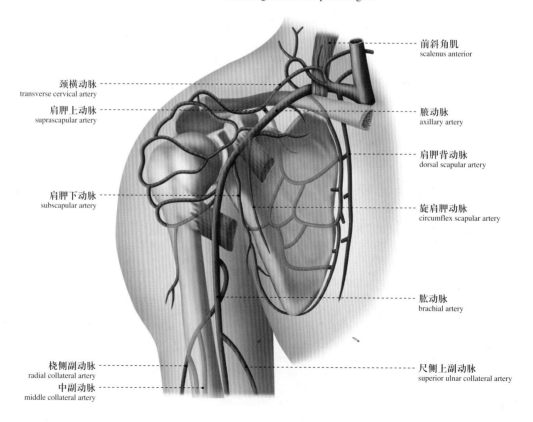

颈横动脉
transverse cervical artery

肩胛上动脉
suprascapular artery

肩胛下动脉
subscapular artery

桡侧副动脉
radial collateral artery

中副动脉
middle collateral artery

前斜角肌
scalenus anterior

腋动脉
axillary artery

肩胛背动脉
dorsal scapular artery

旋肩胛动脉
circumflex scapular artery

肱动脉
brachial artery

尺侧上副动脉
superior ulnar collateral artery

图 334　肩胛动脉网
Scapular arterial network

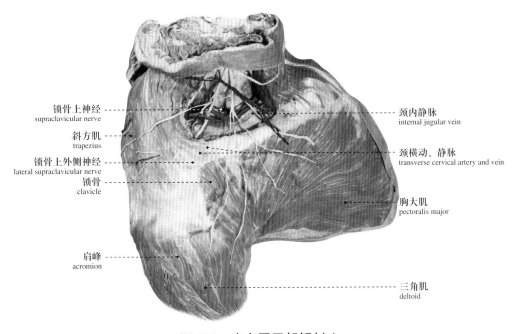

锁骨上神经
supraclavicular nerve

斜方肌
trapezius

锁骨上外侧神经
lateral supraclavicular nerve

锁骨
clavicle

肩峰
acromion

颈内静脉
internal jugular vein

颈横动、静脉
transverse cervical artery and vein

胸大肌
pectoralis major

三角肌
deltoid

图 335　肩上区局部解剖 1
Topography of superior region of the shoulder 1

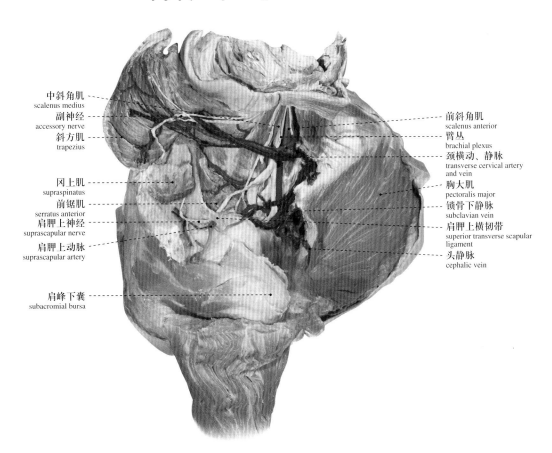

中斜角肌
scalenus medius

副神经
accessory nerve

斜方肌
trapezius

冈上肌
supraspinatus

前锯肌
serratus anterior

肩胛上神经
suprascapular nerve

肩胛上动脉
suprascapular artery

肩峰下囊
subacromial bursa

前斜角肌
scalenus anterior

臂丛
brachial plexus

颈横动、静脉
transverse cervical artery
and vein

胸大肌
pectoralis major

锁骨下静脉
subclavian vein

肩胛上横韧带
superior transverse scapular
ligament

头静脉
cephalic vein

图 336　肩上区局部解剖 2
Topography of superior region of the shoulder 2

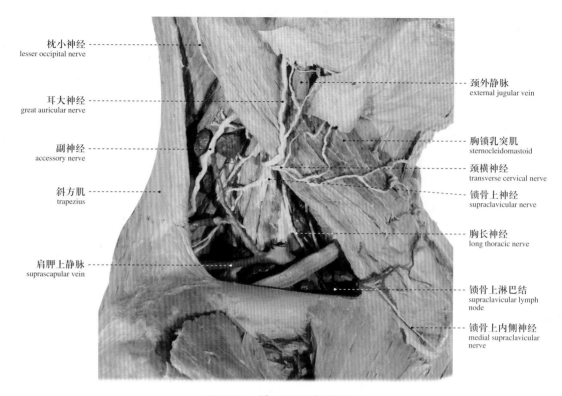

枕小神经
lesser occipital nerve

耳大神经
great auricular nerve

副神经
accessory nerve

斜方肌
trapezius

肩胛上静脉
suprascapular vein

颈外静脉
external jugular vein

胸锁乳突肌
sternocleidomastoid

颈横神经
transverse cervical nerve

锁骨上神经
supraclavicular nerve

胸长神经
long thoracic nerve

锁骨上淋巴结
supraclavicular lymph node

锁骨上内侧神经
medial supraclavicular nerve

图 337　锁骨区局部解剖 1
Topography of the clavicular region 1

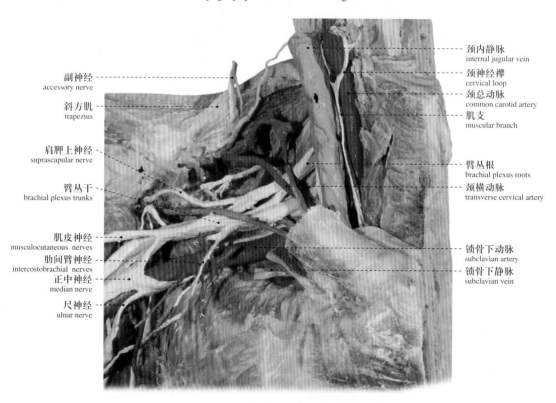

副神经
accessory nerve

斜方肌
trapezius

肩胛上神经
suprascapular nerve

臂丛干
brachial plexus trunks

肌皮神经
musculocutaneous nerves

肋间臂神经
intercostobrachial nerves

正中神经
median nerve

尺神经
ulnar nerve

颈内静脉
internal jugular vein

颈神经襻
cervical loop

颈总动脉
common carotid artery

肌支
muscular branch

臂丛根
brachial plexus roots

颈横动脉
transverse cervical artery

锁骨下动脉
subclavian artery

锁骨下静脉
subclavian vein

图 338　锁骨区局部解剖 2
Topography of the clavicular region 2

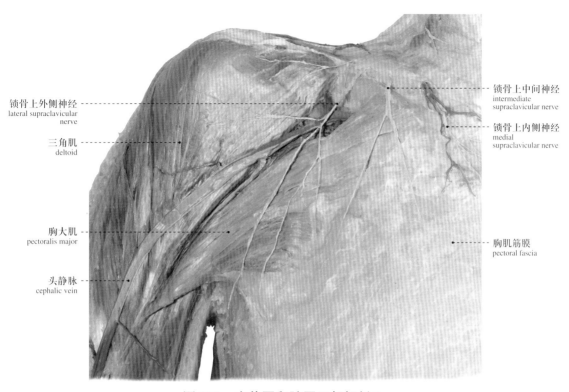

锁骨上外侧神经
lateral supraclavicular
nerve

三角肌
deltoid

胸大肌
pectoralis major

头静脉
cephalic vein

锁骨上中间神经
intermediate
supraclavicular nerve

锁骨上内侧神经
medial
supraclavicular nerve

胸肌筋膜
pectoral fascia

图 339　肩前区和腋区局部解剖 1

Topography of anterior region of the shoulder and the axillary region 1

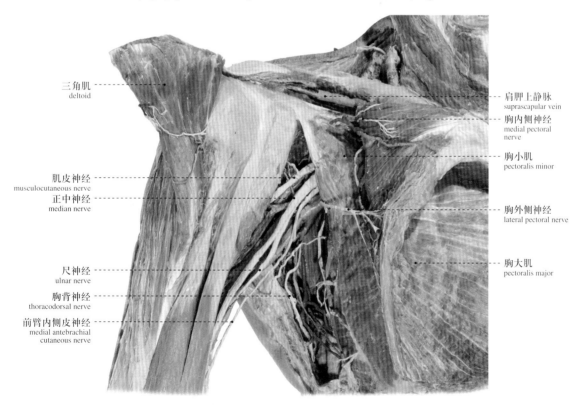

三角肌
deltoid

肌皮神经
musculocutaneous nerve

正中神经
median nerve

尺神经
ulnar nerve

胸背神经
thoracodorsal nerve

前臂内侧皮神经
medial antebrachial
cutaneous nerve

肩胛上静脉
suprascapular vein

胸内侧神经
medial pectoral
nerve

胸小肌
pectoralis minor

胸外侧神经
lateral pectoral nerve

胸大肌
pectoralis major

图 340　肩前区和腋区局部解剖 2

Topography of anterior region of the shoulder and the axillary region 2

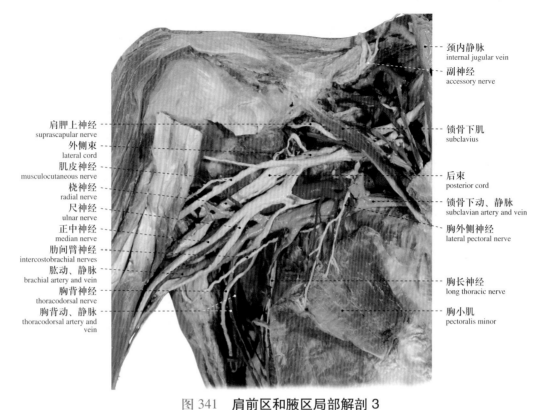

肩胛上神经
suprascapular nerve
外侧束
lateral cord
肌皮神经
musculocutaneous nerve
桡神经
radial nerve
尺神经
ulnar nerve
正中神经
median nerve
肋间臂神经
intercostobrachial nerves
肱动、静脉
brachial artery and vein
胸背神经
thoracodorsal nerve
胸背动、静脉
thoracodorsal artery and vein

颈内静脉
internal jugular vein
副神经
accessory nerve
锁骨下肌
subclavius
后束
posterior cord
锁骨下动、静脉
subclavian artery and vein
胸外侧神经
lateral pectoral nerve
胸长神经
long thoracic nerve
胸小肌
pectoralis minor

图 341　肩前区和腋区局部解剖 3
Topography of anterior region of the shoulder and the axillary region 3

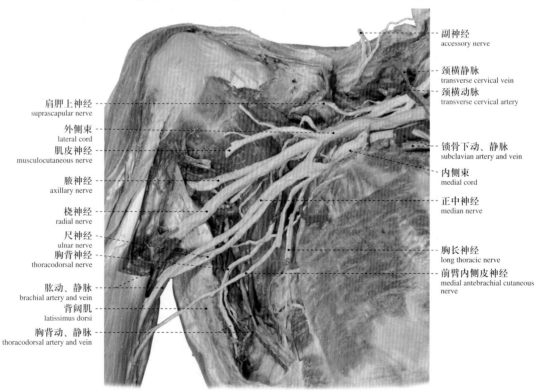

肩胛上神经
suprascapular nerve
外侧束
lateral cord
肌皮神经
musculocutaneous nerve
腋神经
axillary nerve
桡神经
radial nerve
尺神经
ulnar nerve
胸背神经
thoracodorsal nerve
肱动、静脉
brachial artery and vein
背阔肌
latissimus dorsi
胸背动、静脉
thoracodorsal artery and vein

副神经
accessory nerve
颈横静脉
transverse cervical vein
颈横动脉
transverse cervical artery
锁骨下动、静脉
subclavian artery and vein
内侧束
medial cord
正中神经
median nerve
胸长神经
long thoracic nerve
前臂内侧皮神经
medial antebrachial cutaneous nerve

图 342　肩前区和腋区局部解剖 4
Topography of anterior region of the shoulder and the axillary region 4

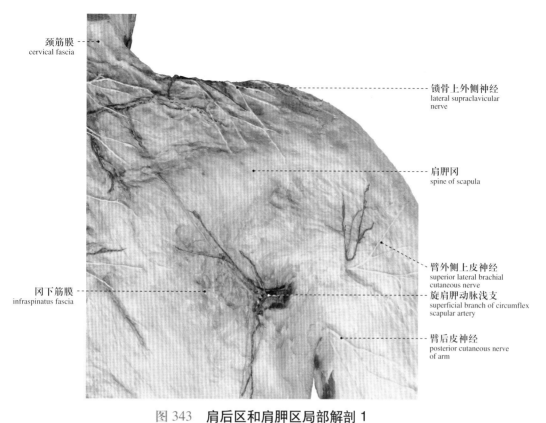

颈筋膜
cervical fascia

锁骨上外侧神经
lateral supraclavicular
nerve

肩胛冈
spine of scapula

臂外侧上皮神经
superior lateral brachial
cutaneous nerve

旋肩胛动脉浅支
superficial branch of circumflex
scapular artery

冈下筋膜
infraspinatus fascia

臂后皮神经
posterior cutaneous nerve
of arm

图 343　肩后区和肩胛区局部解剖 1

Topography of posterior region of the shoulder and the scapular region 1

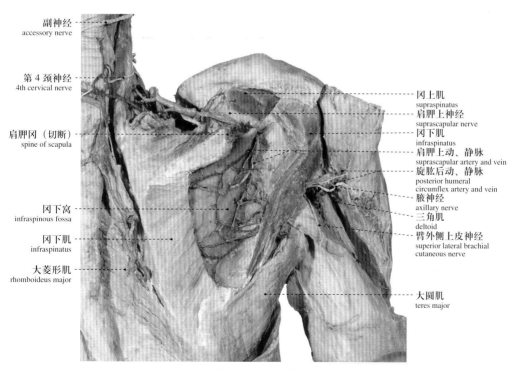

副神经
accessory nerve

第 4 颈神经
4th cervical nerve

冈上肌
supraspinatus

肩胛上神经
suprascapular nerve

冈下肌
infraspinatus

肩胛冈（切断）
spine of scapula

肩胛上动、静脉
suprascapular artery and vein

旋肱后动、静脉
posterior humeral
circumflex artery and vein

腋神经
axillary nerve

冈下窝
infraspinous fossa

三角肌
deltoid

臂外侧上皮神经
superior lateral brachial
cutaneous nerve

冈下肌
infraspinatus

大菱形肌
rhomboideus major

大圆肌
teres major

图 344　肩后区和肩胛区局部解剖 2

Topography of posterior region of the shoulder and the scapular region 2

臂 部

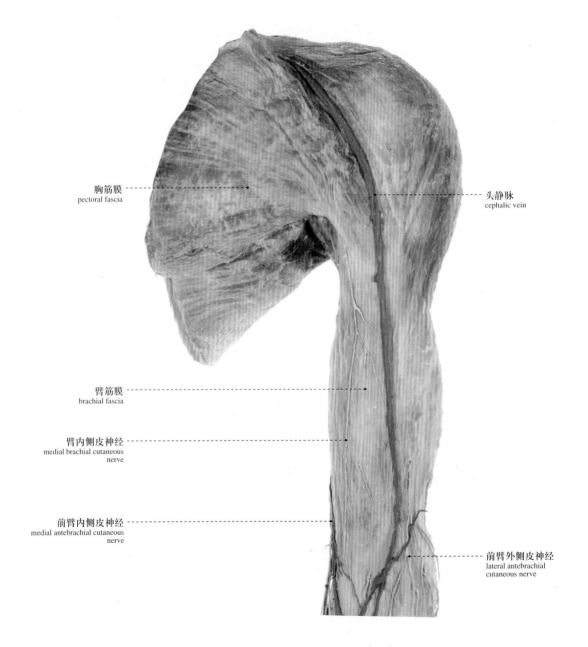

胸筋膜
pectoral fascia

头静脉
cephalic vein

臂筋膜
brachial fascia

臂内侧皮神经
medial brachial cutaneous
nerve

前臂内侧皮神经
medial antebrachial cutaneous
nerve

前臂外侧皮神经
lateral antebrachial
cutaneous nerve

图 345　臂部浅层静脉和神经
Veins and nerves of the superficial layer of the arm

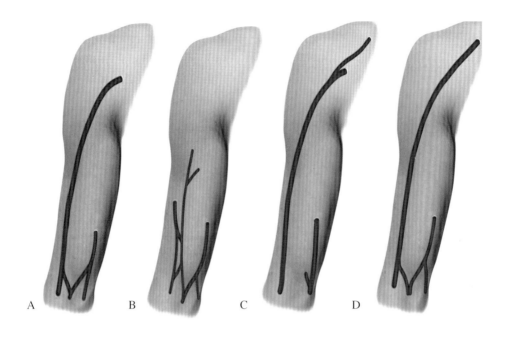

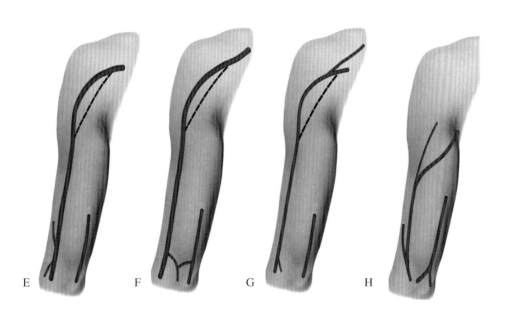

图 346　头静脉干肩部的分型

Forms of the cephalic vein on the shoulder region

A. 正常型（占 65.7%）；B. 头静脉于臂、肩部缺如或极细；C. 注入前发分支入颈外静脉；D. 越锁骨直入颈外静脉；
E. 经三角胸肌沟外侧；F. 经三角胸肌沟外侧越锁骨入颈外静脉；G. 经三角胸肌沟外侧，于锁骨下窝分两支，
一支入腋静脉，一支入颈外静脉；H. 于三角肌止点附近内上行，入腋静脉下段

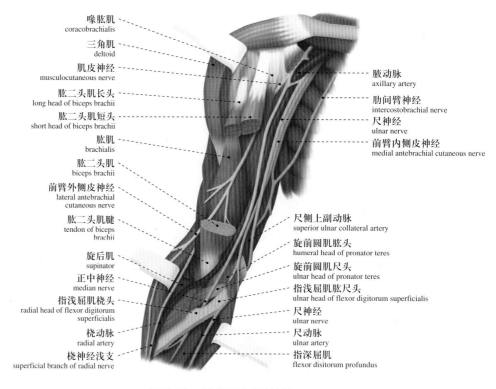

喙肱肌
coracobrachialis

三角肌
deltoid

肌皮神经
musculocutaneous nerve

肱二头肌长头
long head of biceps brachii

肱二头肌短头
short head of biceps brachii

肱肌
brachialis

肱二头肌
biceps brachii

前臂外侧皮神经
lateral antebrachial cutaneous nerve

肱二头肌腱
tendon of biceps brachii

旋后肌
supinator

正中神经
median nerve

指浅屈肌桡头
radial head of flexor digitorum superficialis

桡动脉
radial artery

桡神经浅支
superficial branch of radial nerve

腋动脉
axillary artery

肋间臂神经
intercostobrachial nerve

尺神经
ulnar nerve

前臂内侧皮神经
medial antebrachial cutaneous nerve

尺侧上副动脉
superior ulnar collateral artery

旋前圆肌肱头
humeral head of pronator teres

旋前圆肌尺头
ulnar head of pronator teres

指浅屈肌肱尺头
ulnar head of flexor digitorum superficialis

尺神经
ulnar nerve

尺动脉
ulnar artery

指深屈肌
flexor disitorum profundus

图 347 臂前区深层结构
Deep structure of anterior region of arm

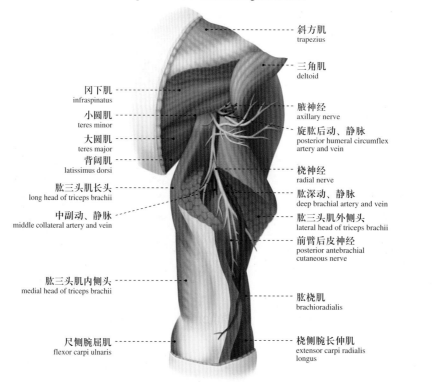

冈下肌
infraspinatus

小圆肌
teres minor

大圆肌
teres major

背阔肌
latissimus dorsi

肱三头肌长头
long head of triceps brachii

中副动、静脉
middle collateral artery and vein

肱三头肌内侧头
medial head of triceps brachii

尺侧腕屈肌
flexor carpi ulnaris

斜方肌
trapezius

三角肌
deltoid

腋神经
axillary nerve

旋肱后动、静脉
posterior humeral circumflex artery and vein

桡神经
radial nerve

肱深动、静脉
deep brachial artery and vein

肱三头肌外侧头
lateral head of triceps brachii

前臂后皮神经
posterior antebrachial cutaneous nerve

肱桡肌
brachioradialis

桡侧腕长伸肌
extensor carpi radialis longus

图 348 臂后区深层结构
Deep structure of posterior brachial region

第三节

肘 部

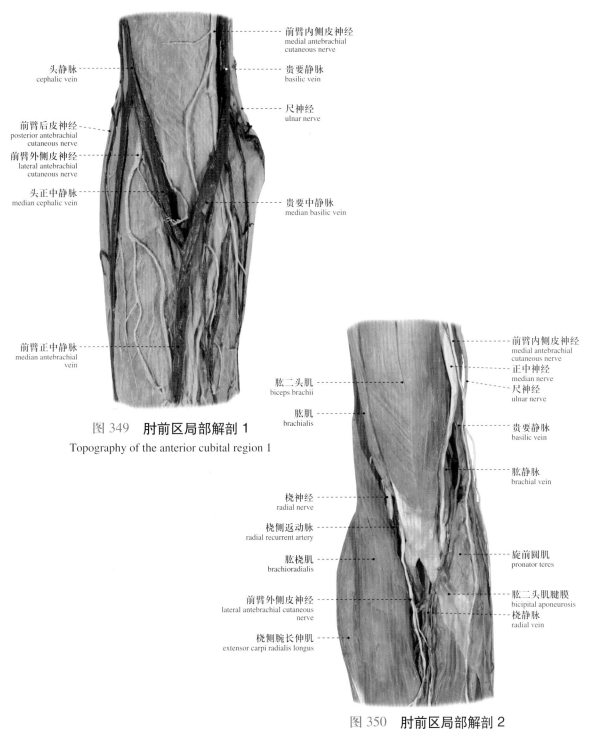

图 349　肘前区局部解剖 1
Topography of the anterior cubital region 1

图 349 labels:
- 前臂内侧皮神经 medial antebrachial cutaneous nerve
- 头静脉 cephalic vein
- 贵要静脉 basilic vein
- 尺神经 ulnar nerve
- 前臂后皮神经 posterior antebrachial cutaneous nerve
- 前臂外侧皮神经 lateral antebrachial cutaneous nerve
- 头正中静脉 median cephalic vein
- 贵要中静脉 median basilic vein
- 前臂正中静脉 median antebrachial vein

图 350　肘前区局部解剖 2
Topography of the anterior cubital region 2

图 350 labels:
- 前臂内侧皮神经 medial antebrachial cutaneous nerve
- 正中神经 median nerve
- 尺神经 ulnar nerve
- 肱二头肌 biceps brachii
- 肱肌 brachialis
- 贵要静脉 basilic vein
- 肱静脉 brachial vein
- 桡神经 radial nerve
- 桡侧返动脉 radial recurrent artery
- 肱桡肌 brachioradialis
- 旋前圆肌 pronator teres
- 前臂外侧皮神经 lateral antebrachial cutaneous nerve
- 肱二头肌腱膜 bicipital aponeurosis
- 桡静脉 radial vein
- 桡侧腕长伸肌 extensor carpi radialis longus

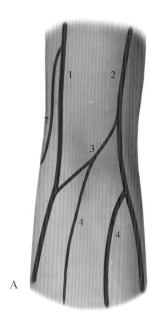

A

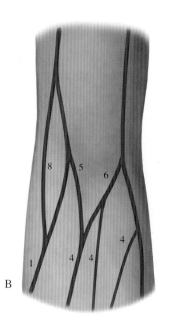

B

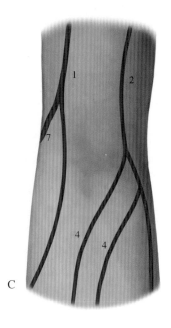

C

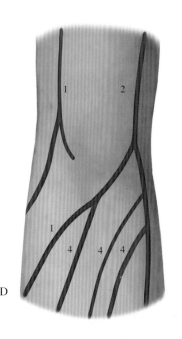

D

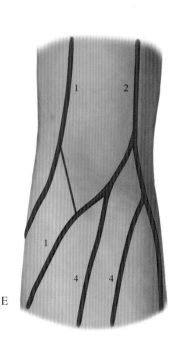

E

1. 头静脉
cephalic vein

2. 贵要静脉
basilic vein

3. 肘正中静脉
median cubital vein

4. 前臂正中静脉
median vein of forearm

5. 头正中静脉
median cephalic vein

6. 贵要正中静脉
median basilic vein

7. 副头静脉
accessory cephalic vein

8. 岛头静脉
island cephalic vein

图 351　肘浅静脉分型
Forms of the cubital superficial veins

A. 头静脉借一条肘正中静脉与贵要静脉相连；B. 头静脉借 Y 型肘正中静脉与贵要静脉相连，Y 型的两臂分别称头正中静脉和贵要静脉；C. 头静脉与贵要静脉与肘浅部无静脉交通；D. 头静脉在肘前直入贵要静脉，臂部头静脉来源于肘部深静脉，或臂部头静脉细小；E. 前臂头静脉主干斜过肘窝入贵要静脉，但有细支与臂部头静脉相连

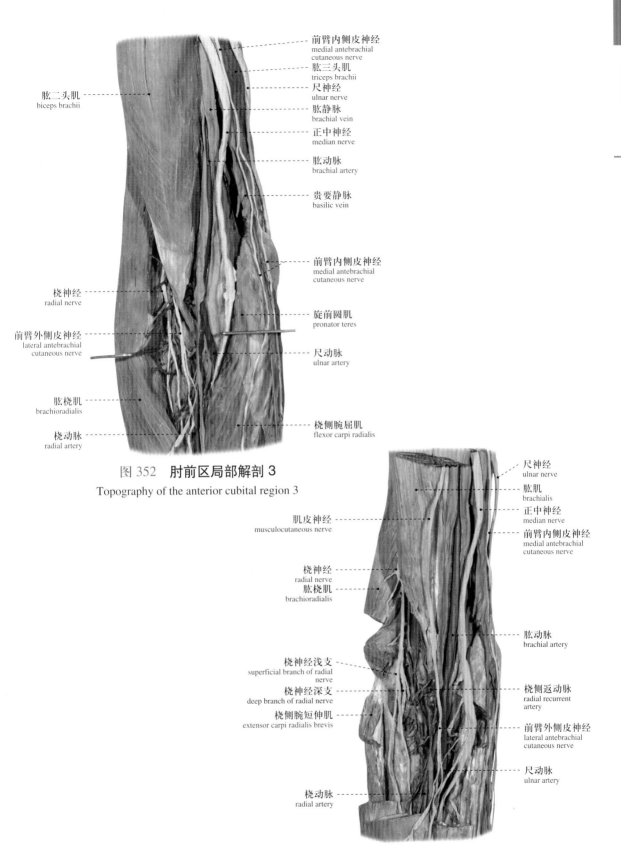

肱二头肌
biceps brachii

前臂内侧皮神经
medial antebrachial
cutaneous nerve

肱三头肌
triceps brachii

尺神经
ulnar nerve

肱静脉
brachial vein

正中神经
median nerve

肱动脉
brachial artery

贵要静脉
basilic vein

前臂内侧皮神经
medial antebrachial
cutaneous nerve

旋前圆肌
pronator teres

尺动脉
ulnar artery

桡神经
radial nerve

前臂外侧皮神经
lateral antebrachial
cutaneous nerve

肱桡肌
brachioradialis

桡动脉
radial artery

桡侧腕屈肌
flexor carpi radialis

图 352 肘前区局部解剖 3
Topography of the anterior cubital region 3

肌皮神经
musculocutaneous nerve

桡神经
radial nerve

肱桡肌
brachioradialis

桡神经浅支
superficial branch of radial
nerve

桡神经深支
deep branch of radial nerve

桡侧腕短伸肌
extensor carpi radialis brevis

桡动脉
radial artery

尺神经
ulnar nerve

肱肌
brachialis

正中神经
median nerve

前臂内侧皮神经
medial antebrachial
cutaneous nerve

肱动脉
brachial artery

桡侧返动脉
radial recurrent
artery

前臂外侧皮神经
lateral antebrachial
cutaneous nerve

尺动脉
ulnar artery

图 353 肘前区局部解剖 4
Topography of the anterior cubital region 4

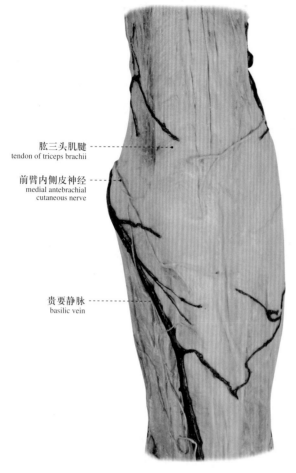

肱三头肌腱
tendon of triceps brachii

前臂内侧皮神经
medial antebrachial
cutaneous nerve

贵要静脉
basilic vein

图 354　肘后区局部解剖 1
Topography of the posterior cubital region 1

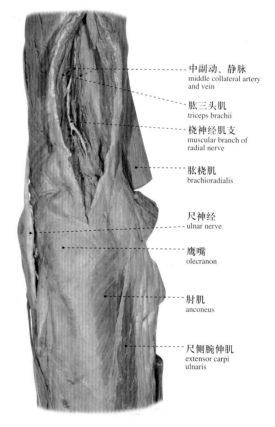

中副动、静脉
middle collateral artery
and vein

肱三头肌
triceps brachii

桡神经肌支
muscular branch of
radial nerve

肱桡肌
brachioradialis

尺神经
ulnar nerve

鹰嘴
olecranon

肘肌
anconeus

尺侧腕伸肌
extensor carpi
ulnaris

图 355　肘后区局部解剖 2
Topography of the posterior cubital region 2

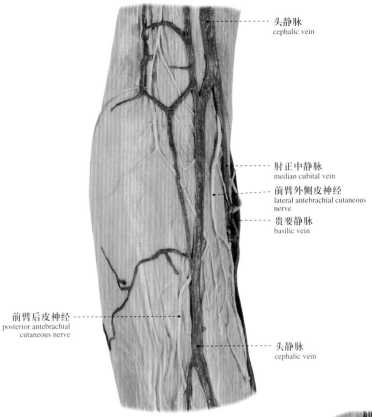

头静脉
cephalic vein

肘正中静脉
median cubital vein

前臂外侧皮神经
lateral antebrachial cutaneous
nerve

贵要静脉
basilic vein

前臂后皮神经
posterior antebrachial
cutaneous nerve

头静脉
cephalic vein

图 356 肘外侧面局部解剖 1
Topography of the lateral cubital aspect 1

肱二头肌
biceps brachii

肱肌
brachialis

桡神经
radial nerve

肌支
muscular branch

前臂外侧皮神经
lateral antebrachial
cutaneous nerve

肱桡肌
brachioradialis

桡侧腕长伸肌
extensor carpi radialis
longus

桡静脉
radial vein

图 357 肘外侧面局部解剖 2
Topography of the lateral cubital aspect 2

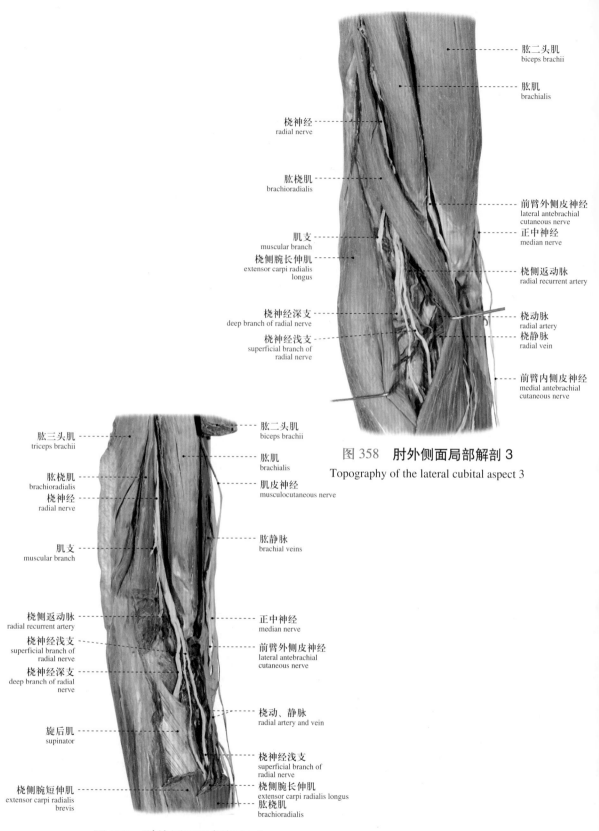

桡神经
radial nerve

肱桡肌
brachioradialis

肌支
muscular branch

桡侧腕长伸肌
extensor carpi radialis longus

桡神经深支
deep branch of radial nerve

桡神经浅支
superficial branch of radial nerve

肱二头肌
biceps brachii

肱肌
brachialis

前臂外侧皮神经
lateral antebrachial cutaneous nerve

正中神经
median nerve

桡侧返动脉
radial recurrent artery

桡动脉
radial artery

桡静脉
radial vein

前臂内侧皮神经
medial antebrachial cutaneous nerve

图 358　肘外侧面局部解剖 3
Topography of the lateral cubital aspect 3

肱三头肌
triceps brachii

肱桡肌
brachioradialis

桡神经
radial nerve

肌支
muscular branch

桡侧返动脉
radial recurrent artery

桡神经浅支
superficial branch of radial nerve

桡神经深支
deep branch of radial nerve

旋后肌
supinator

桡侧腕短伸肌
extensor carpi radialis brevis

肱二头肌
biceps brachii

肱肌
brachialis

肌皮神经
musculocutaneous nerve

肱静脉
brachial veins

正中神经
median nerve

前臂外侧皮神经
lateral antebrachial cutaneous nerve

桡动、静脉
radial artery and vein

桡神经浅支
superficial branch of radial nerve

桡侧腕长伸肌
extensor carpi radialis longus

肱桡肌
brachioradialis

图 359　肘外侧面局部解剖 4
Topography of the lateral cubital aspect 4

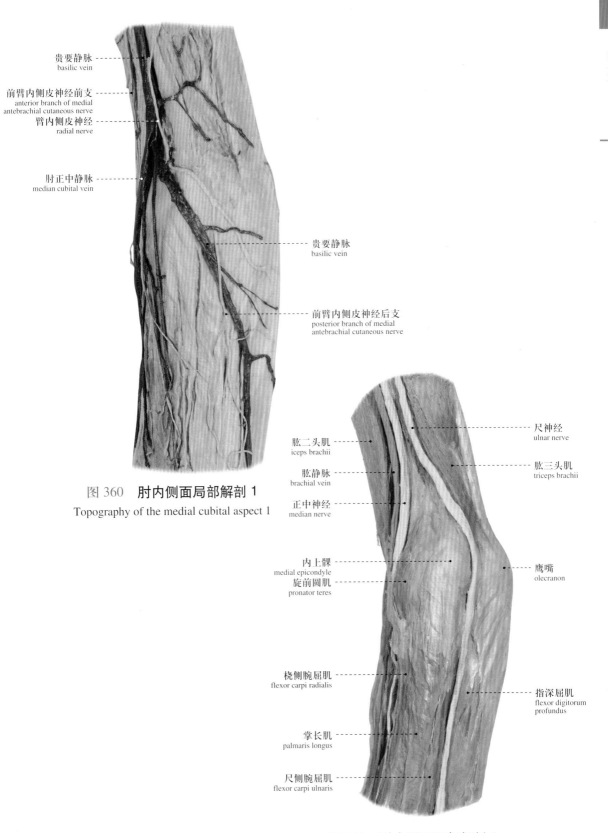

贵要静脉
basilic vein

前臂内侧皮神经前支
anterior branch of medial
antebrachial cutaneous nerve

臂内侧皮神经
radial nerve

肘正中静脉
median cubital vein

贵要静脉
basilic vein

前臂内侧皮神经后支
posterior branch of medial
antebrachial cutaneous nerve

图 360　肘内侧面局部解剖 1
Topography of the medial cubital aspect 1

肱二头肌
iceps brachii

肱静脉
brachial vein

正中神经
median nerve

尺神经
ulnar nerve

肱三头肌
triceps brachii

内上髁
medial epicondyle

旋前圆肌
pronator teres

鹰嘴
olecranon

桡侧腕屈肌
flexor carpi radialis

指深屈肌
flexor digitorum
profundus

掌长肌
palmaris longus

尺侧腕屈肌
flexor carpi ulnaris

图 361　肘内侧面局部解剖 2
Topography of the medial cubital aspect 2

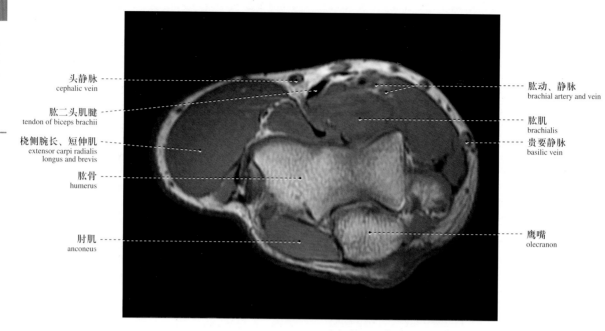

头静脉
cephalic vein

肱二头肌腱
tendon of biceps brachii

桡侧腕长、短伸肌
extensor carpi radialis
longus and brevis

肱骨
humerus

肘肌
anconeus

肱动、静脉
brachial artery and vein

肱肌
brachialis

贵要静脉
basilic vein

鹰嘴
olecranon

图 362　肘部磁共振成像（轴位）
MRI of the elbow (axial view)

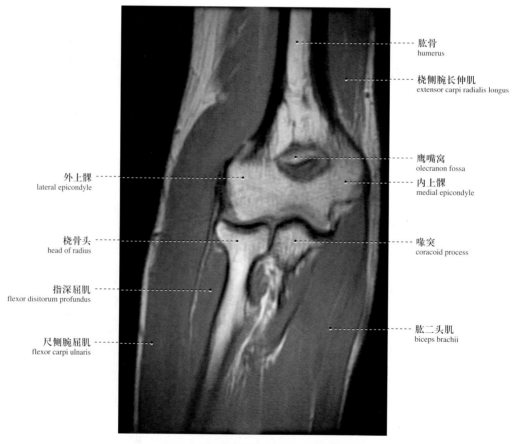

肱骨
humerus

桡侧腕长伸肌
extensor carpi radialis longus

鹰嘴窝
olecranon fossa

内上髁
medial epicondyle

喙突
coracoid process

肱二头肌
biceps brachii

外上髁
lateral epicondyle

桡骨头
head of radius

指深屈肌
flexor disitorum profundus

尺侧腕屈肌
flexor carpi ulnaris

图 363　肘部磁共振成像（冠状位）
MRI of the elbow (coronal view)

第四节

前臂部

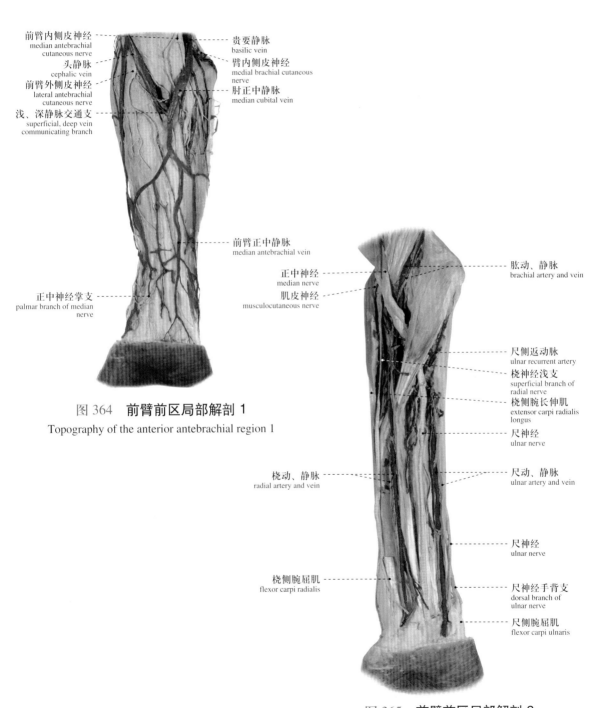

前臂内侧皮神经
median antebrachial cutaneous nerve

头静脉
cephalic vein

前臂外侧皮神经
lateral antebrachial cutaneous nerve

浅、深静脉交通支
superficial, deep vein communicating branch

贵要静脉
basilic vein

臂内侧皮神经
medial brachial cutaneous nerve

肘正中静脉
median cubital vein

前臂正中静脉
median antebrachial vein

正中神经掌支
palmar branch of median nerve

正中神经
median nerve

肌皮神经
musculocutaneous nerve

桡动、静脉
radial artery and vein

桡侧腕屈肌
flexor carpi radialis

肱动、静脉
brachial artery and vein

尺侧返动脉
ulnar recurrent artery

桡神经浅支
superficial branch of radial nerve

桡侧腕长伸肌
extensor carpi radialis longus

尺神经
ulnar nerve

尺动、静脉
ulnar artery and vein

尺神经
ulnar nerve

尺神经手背支
dorsal branch of ulnar nerve

尺侧腕屈肌
flexor carpi ulnaris

图 364　前臂前区局部解剖 1
Topography of the anterior antebrachial region 1

图 365　前臂前区局部解剖 2
Topography of the anterior antebrachial region 2

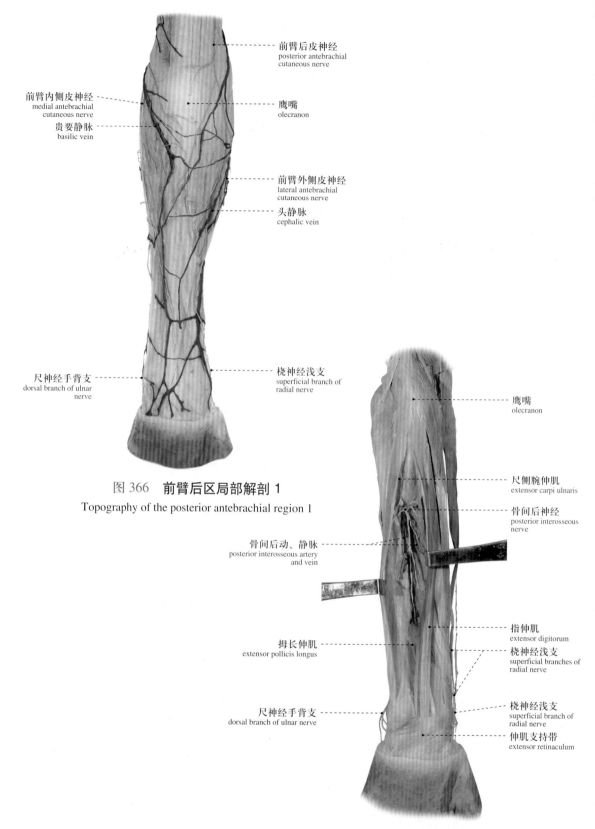

前臂后皮神经
posterior antebrachial
cutaneous nerve

前臂内侧皮神经
medial antebrachial
cutaneous nerve

贵要静脉
basilic vein

鹰嘴
olecranon

前臂外侧皮神经
lateral antebrachial
cutaneous nerve

头静脉
cephalic vein

尺神经手背支
dorsal branch of ulnar
nerve

桡神经浅支
superficial branch of
radial nerve

图 366　前臂后区局部解剖 1
Topography of the posterior antebrachial region 1

鹰嘴
olecranon

尺侧腕伸肌
extensor carpi ulnaris

骨间后神经
posterior interosseous
nerve

骨间后动、静脉
posterior interosseous artery
and vein

指伸肌
extensor digitorum

桡神经浅支
superficial branches of
radial nerve

拇长伸肌
extensor pollicis longus

桡神经浅支
superficial branch of
radial nerve

尺神经手背支
dorsal branch of ulnar nerve

伸肌支持带
extensor retinaculum

图 367　前臂后区局部解剖 2
Topography of the posterior antebrachial region 2

第五节

腕和手

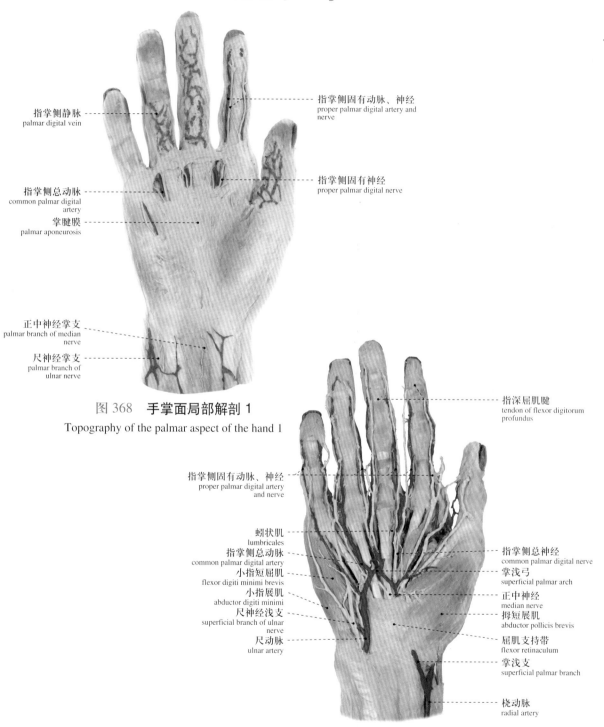

指掌侧静脉
palmar digital vein

指掌侧总动脉
common palmar digital artery

掌腱膜
palmar aponeurosis

正中神经掌支
palmar branch of median nerve

尺神经掌支
palmar branch of ulnar nerve

指掌侧固有动脉、神经
proper palmar digital artery and nerve

指掌侧固有神经
proper palmar digital nerve

图 368　手掌面局部解剖 1
Topography of the palmar aspect of the hand 1

指掌侧固有动脉、神经
proper palmar digital artery and nerve

蚓状肌
lumbricales

指掌侧总动脉
common palmar digital artery

小指短屈肌
flexor digiti minimi brevis

小指展肌
abductor digiti minimi

尺神经浅支
superficial branch of ulnar nerve

尺动脉
ulnar artery

指深屈肌腱
tendon of flexor digitorum profundus

指掌侧总神经
common palmar digital nerve

掌浅弓
superficial palmar arch

正中神经
median nerve

拇短展肌
abductor pollicis brevis

屈肌支持带
flexor retinaculum

掌浅支
superficial palmar branch

桡动脉
radial artery

图 369　手掌面局部解剖 2
Topography of the palmar aspect of the hand 2

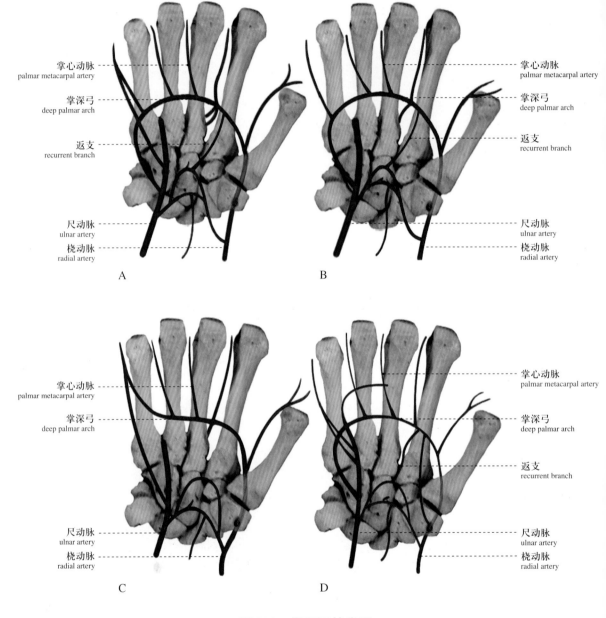

掌心动脉
palmar metacarpal artery

掌深弓
deep palmar arch

返支
recurrent branch

尺动脉
ulnar artery

桡动脉
radial artery

掌心动脉
palmar metacarpal artery

掌深弓
deep palmar arch

返支
recurrent branch

尺动脉
ulnar artery

桡动脉
radial artery

A

B

掌心动脉
palmar metacarpal artery

掌深弓
deep palmar arch

尺动脉
ulnar artery

桡动脉
radial artery

掌心动脉
palmar metacarpal artery

掌深弓
deep palmar arch

返支
recurrent branch

尺动脉
ulnar artery

桡动脉
radial artery

C

D

图 370 掌深弓的类型

Patterns of the deep palmar arch

A. 完全成弓型；B. 完全成弓型；C. 不完全成弓型；D 不完全成弓型，掌深弓由尺动脉掌深支形成

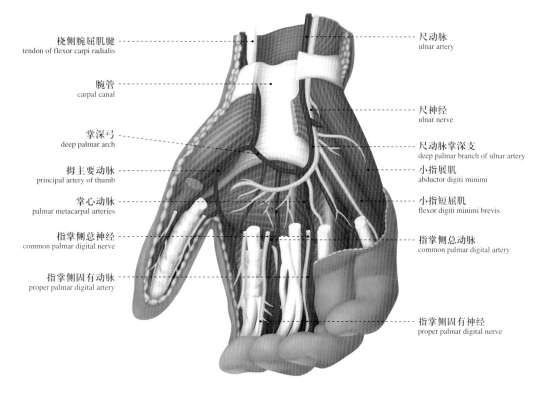

桡侧腕屈肌腱
tendon of flexor carpi radialis

腕管
carpal canal

掌深弓
deep palmar arch

拇主要动脉
principal artery of thumb

掌心动脉
palmar metacarpal arteries

指掌侧总神经
common palmar digital nerve

指掌侧固有动脉
proper palmar digital artery

尺动脉
ulnar artery

尺神经
ulnar nerve

尺动脉掌深支
deep palmar branch of ulnar artery

小指展肌
abductor digiti minimi

小指短屈肌
flexor digiti minimi brevis

指掌侧总动脉
common palmar digital artery

指掌侧固有神经
proper palmar digital nerve

图 371　掌深弓、尺神经及其分支
Deep palmar arch, the ulnar nerve and its branches

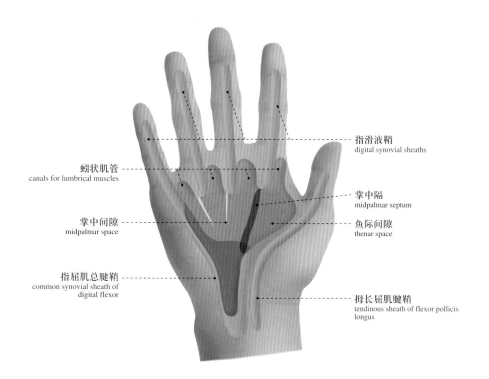

蚓状肌管
canals for lumbrical muscles

掌中间隙
midpalmar space

指屈肌总腱鞘
common synovial sheath of digital flexor

指滑液鞘
digital synovial sheaths

掌中隔
midpalmar septum

鱼际间隙
thenar space

拇长屈肌腱鞘
tendinous sheath of flexor pollicis longus

图 372　筋膜间隙和腱滑液鞘
Fascial spaces and the synovial sheaths of the tendon

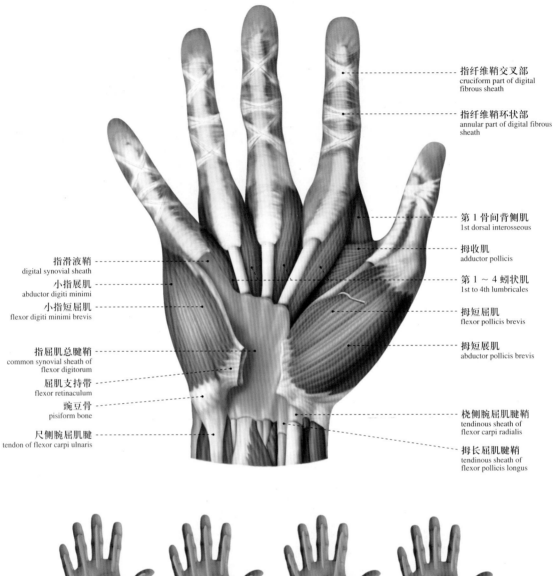

指纤维鞘交叉部
cruciform part of digital fibrous sheath

指纤维鞘环状部
annular part of digital fibrous sheath

第 1 骨间背侧肌
1st dorsal interosseous

拇收肌
adductor pollicis

第 1～4 蚓状肌
1st to 4th lumbricales

拇短屈肌
flexor pollicis brevis

拇短展肌
abductor pollicis brevis

桡侧腕屈肌腱鞘
tendinous sheath of flexor carpi radialis

拇长屈肌腱鞘
tendinous sheath of flexor pollicis longus

指滑液鞘
digital synovial sheath

小指展肌
abductor digiti minimi

小指短屈肌
flexor digiti minimi brevis

指屈肌总腱鞘
common synovial sheath of flexor digitorum

屈肌支持带
flexor retinaculum

豌豆骨
pisiform bone

尺侧腕屈肌腱
tendon of flexor carpi ulnaris

图 373　手腱滑液鞘及分型（掌面）
Synovial sheaths of the tendons and its patterns of the hand (palmar aspect)

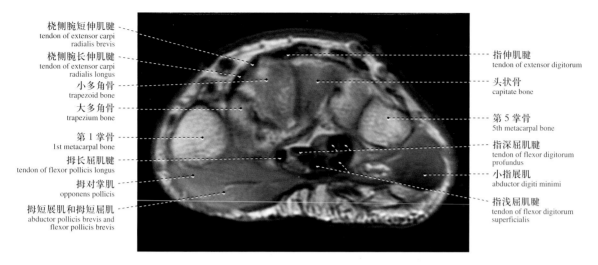

桡侧腕短伸肌腱
tendon of extensor carpi radialis brevis

桡侧腕长伸肌腱
tendon of extensor carpi radialis longus

小多角骨
trapezoid bone

大多角骨
trapezium bone

第 1 掌骨
1st metacarpal bone

拇长屈肌腱
tendon of flexor pollicis longus

拇对掌肌
opponens pollicis

拇短展肌和拇短屈肌
abductor pollicis brevis and flexor pollicis brevis

指伸肌腱
tendon of extensor digitorum

头状骨
capitate bone

第 5 掌骨
5th metacarpal bone

指深屈肌腱
tendon of flexor digitorum profundus

小指展肌
abductor digiti minimi

指浅屈肌腱
tendon of flexor digitorum superficialis

图 374　腕部磁共振成像（轴位）
MRI of the wrist（axial view）

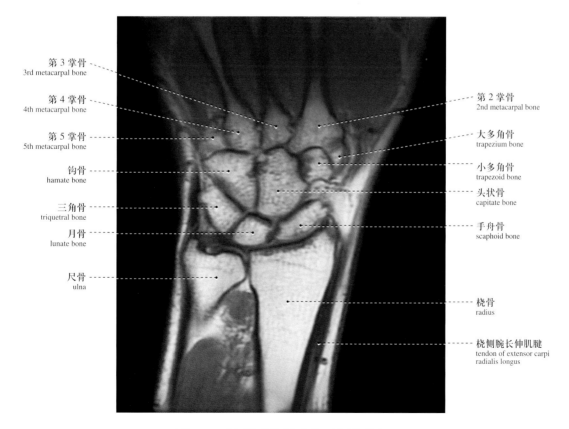

第 3 掌骨
3rd metacarpal bone

第 4 掌骨
4th metacarpal bone

第 5 掌骨
5th metacarpal bone

钩骨
hamate bone

三角骨
triquetral bone

月骨
lunate bone

尺骨
ulna

第 2 掌骨
2nd metacarpal bone

大多角骨
trapezium bone

小多角骨
trapezoid bone

头状骨
capitate bone

手舟骨
scaphoid bone

桡骨
radius

桡侧腕长伸肌腱
tendon of extensor carpi radialis longus

图 375　腕部磁共振成像（冠状位）
MRI of the wrist (coronal view)

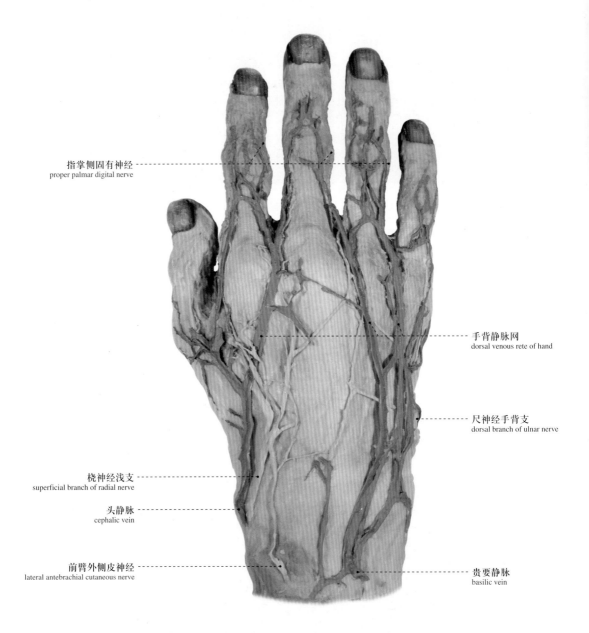

指掌侧固有神经
proper palmar digital nerve

手背静脉网
dorsal venous rete of hand

尺神经手背支
dorsal branch of ulnar nerve

桡神经浅支
superficial branch of radial nerve

头静脉
cephalic vein

前臂外侧皮神经
lateral antebrachial cutaneous nerve

贵要静脉
basilic vein

图 376　手背面局部解剖 1
Topography of the dorsal aspect of the hand 1

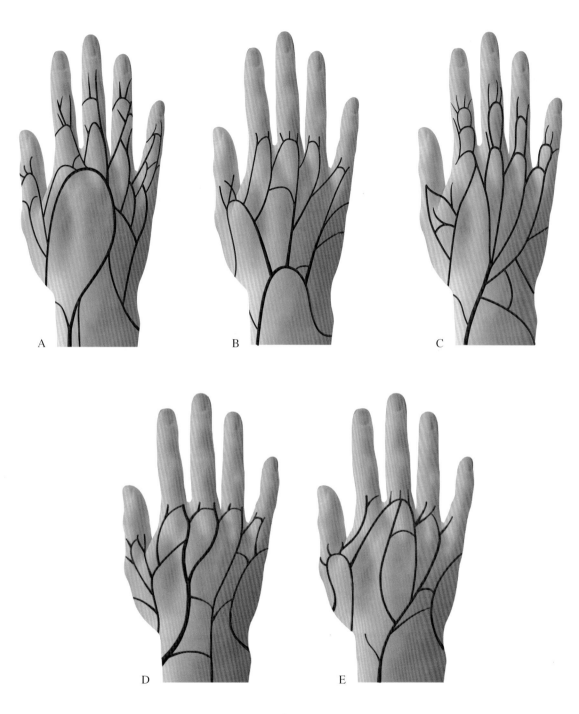

图 377　手背浅静脉的主要分型

Chief forms of the superficial veins on the dorsum of the hand

A. 弓型：掌背静脉于手背形成一大静脉弓，此型较多；B. 弓型：掌背静脉于腕背面形成一较大静脉弓，有时于手背形成 2、3 排静脉弓，此型亦较多；C. 网型：第 2～4 掌背静脉较粗，向近侧逐渐会合，形成一粗静脉干；D. 网型：第 2、3 掌背静脉较粗，形成一粗静脉干，其余静脉较细，呈网状；E. 网型：第 3、4 掌背静脉较粗，向近侧合成一条大静脉干，其余细小

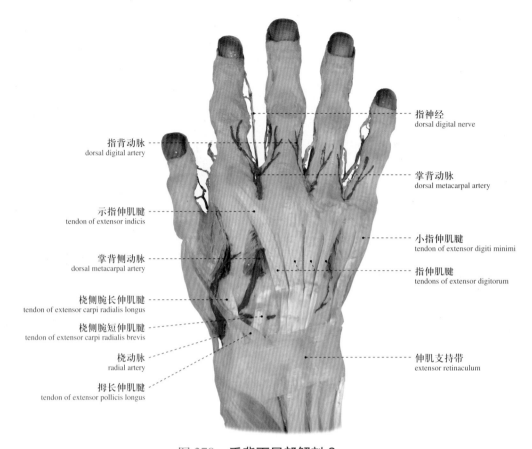

指神经
dorsal digital nerve

指背动脉
dorsal digital artery

掌背动脉
dorsal metacarpal artery

示指伸肌腱
tendon of extensor indicis

小指伸肌腱
tendon of extensor digiti minimi

掌背侧动脉
dorsal metacarpal artery

指伸肌腱
tendons of extensor digitorum

桡侧腕长伸肌腱
tendon of extensor carpi radialis longus

桡侧腕短伸肌腱
tendon of extensor carpi radialis brevis

桡动脉
radial artery

伸肌支持带
extensor retinaculum

拇长伸肌腱
tendon of extensor pollicis longus

图 378　手背面局部解剖 2
Topography of the dorsal aspect of the hand 2

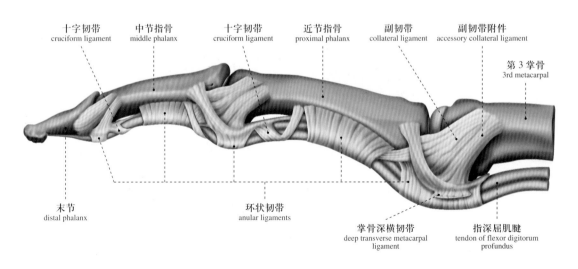

十字韧带
cruciform ligament

中节指骨
middle phalanx

十字韧带
cruciform ligament

近节指骨
proximal phalanx

副韧带
collateral ligament

副韧带附件
accessory collateral ligament

第 3 掌骨
3rd metacarpal

末节
distal phalanx

环状韧带
anular ligaments

掌骨深横韧带
deep transverse metacarpal ligament

指深屈肌腱
tendon of flexor digitorum profundus

图 379　手指的韧带
Finger ligaments

第一节

臀　部

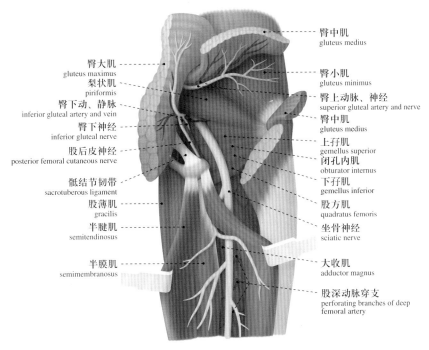

臀中肌
gluteus medius

臀大肌
gluteus maximus

臀小肌
gluteus minimus

梨状肌
piriformis

臀上动脉、神经
superior gluteal artery and nerve

臀下动、静脉
inferior gluteal artery and vein

臀中肌
gluteus medius

臀下神经
inferior gluteal nerve

上孖肌
gemellus superior

股后皮神经
posterior femoral cutaneous nerve

闭孔内肌
obturator internus

骶结节韧带
sacrotuberous ligament

下孖肌
gemellus inferior

股薄肌
gracilis

股方肌
quadratus femoris

半腱肌
semitendinosus

坐骨神经
sciatic nerve

半膜肌
semimembranosus

大收肌
adductor magnus

股深动脉穿支
perforating branches of deep femoral artery

图 380　臀部及大腿的肌肉、动脉和神经

Muscles, arteries, nerves of the hip and thigh

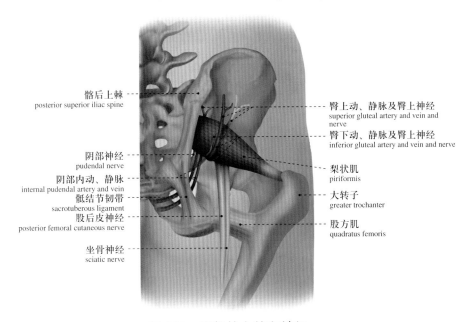

髂后上棘
posterior superior iliac spine

臀上动、静脉及臀上神经
superior gluteal artery and vein and nerve

臀下动、静脉及臀上神经
inferior gluteal artery and vein and nerve

阴部神经
pudendal nerve

梨状肌
piriformis

阴部内动、静脉
internal pudendal artery and vein

大转子
greater trochanter

骶结节韧带
sacrotuberous ligament

股后皮神经
posterior femoral cutaneous nerve

股方肌
quadratus femoris

坐骨神经
sciatic nerve

图 381　臀部的血管和神经

Blood vessels and nerves of the hip

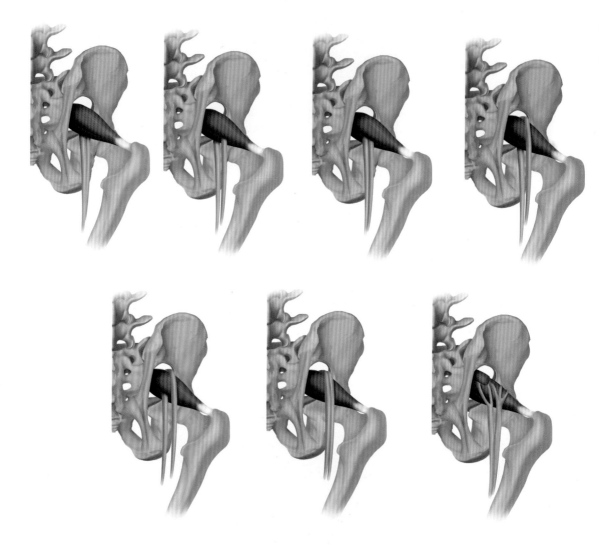

图 382　坐骨神经与梨状肌的关系
Relationship between sciatic nerve and piriformis muscle

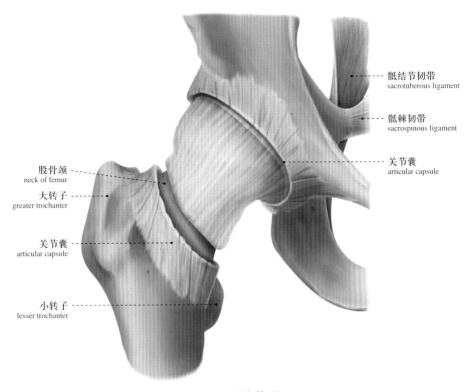

图 383　髋关节囊
Capsule of the hip joint

骶结节韧带
sacrotuberous ligament

骶棘韧带
sacrospinous ligament

关节囊
articular capsule

股骨颈
neck of femur

大转子
greater trochanter

关节囊
articular capsule

小转子
lesser trochanter

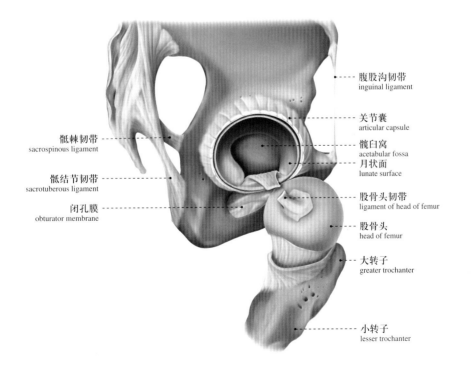

图 384　髋关节（内面观）
Hip joint (internal aspect)

腹股沟韧带
inguinal ligament

关节囊
articular capsule

髋臼窝
acetabular fossa

月状面
lunate surface

股骨头韧带
ligament of head of femur

股骨头
head of femur

大转子
greater trochanter

小转子
lesser trochanter

骶棘韧带
sacrospinous ligament

骶结节韧带
sacrotuberous ligament

闭孔膜
obturator membrane

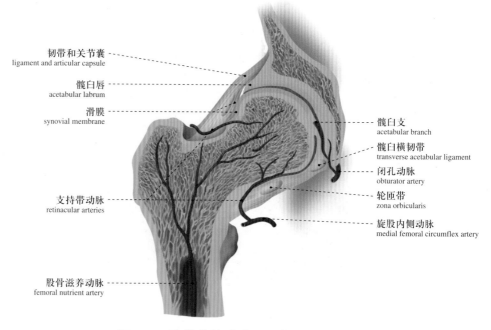

韧带和关节囊
ligament and articular capsule

髋臼唇
acetabular labrum

滑膜
synovial membrane

支持带动脉
retinacular arteries

股骨滋养动脉
femoral nutrient artery

髋臼支
acetabular branch

髋臼横韧带
transverse acetabular ligament

闭孔动脉
obturator artery

轮匝带
zona orbicularis

旋股内侧动脉
medial femoral circumflex artery

图 385 髋关节的动脉（冠状切面）
Arteries of the hip joint (coronal section)

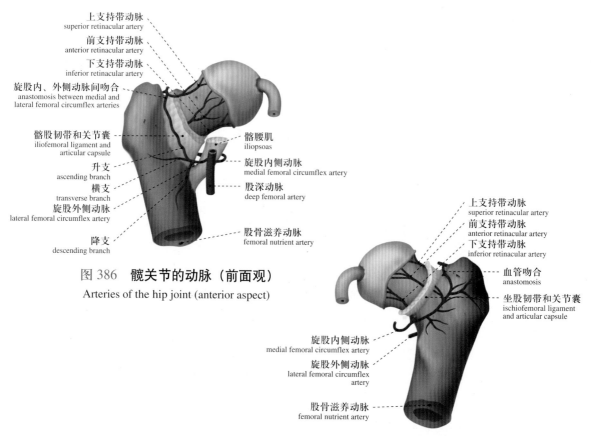

上支持带动脉
superior retinacular artery

前支持带动脉
anterior retinacular artery

下支持带动脉
inferior retinacular artery

旋股内、外侧动脉间吻合
anastomosis between medial and lateral femoral circumflex arteries

髂股韧带和关节囊
iliofemoral ligament and articular capsule

升支
ascending branch

横支
transverse branch

旋股外侧动脉
lateral femoral circumflex artery

降支
descending branch

髂腰肌
iliopsoas

旋股内侧动脉
medial femoral circumflex artery

股深动脉
deep femoral artery

股骨滋养动脉
femoral nutrient artery

图 386 髋关节的动脉（前面观）
Arteries of the hip joint (anterior aspect)

上支持带动脉
superior retinacular artery

前支持带动脉
anterior retinacular artery

下支持带动脉
inferior retinacular artery

血管吻合
anastomosis

坐股韧带和关节囊
ischiofemoral ligament and articular capsule

旋股内侧动脉
medial femoral circumflex artery

旋股外侧动脉
lateral femoral circumflex artery

股骨滋养动脉
femoral nutrient artery

图 387 髋关节的动脉（后面观）
Arteries of the hip joint (posterior section)

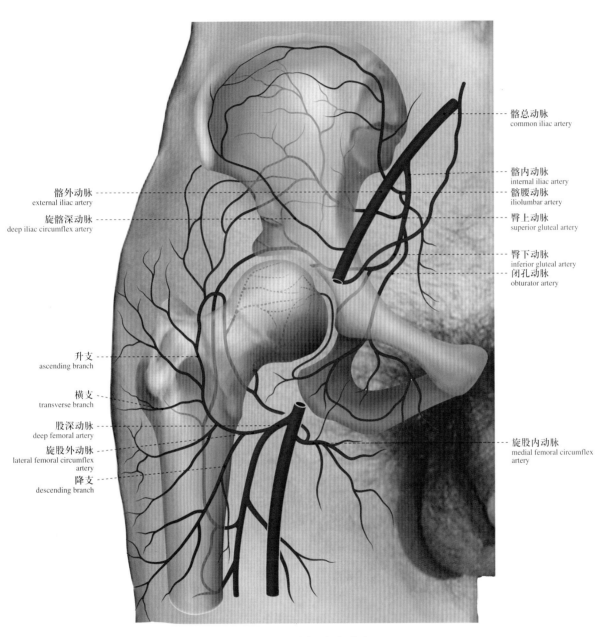

髂外动脉
external iliac artery

旋髂深动脉
deep iliac circumflex artery

升支
ascending branch

横支
transverse branch

股深动脉
deep femoral artery

旋股外动脉
lateral femoral circumflex artery

降支
descending branch

髂总动脉
common iliac artery

髂内动脉
internal iliac artery

髂腰动脉
iliolumbar artery

臀上动脉
superior gluteal artery

臀下动脉
inferior gluteal artery

闭孔动脉
obturator artery

旋股内动脉
medial femoral circumflex artery

图 388　髋部动脉分布

Arterial distribution in the hip region

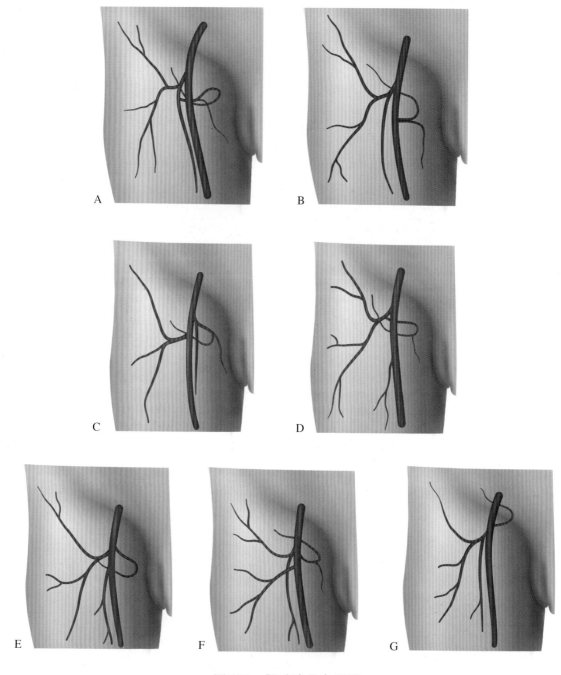

图 389　股动脉分支类型

Branch type of the femoral artery

A. 深全干型：旋股内、外侧动脉皆发自股深动脉，为常见型；B. 深外干型：旋股外侧动脉起自股深动脉，旋股内侧动脉起自股动脉；C. 深内干型：旋股内侧动脉起自股深动脉，旋股外侧动脉起自股动脉；D. 旋股内、外侧动脉以一总干从股动脉发出；E. 旋股内、外侧动脉和股深动脉分别由股动脉发出；F. 旋股外侧动脉升支发自股深动脉，降支发自股动脉；G. 旋股外侧动脉起自股深动脉，旋股内侧动脉缺如，由闭孔动脉代替

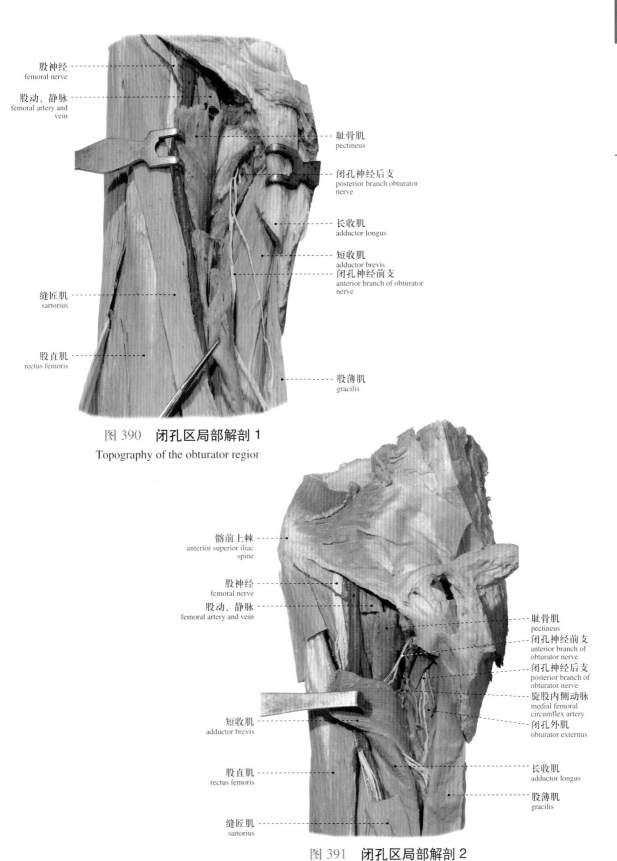

股神经
femoral nerve

股动、静脉
femoral artery and vein

耻骨肌
pectineus

闭孔神经后支
posterior branch obturator nerve

长收肌
adductor longus

短收肌
adductor brevis

闭孔神经前支
anterior branch of obturator nerve

缝匠肌
sartorius

股直肌
rectus femoris

股薄肌
gracilis

图 390　闭孔区局部解剖 1
Topography of the obturator regior

髂前上棘
anterior superior iliac spine

股神经
femoral nerve

股动、静脉
femoral artery and vein

耻骨肌
pectineus

闭孔神经前支
anterior branch of obturator nerve

闭孔神经后支
posterior branch of obturator nerve

旋股内侧动脉
medial femoral circumflex artery

闭孔外肌
obturator externus

短收肌
adductor brevis

股直肌
rectus femoris

长收肌
adductor longus

股薄肌
gracilis

缝匠肌
sartorius

图 391　闭孔区局部解剖 2
Topography of the obturator region 2

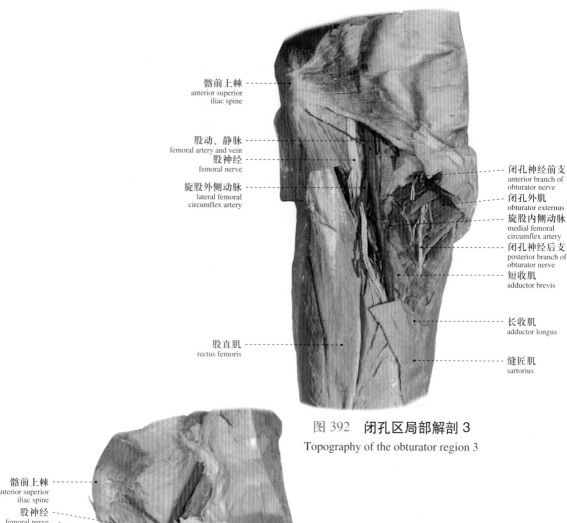

髂前上棘
anterior superior
iliac spine

股动、静脉
femoral artery and vein
股神经
femoral nerve

旋股外侧动脉
lateral femoral
circumflex artery

股直肌
rectus femoris

闭孔神经前支
anterior branch of
obturator nerve
闭孔外肌
obturator externus
旋股内侧动脉
medial femoral
circumflex artery
闭孔神经后支
posterior branch of
obturator nerve
短收肌
adductor brevis

长收肌
adductor longus

缝匠肌
sartorius

图 392　闭孔区局部解剖 3
Topography of the obturator region 3

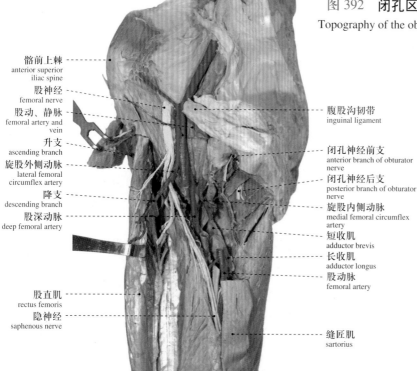

髂前上棘
anterior superior
iliac spine
股神经
femoral nerve
股动、静脉
femoral artery and
vein
升支
ascending branch
旋股外侧动脉
lateral femoral
circumflex artery
降支
descending branch
股深动脉
deep femoral artery

股直肌
rectus femoris
隐神经
saphenous nerve

腹股沟韧带
inguinal ligament

闭孔神经前支
anterior branch of obturator
nerve
闭孔神经后支
posterior branch of obturator
nerve
旋股内侧动脉
medial femoral circumflex
artery
短收肌
adductor brevis
长收肌
adductor longus
股动脉
femoral artery

缝匠肌
sartorius

图 393　闭孔区局部解剖 4
Topography of the obturator region 4

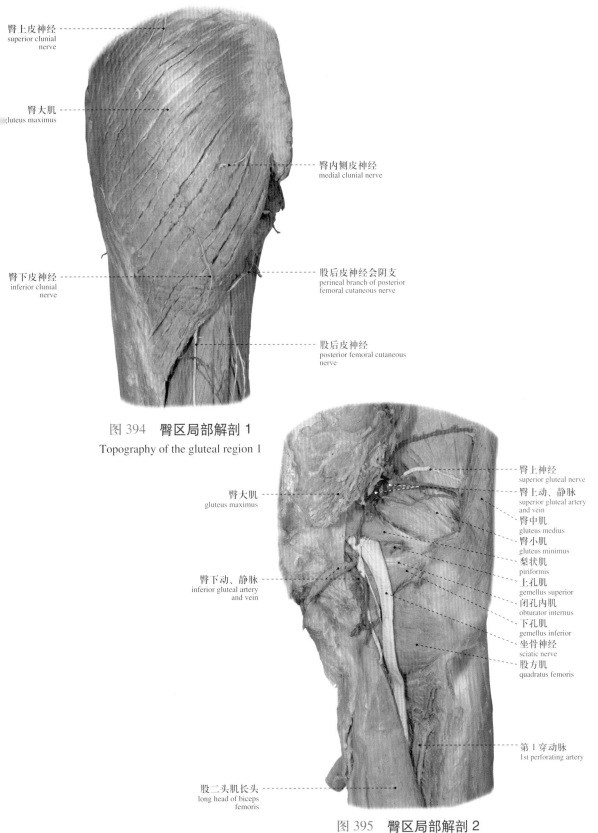

臀上皮神经
superior clunial
nerve

臀大肌
gluteus maximus

臀内侧皮神经
medial clunial nerve

臀下皮神经
inferior clunial
nerve

股后皮神经会阴支
perineal branch of posterior
femoral cutaneous nerve

股后皮神经
posterior femoral cutaneous
nerve

图 394　臀区局部解剖 1
Topography of the gluteal region 1

臀大肌
gluteus maximus

臀下动、静脉
inferior gluteal artery
and vein

臀上神经
superior gluteal nerve

臀上动、静脉
superior gluteal artery
and vein

臀中肌
gluteus medius

臀小肌
gluteus minimus

梨状肌
piriformis

上孔肌
gemellus superior

闭孔内肌
obturator internus

下孔肌
gemellus inferior

坐骨神经
sciatic nerve

股方肌
quadratus femoris

第 1 穿动脉
1st perforating artery

股二头肌长头
long head of biceps
femoris

图 395　臀区局部解剖 2
Topography of the gluteal region 2

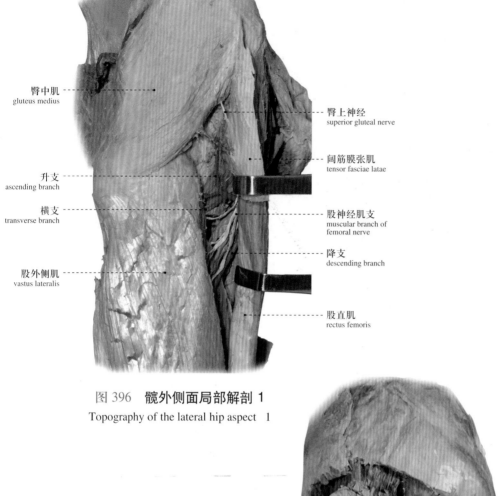

臀中肌
gluteus medius

臀上神经
superior gluteal nerve

阔筋膜张肌
tensor fasciae latae

升支
ascending branch

横支
transverse branch

股神经肌支
muscular branch of
femoral nerve

降支
descending branch

股外侧肌
vastus lateralis

股直肌
rectus femoris

图 396　髋外侧面局部解剖 1
Topography of the lateral hip aspect　1

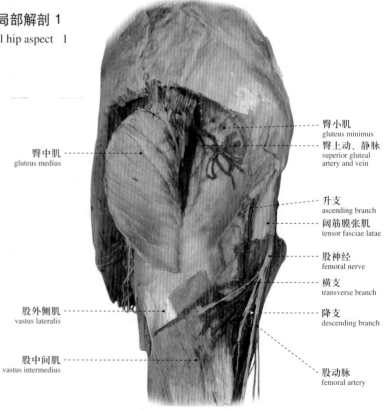

臀中肌
gluteus medius

臀小肌
gluteus minimus

臀上动、静脉
superior gluteal
artery and vein

升支
ascending branch

阔筋膜张肌
tensor fasciae latae

股神经
femoral nerve

横支
transverse branch

降支
descending branch

股外侧肌
vastus lateralis

股中间肌
vastus intermedius

股动脉
femoral artery

图 397　髋外侧面局部解剖 2
Topography of the lateral hip aspect　2

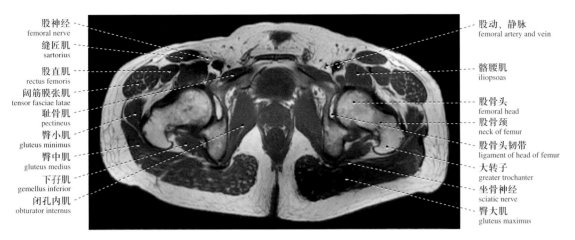

股神经
femoral nerve

缝匠肌
sartorius

股直肌
rectus femoris

阔筋膜张肌
tensor fasciae latae

耻骨肌
pectineus

臀小肌
gluteus minimus

臀中肌
gluteus medius

下孖肌
gemellus inferior

闭孔内肌
obturator internus

股动、静脉
femoral artery and vein

髂腰肌
iliopsoas

股骨头
femoral head

股骨颈
neck of femur

股骨头韧带
ligament of head of femur

大转子
greater trochanter

坐骨神经
sciatic nerve

臀大肌
gluteus maximus

图 398　髋部磁共振成像（轴位）
MRI of the hip (axial view)

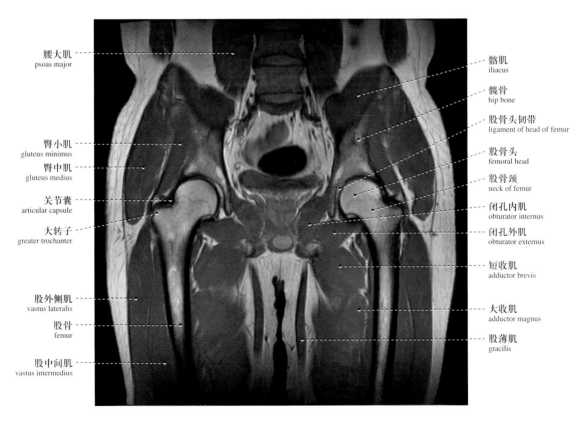

腰大肌
psoas major

臀小肌
gluteus minimus

臀中肌
gluteus medius

关节囊
articular capsule

大转子
greater trochanter

股外侧肌
vastus lateralis

股骨
femur

股中间肌
vastus intermedius

髂肌
iliacus

髋骨
hip bone

股骨头韧带
ligament of head of femur

股骨头
femoral head

股骨颈
neck of femur

闭孔内肌
obturator internus

闭孔外肌
obturator externus

短收肌
adductor brevis

大收肌
adductor magnus

股薄肌
gracilis

图 399　髋部磁共振成像（冠状位）
MRI of the hip (coronal view)

股 部

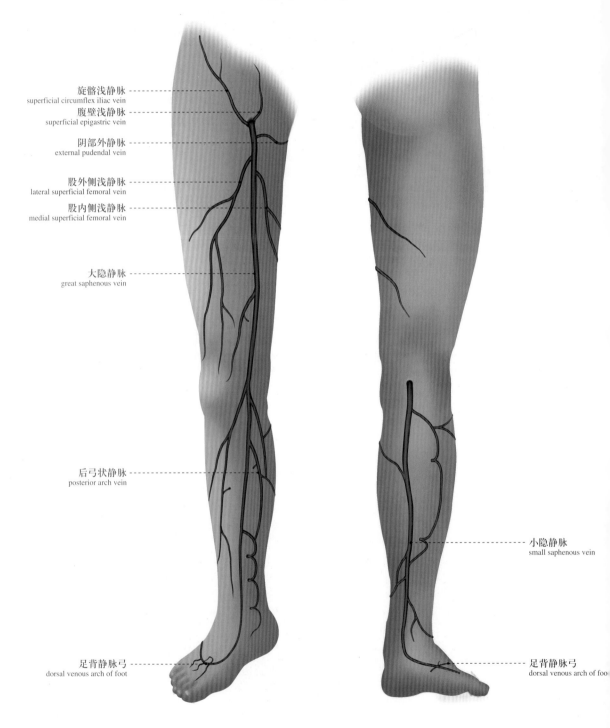

旋髂浅静脉
superficial circumflex iliac vein

腹壁浅静脉
superficial epigastric vein

阴部外静脉
external pudendal vein

股外侧浅静脉
lateral superficial femoral vein

股内侧浅静脉
medial superficial femoral vein

大隐静脉
great saphenous vein

后弓状静脉
posterior arch vein

小隐静脉
small saphenous vein

足背静脉弓
dorsal venous arch of foot

足背静脉弓
dorsal venous arch of foot

图 400　大、小隐静脉及其属支
Great and small saphenous veins and its tributaries

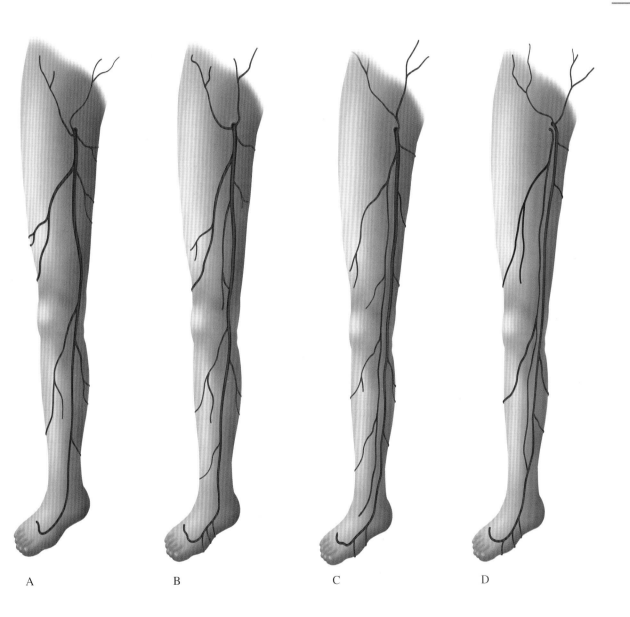

图 401　大隐静脉干类型

Types of the trunk of the great saphenous vein

A. 单干型；B. 岛型；C. 副隐型；D. 双大隐型

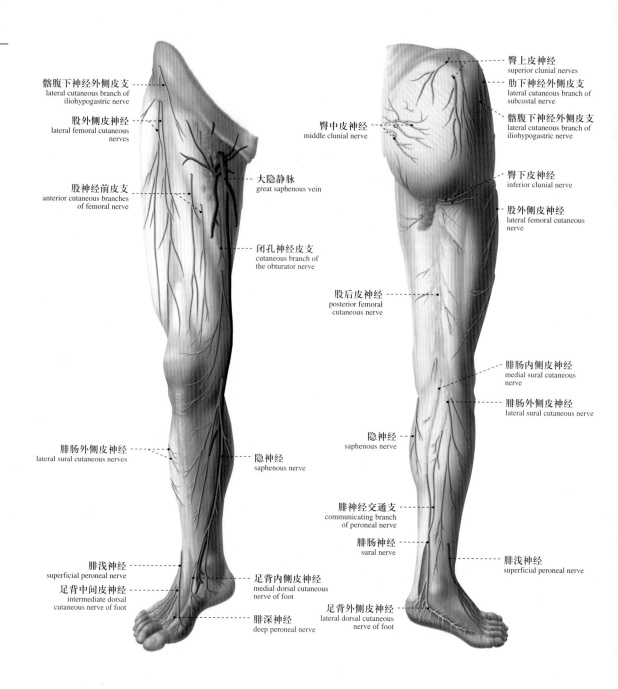

髂腹下神经外侧皮支
lateral cutaneous branch of
iliohypogastric nerve

股外侧皮神经
lateral femoral cutaneous
nerves

股神经前皮支
anterior cutaneous branches
of femoral nerve

腓肠外侧皮神经
lateral sural cutaneous nerves

腓浅神经
superficial peroneal nerve

足背中间皮神经
intermediate dorsal
cutaneous nerve of foot

大隐静脉
great saphenous vein

闭孔神经皮支
cutaneous branch of
the obturator nerve

隐神经
saphenous nerve

足背内侧皮神经
medial dorsal cutaneous
nerve of foot

腓深神经
deep peroneal nerve

臀上皮神经
superior clunial nerves

肋下神经外侧皮支
lateral cutaneous branch of
subcostal nerve

髂腹下神经外侧皮支
lateral cutaneous branch of
iliohypogastric nerve

臀中皮神经
middle clunial nerve

臀下皮神经
inferior clunial nerve

股外侧皮神经
lateral femoral cutaneous
nerve

股后皮神经
posterior femoral
cutaneous nerve

腓肠内侧皮神经
medial sural cutaneous
nerve

腓肠外侧皮神经
lateral sural cutaneous nerve

隐神经
saphenous nerve

腓神经交通支
communicating branch
of peroneal nerve

腓肠神经
sural nerve

腓浅神经
superficial peroneal nerve

足背外侧皮神经
lateral dorsal cutaneous
nerve of foot

图 402　下肢皮神经
Cutaneous nerves of lower limb

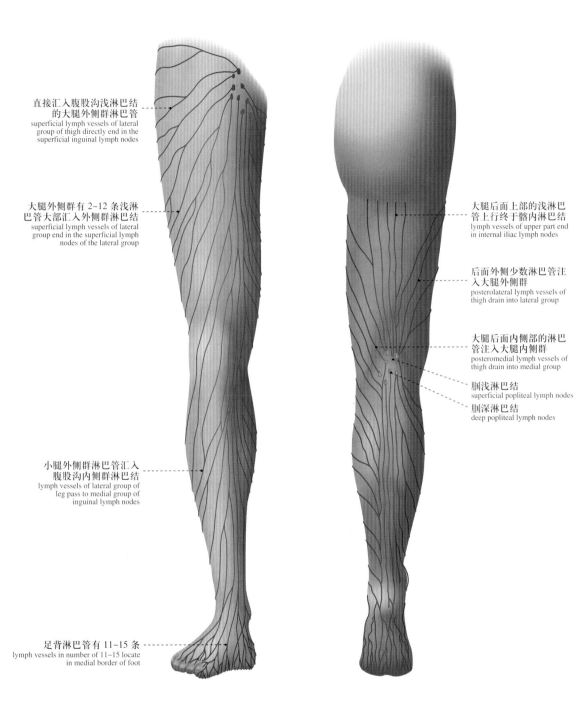

直接汇入腹股沟浅淋巴结
的大腿外侧群淋巴管
superficial lymph vessels of lateral
group of thigh directly end in the
superficial inguinal lymph nodes

大腿外侧群有 2~12 条浅淋
巴管大部汇入外侧群淋巴结
superficial lymph vessels of lateral
group end in the superficial lymph
nodes of the lateral group

小腿外侧群淋巴管汇入
腹股沟内侧群淋巴结
lymph vessels of lateral group of
leg pass to medial group of
inguinal lymph nodes

足背淋巴管有 11~15 条
lymph vessels in number of 11~15 locate
in medial border of foot

大腿后面上部的浅淋巴
管上行终于髂内淋巴结
lymph vessels of upper part end
in internal iliac lymph nodes

后面外侧少数淋巴管注
入大腿外侧群
posterolateral lymph vessels of
thigh drain into lateral group

大腿后面内侧部的淋巴
管注入大腿内侧群
posteromedial lymph vessels of
thigh drain into medial group

腘浅淋巴结
superficial popliteal lymph nodes

腘深淋巴结
deep popliteal lymph nodes

图 403　下肢的淋巴（前面观）
Lymphs of the lower limb (anterior aspect)

图 404　下肢的淋巴（后面观）
Lymphs of the lower limb (posterior aspect)

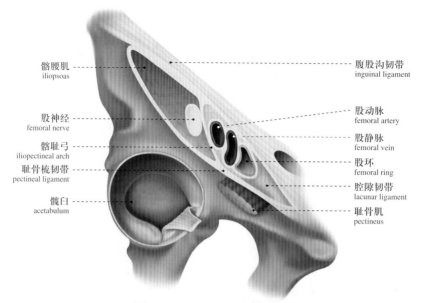

髂腰肌
iliopsoas

股神经
femoral nerve

髂耻弓
iliopectineal arch

耻骨梳韧带
pectineal ligament

髋臼
acetabulum

腹股沟韧带
inguinal ligament

股动脉
femoral artery

股静脉
femoral vein

股环
femoral ring

腔隙韧带
lacunar ligament

耻骨肌
pectineus

图 405　肌腔隙和血管腔隙

Muscular lacuna and vascular lacuna

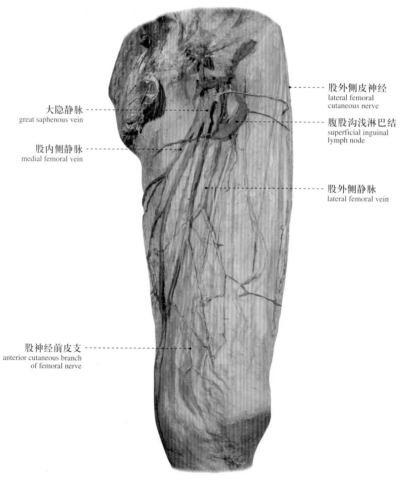

大隐静脉
great saphenous vein

股内侧静脉
medial femoral vein

股神经前皮支
anterior cutaneous branch
of femoral nerve

股外侧皮神经
lateral femoral
cutaneous nerve

腹股沟浅淋巴结
superficial inguinal
lymph node

股外侧静脉
lateral femoral vein

图 406　股前区局部解剖 1

Topography of the anterior femoral region 1

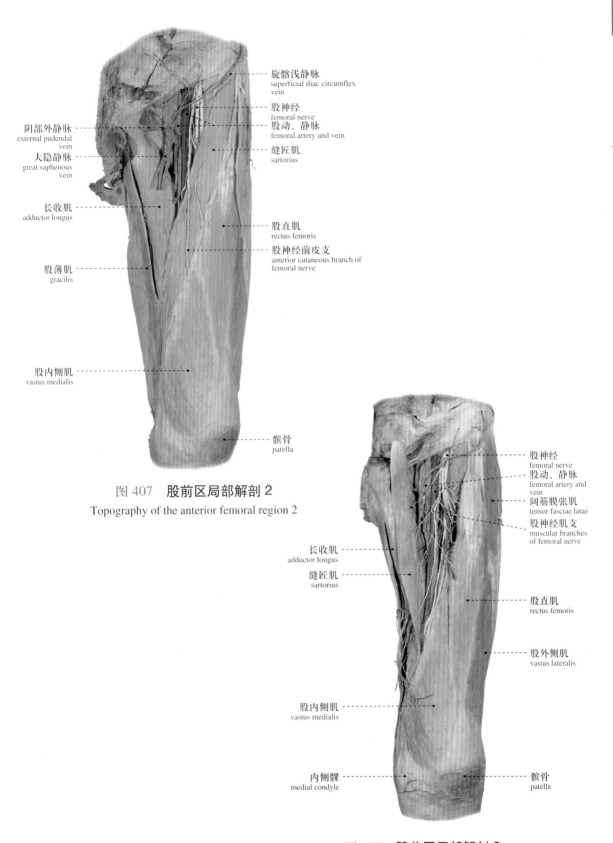

旋髂浅静脉
superficial iliac circumflex vein

股神经
femoral nerve

股动、静脉
femoral artery and vein

缝匠肌
sartorius

阴部外静脉
external pudendal vein

大隐静脉
great saphenous vein

长收肌
adductor longus

股直肌
rectus femoris

股神经前皮支
anterior cutaneous branch of femoral nerve

股薄肌
gracilis

股内侧肌
vastus medialis

髌骨
patella

图 407　股前区局部解剖 2
Topography of the anterior femoral region 2

股神经
femoral nerve

股动、静脉
femoral artery and vein

阔筋膜张肌
tensor fasciae latae

股神经肌支
muscular branches of femoral nerve

长收肌
adductor longus

缝匠肌
sartorius

股直肌
rectus femoris

股外侧肌
vastus lateralis

股内侧肌
vastus medialis

内侧髁
medial condyle

髌骨
patella

图 408　股前区局部解剖 3
Topography of the anterior femoral region 3

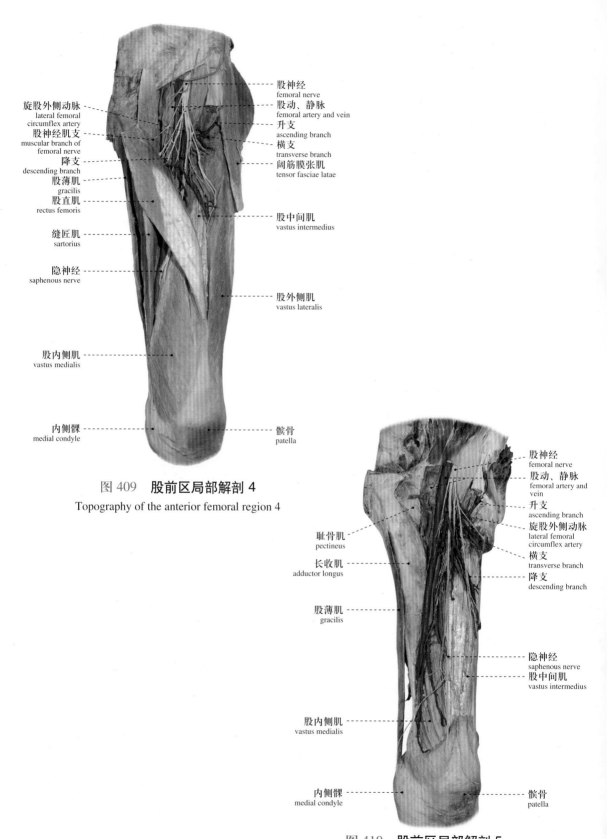

旋股外侧动脉
lateral femoral
circumflex artery

股神经肌支
muscular branch of
femoral nerve

降支
descending branch

股薄肌
gracilis

股直肌
rectus femoris

缝匠肌
sartorius

隐神经
saphenous nerve

股内侧肌
vastus medialis

内侧髁
medial condyle

股神经
femoral nerve

股动、静脉
femoral artery and vein

升支
ascending branch

横支
transverse branch

阔筋膜张肌
tensor fasciae latae

股中间肌
vastus intermedius

股外侧肌
vastus lateralis

髌骨
patella

图 409　股前区局部解剖 4
Topography of the anterior femoral region 4

耻骨肌
pectineus

长收肌
adductor longus

股薄肌
gracilis

股内侧肌
vastus medialis

内侧髁
medial condyle

股神经
femoral nerve

股动、静脉
femoral artery and
vein

升支
ascending branch

旋股外侧动脉
lateral femoral
circumflex artery

横支
transverse branch

降支
descending branch

隐神经
saphenous nerve

股中间肌
vastus intermedius

髌骨
patella

图 410　股前区局部解剖 5
Topography of the anterior femoral region 5

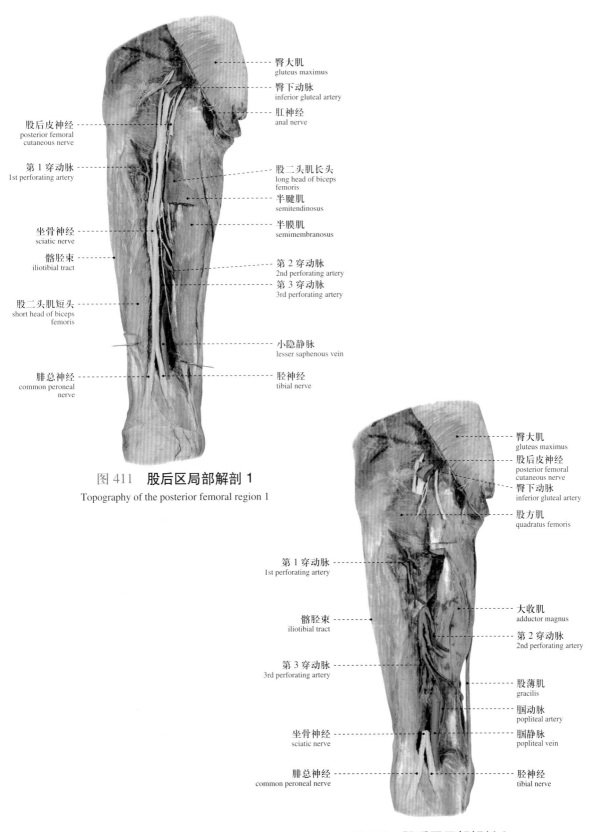

臀大肌
gluteus maximus

臀下动脉
inferior gluteal artery

肛神经
anal nerve

股后皮神经
posterior femoral
cutaneous nerve

第 1 穿动脉
1st perforating artery

股二头肌长头
long head of biceps
femoris

半腱肌
semitendinosus

半膜肌
semimembranosus

坐骨神经
sciatic nerve

髂胫束
iliotibial tract

第 2 穿动脉
2nd perforating artery

第 3 穿动脉
3rd perforating artery

股二头肌短头
short head of biceps
femoris

小隐静脉
lesser saphenous vein

腓总神经
common peroneal
nerve

胫神经
tibial nerve

图 411 股后区局部解剖 1
Topography of the posterior femoral region 1

臀大肌
gluteus maximus

股后皮神经
posterior femoral
cutaneous nerve

臀下动脉
inferior gluteal artery

股方肌
quadratus femoris

第 1 穿动脉
1st perforating artery

髂胫束
iliotibial tract

大收肌
adductor magnus

第 2 穿动脉
2nd perforating artery

第 3 穿动脉
3rd perforating artery

股薄肌
gracilis

腘动脉
popliteal artery

坐骨神经
sciatic nerve

腘静脉
popliteal vein

腓总神经
common peroneal nerve

胫神经
tibial nerve

图 412 股后区局部解剖 2
Topography of the posterior femoral region 2

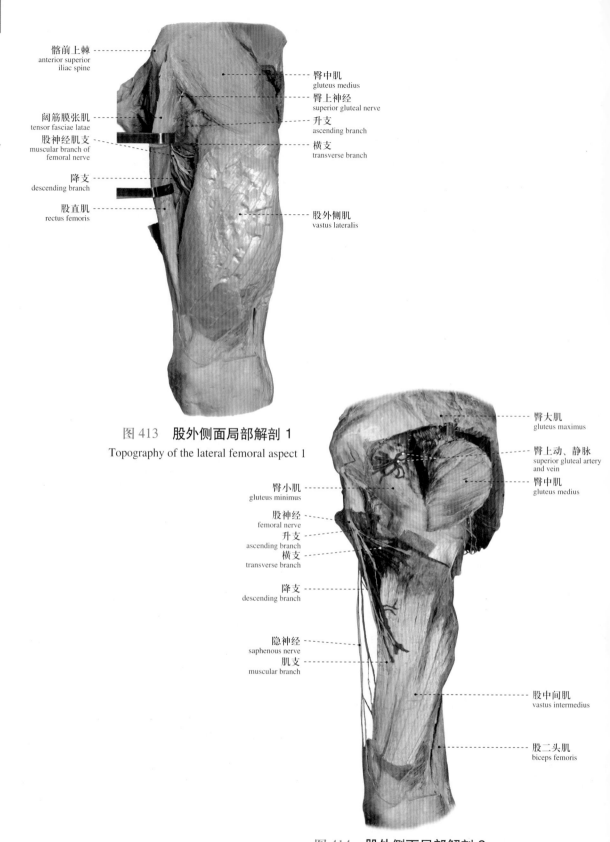

髂前上棘
anterior superior
iliac spine

阔筋膜张肌
tensor fasciae latae

股神经肌支
muscular branch of
femoral nerve

降支
descending branch

股直肌
rectus femoris

臀中肌
gluteus medius

臀上神经
superior gluteal nerve

升支
ascending branch

横支
transverse branch

股外侧肌
vastus lateralis

图 413　股外侧面局部解剖 1
Topography of the lateral femoral aspect 1

臀小肌
gluteus minimus

股神经
femoral nerve

升支
ascending branch

横支
transverse branch

降支
descending branch

隐神经
saphenous nerve

肌支
muscular branch

臀大肌
gluteus maximus

臀上动、静脉
superior gluteal artery
and vein

臀中肌
gluteus medius

股中间肌
vastus intermedius

股二头肌
biceps femoris

图 414　股外侧面局部解剖 2
Topography of the lateral femoral aspect 2

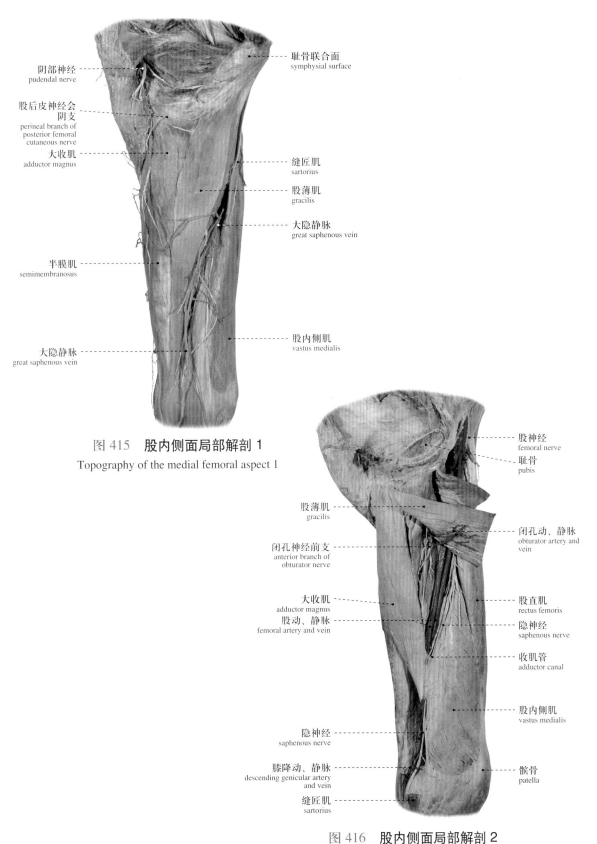

阴部神经
pudendal nerve

股后皮神经会阴支
perineal branch of posterior femoral cutaneous nerve

大收肌
adductor magnus

半膜肌
semimembranosus

大隐静脉
great saphenous vein

耻骨联合面
symphysial surface

缝匠肌
sartorius

股薄肌
gracilis

大隐静脉
great saphenous vein

股内侧肌
vastus medialis

图 415　股内侧面局部解剖 1
Topography of the medial femoral aspect 1

股薄肌
gracilis

闭孔神经前支
anterior branch of obturator nerve

大收肌
adductor magnus

股动、静脉
femoral artery and vein

隐神经
saphenous nerve

膝降动、静脉
descending genicular artery and vein

缝匠肌
sartorius

股神经
femoral nerve

耻骨
pubis

闭孔动、静脉
obturator artery and vein

股直肌
rectus femoris

隐神经
saphenous nerve

收肌管
adductor canal

股内侧肌
vastus medialis

髌骨
patella

图 416　股内侧面局部解剖 2
Topography of the medial femoral aspect 2

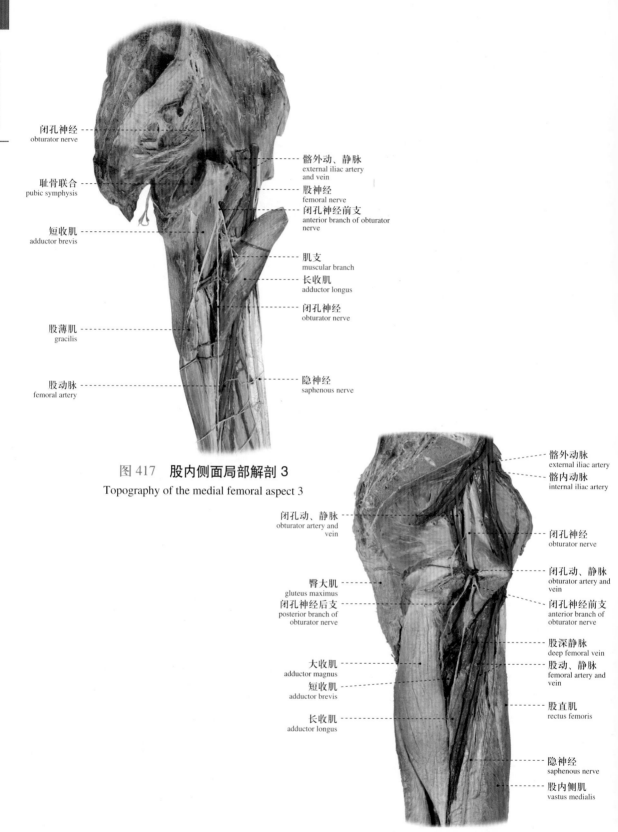

闭孔神经
obturator nerve

耻骨联合
pubic symphysis

短收肌
adductor brevis

股薄肌
gracilis

股动脉
femoral artery

髂外动、静脉
external iliac artery
and vein

股神经
femoral nerve

闭孔神经前支
anterior branch of obturator
nerve

肌支
muscular branch

长收肌
adductor longus

闭孔神经
obturator nerve

隐神经
saphenous nerve

图 417　股内侧面局部解剖 3

Topography of the medial femoral aspect 3

闭孔动、静脉
obturator artery and
vein

臀大肌
gluteus maximus

闭孔神经后支
posterior branch of
obturator nerve

大收肌
adductor magnus

短收肌
adductor brevis

长收肌
adductor longus

髂外动脉
external iliac artery

髂内动脉
internal iliac artery

闭孔神经
obturator nerve

闭孔动、静脉
obturator artery and
vein

闭孔神经前支
anterior branch of
obturator nerve

股深静脉
deep femoral vein

股动、静脉
femoral artery and
vein

股直肌
rectus femoris

隐神经
saphenous nerve

股内侧肌
vastus medialis

图 418　股内侧面局部解剖 4

Topography of the medial femoral aspect 4

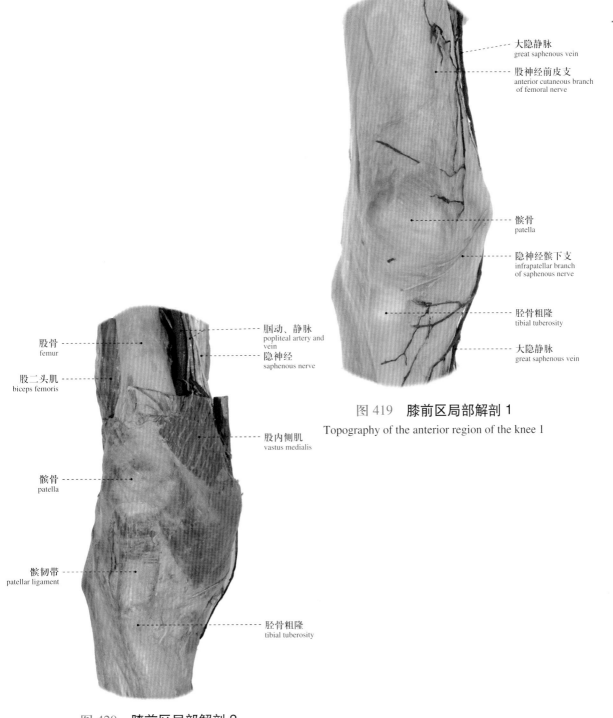

第三节

膝 部

大隐静脉
great saphenous vein

股神经前皮支
anterior cutaneous branch
of femoral nerve

髌骨
patella

隐神经髌下支
infrapatellar branch
of saphenous nerve

胫骨粗隆
tibial tuberosity

大隐静脉
great saphenous vein

图 419　膝前区局部解剖 1
Topography of the anterior region of the knee 1

股骨
femur

股二头肌
biceps femoris

腘动、静脉
popliteal artery and
vein

隐神经
saphenous nerve

股内侧肌
vastus medialis

髌骨
patella

髌韧带
patellar ligament

胫骨粗隆
tibial tuberosity

图 420　膝前区局部解剖 2
Topography of the anterior region of the knee 2

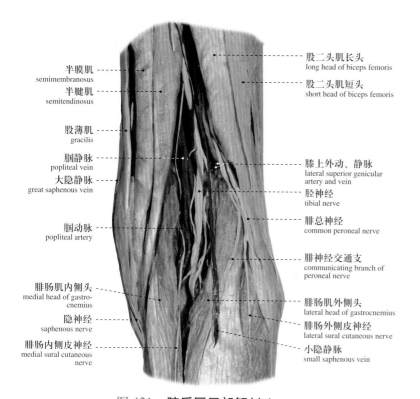

半膜肌
semimembranosus

半腱肌
semitendinosus

股薄肌
gracilis

腘静脉
popliteal vein

大隐静脉
great saphenous vein

腘动脉
popliteal artery

腓肠肌内侧头
medial head of gastro-
cnemius

隐神经
saphenous nerve

腓肠内侧皮神经
medial sural cutaneous
nerve

股二头肌长头
long head of biceps femoris

股二头肌短头
short head of biceps femoris

膝上外动、静脉
lateral superior genicular
artery and vein

胫神经
tibial nerve

腓总神经
common peroneal nerve

腓神经交通支
communicating branch of
peroneal nerve

腓肠肌外侧头
lateral head of gastrocnemius

腓肠外侧皮神经
lateral sural cutaneous nerve

小隐静脉
small saphenous vein

图 421　膝后区局部解剖 1
Topography of the anterior region of the knee 1

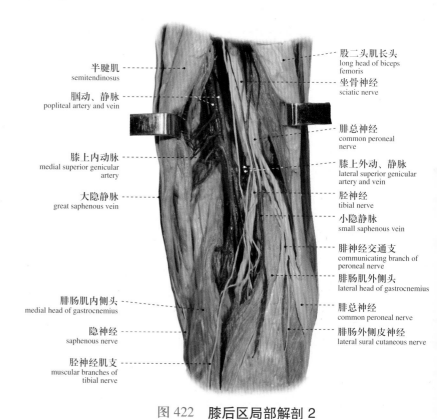

半腱肌
semitendinosus

腘动、静脉
popliteal artery and vein

膝上内动脉
medial superior genicular
artery

大隐静脉
great saphenous vein

腓肠肌内侧头
medial head of gastrocnemius

隐神经
saphenous nerve

胫神经肌支
muscular branches of
tibial nerve

股二头肌长头
long head of biceps
femoris

坐骨神经
sciatic nerve

腓总神经
common peroneal
nerve

膝上外动、静脉
lateral superior genicular
artery and vein

胫神经
tibial nerve

小隐静脉
small saphenous vein

腓神经交通支
communicating branch of
peroneal nerve

腓肠肌外侧头
lateral head of gastrocnemius

腓总神经
common peroneal nerve

腓肠外侧皮神经
lateral sural cutaneous nerve

图 422　膝后区局部解剖 2
Topography of the anterior region of the knee 2

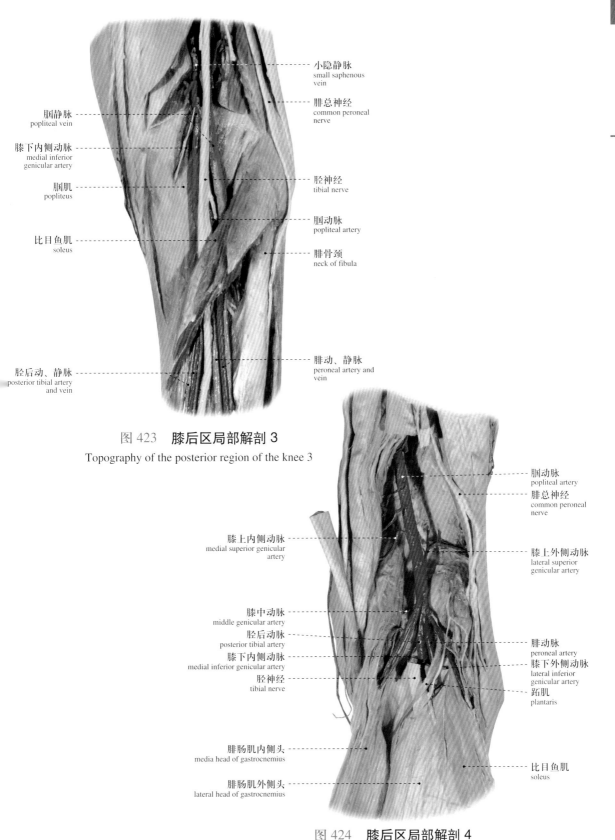

小隐静脉
small saphenous vein

腓总神经
common peroneal nerve

腘静脉
popliteal vein

膝下内侧动脉
medial inferior genicular artery

腘肌
popliteus

比目鱼肌
soleus

胫神经
tibial nerve

腘动脉
popliteal artery

腓骨颈
neck of fibula

胫后动、静脉
posterior tibial artery and vein

腓动、静脉
peroneal artery and vein

图 423　膝后区局部解剖 3
Topography of the posterior region of the knee 3

腘动脉
popliteal artery

腓总神经
common peroneal nerve

膝上内侧动脉
medial superior genicular artery

膝上外侧动脉
lateral superior genicular artery

膝中动脉
middle genicular artery

胫后动脉
posterior tibial artery

膝下内侧动脉
medial inferior genicular artery

胫神经
tibial nerve

腓动脉
peroneal artery

膝下外侧动脉
lateral inferior genicular artery

跖肌
plantaris

腓肠肌内侧头
media head of gastrocnemius

腓肠肌外侧头
lateral head of gastrocnemius

比目鱼肌
soleus

图 424　膝后区局部解剖 4
Topography of the posterior region of the knee 4

241

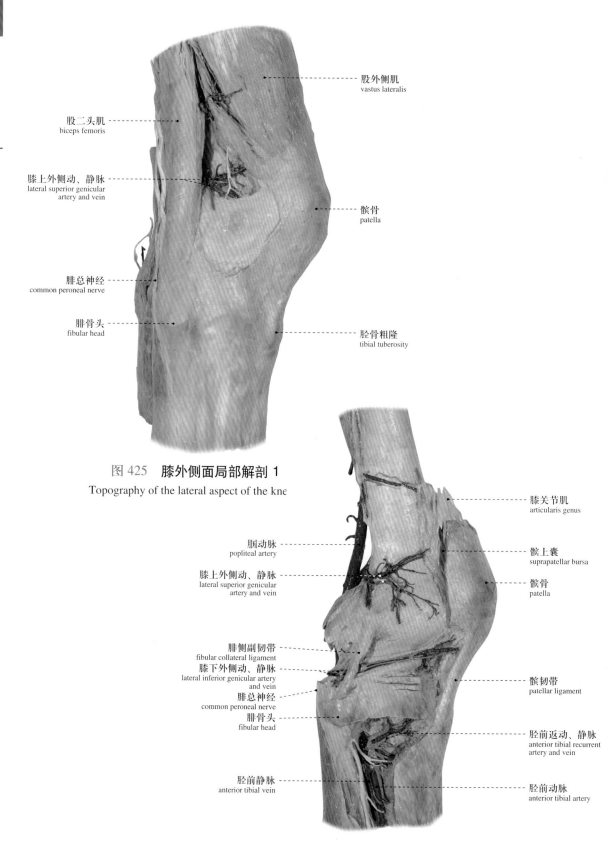

股二头肌
biceps femoris

股外侧肌
vastus lateralis

膝上外侧动、静脉
lateral superior genicular
artery and vein

髌骨
patella

腓总神经
common peroneal nerve

腓骨头
fibular head

胫骨粗隆
tibial tuberosity

图 425 膝外侧面局部解剖 1
Topography of the lateral aspect of the kne

膝关节肌
articularis genus

腘动脉
popliteal artery

髌上囊
suprapatellar bursa

膝上外侧动、静脉
lateral superior genicular
artery and vein

髌骨
patella

腓侧副韧带
fibular collateral ligament

膝下外侧动、静脉
lateral inferior genicular artery
and vein

腓总神经
common peroneal nerve

髌韧带
patellar ligament

腓骨头
fibular head

胫前返动、静脉
anterior tibial recurrent
artery and vein

胫前静脉
anterior tibial vein

胫前动脉
anterior tibial artery

图 426 膝外侧面局部解剖 2
Topography of the lateral aspect of the knee 2

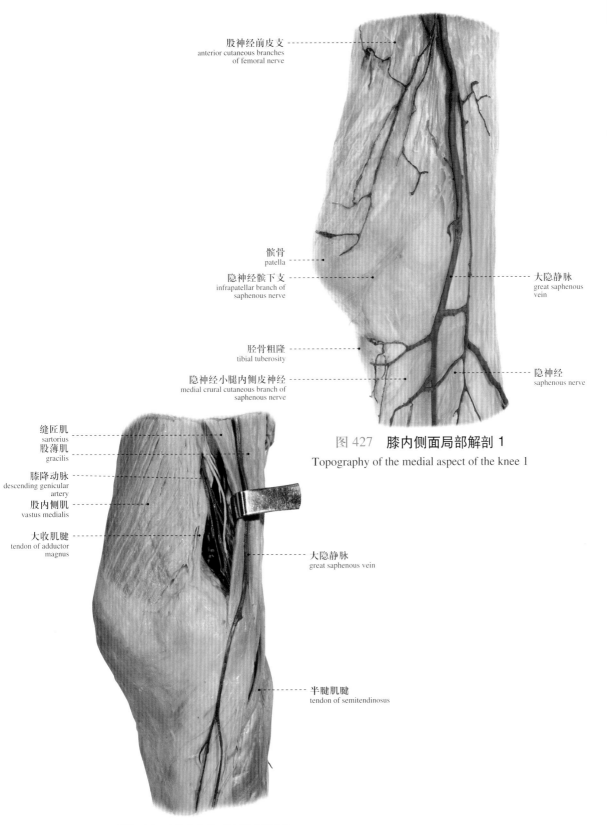

股神经前皮支
anterior cutaneous branches
of femoral nerve

髌骨
patella

隐神经髌下支
infrapatellar branch of
saphenous nerve

大隐静脉
great saphenous
vein

胫骨粗隆
tibial tuberosity

隐神经小腿内侧皮神经
medial crural cutaneous branch of
saphenous nerve

隐神经
saphenous nerve

图 427　膝内侧面局部解剖 1
Topography of the medial aspect of the knee 1

缝匠肌
sartorius

股薄肌
gracilis

膝降动脉
descending genicular
artery

股内侧肌
vastus medialis

大收肌腱
tendon of adductor
magnus

大隐静脉
great saphenous vein

半腱肌腱
tendon of semitendinosus

图 428　膝内侧面局部解剖 2
Topography of the medial aspect of the knee 2

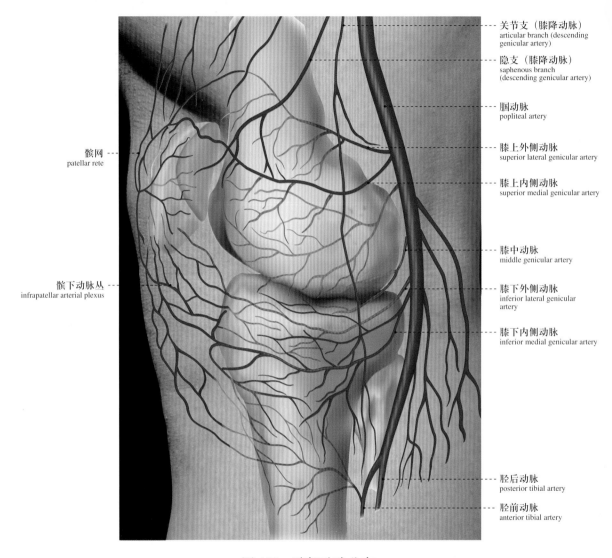

关节支（膝降动脉）
articular branch (descending
genicular artery)

隐支（膝降动脉）
saphenous branch
(descending genicular artery)

腘动脉
popliteal artery

膝上外侧动脉
superior lateral genicular artery

膝上内侧动脉
superior medial genicular artery

膝中动脉
middle genicular artery

膝下外侧动脉
inferior lateral genicular
artery

膝下内侧动脉
inferior medial genicular artery

胫后动脉
posterior tibial artery

胫前动脉
anterior tibial artery

髌网
patellar rete

髌下动脉丛
infrapatellar arterial plexus

图 429　膝部动脉分布
Arterial distribution of the knee region

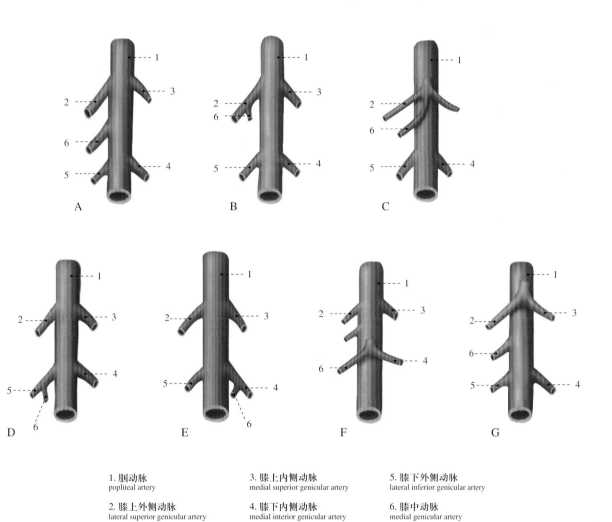

1. 腘动脉
   popliteal artery

3. 膝上内侧动脉
   medial superior genicular artery

5. 膝下外侧动脉
   lateral inferior genicular artery

2. 膝上外侧动脉
   lateral superior genicular artery

4. 膝下内侧动脉
   medial interior genicular artery

6. 膝中动脉
   medial genicular artery

图 430　腘动脉分支类型
Types of branches of the popliteal artery

A. 膝中动脉起自腘动脉；B. 膝中动脉起自膝上外侧动脉；C. 膝上内、外侧动脉共干，并发出膝中动脉；D. 膝中动脉起自膝下外侧动脉；E. 膝中动脉起自膝下内侧动脉；F. 膝下内、外侧动脉共干，膝中动脉起自腘动脉；G. 膝上内、外侧动脉共干，膝中动脉起自腘动脉

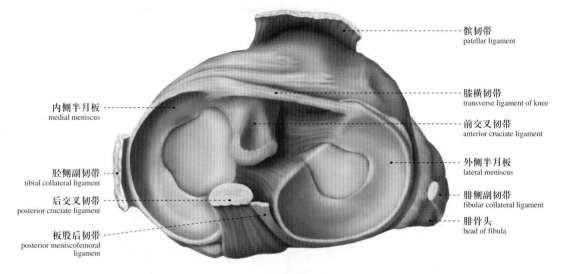

内侧半月板
medial meniscus

髌韧带
patellar ligament

膝横韧带
transverse ligament of knee

前交叉韧带
anterior cruciate ligament

外侧半月板
lateral meniscus

腓侧副韧带
fibular collateral ligament

腓骨头
head of fibula

胫侧副韧带
tibial collateral ligament

后交叉韧带
posterior cruciate ligament

板股后韧带
posterior meniscofemoral ligament

图 431　膝关节半月板
Meniscus of the knee joint

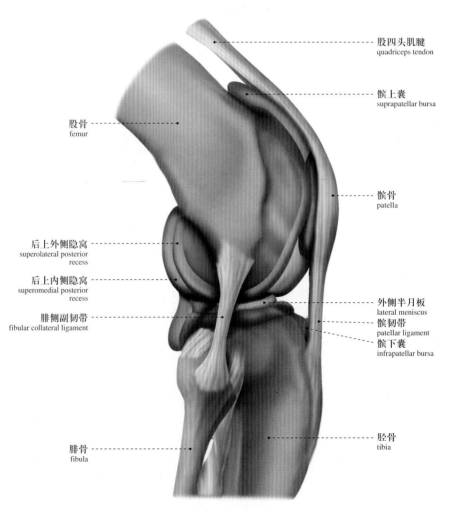

股四头肌腱
quadriceps tendon

髌上囊
suprapatellar bursa

股骨
femur

髌骨
patella

后上外侧隐窝
superolateral posterior recess

后上内侧隐窝
superomedial posterior recess

腓侧副韧带
fibular collateral ligament

外侧半月板
lateral meniscus

髌韧带
patellar ligament

髌下囊
infrapatellar bursa

腓骨
fibula

胫骨
tibia

图 432　膝关节腔
Cavity of the knee joint

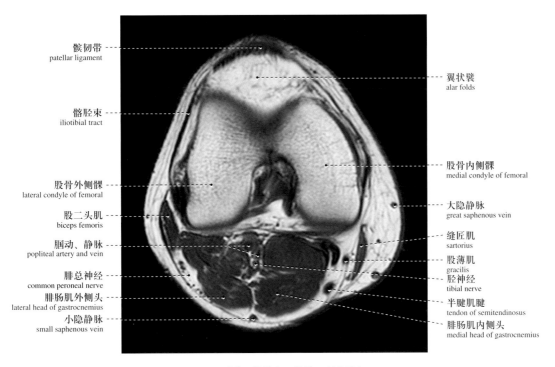

髌韧带
patellar ligament

翼状襞
alar folds

髂胫束
iliotibial tract

股骨内侧髁
medial condyle of femoral

股骨外侧髁
lateral condyle of femoral

大隐静脉
great saphenous vein

股二头肌
biceps femoris

缝匠肌
sartorius

腘动、静脉
popliteal artery and vein

股薄肌
gracilis

腓总神经
common peroneal nerve

胫神经
tibial nerve

腓肠肌外侧头
lateral head of gastrocnemius

半腱肌腱
tendon of semitendinosus

小隐静脉
small saphenous vein

腓肠肌内侧头
medial head of gastrocnemius

图 433　膝部磁共振成像（轴位）
MRI of the knee (axial view)

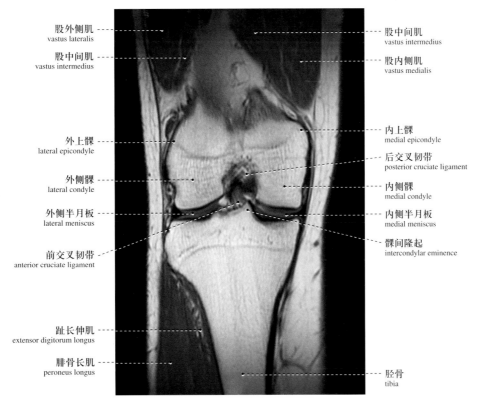

股外侧肌
vastus lateralis

股中间肌
vastus intermedius

股中间肌
vastus intermedius

股内侧肌
vastus medialis

外上髁
lateral epicondyle

内上髁
medial epicondyle

外侧髁
lateral condyle

后交叉韧带
posterior cruciate ligament

外侧半月板
lateral meniscus

内侧髁
medial condyle

前交叉韧带
anterior cruciate ligament

内侧半月板
medial meniscus

髁间隆起
intercondylar eminence

趾长伸肌
extensor digitorum longus

腓骨长肌
peroneus longus

胫骨
tibia

图 434　膝部磁共振成像（冠状位）
MRI of the knee (coronal view)

第四节

小腿部

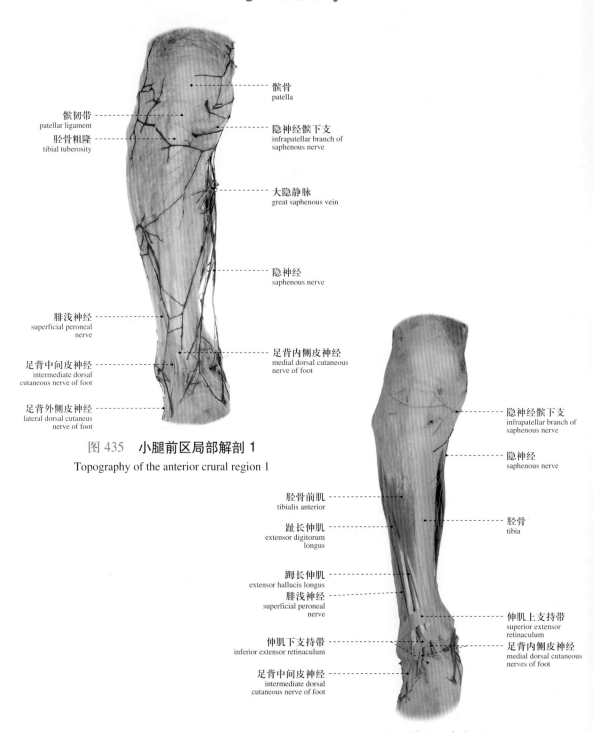

髌骨
patella

髌韧带
patellar ligament

胫骨粗隆
tibial tuberosity

隐神经髌下支
infrapatellar branch of
saphenous nerve

大隐静脉
great saphenous vein

隐神经
saphenous nerve

腓浅神经
superficial peroneal
nerve

足背中间皮神经
intermediate dorsal
cutaneous nerve of foot

足背外侧皮神经
lateral dorsal cutaneus
nerve of foot

足背内侧皮神经
medial dorsal cutaneous
nerve of foot

图 435　小腿前区局部解剖 1
Topography of the anterior crural region 1

隐神经髌下支
infrapatellar branch of
saphenous nerve

隐神经
saphenous nerve

胫骨前肌
tibialis anterior

胫骨
tibia

趾长伸肌
extensor digitorum
longus

蹬长伸肌
extensor hallucis longus

腓浅神经
superficial peroneal
nerve

伸肌上支持带
superior extensor
retinaculum

足背内侧皮神经
medial dorsal cutaneous
nerves of foot

伸肌下支持带
inferior extensor retinaculum

足背中间皮神经
intermediate dorsal
cutaneous nerve of foot

图 436　小腿前区局部解剖 2
Topography of the anterior crural region 2

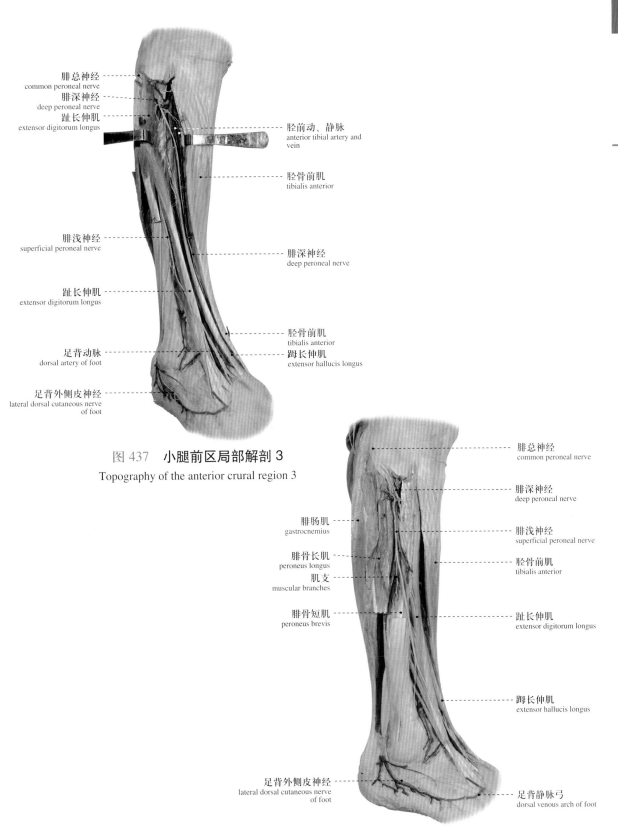

腓总神经
common peroneal nerve

腓深神经
deep peroneal nerve

趾长伸肌
extensor digitorum longus

胫前动、静脉
anterior tibial artery and
vein

胫骨前肌
tibialis anterior

腓浅神经
superficial peroneal nerve

腓深神经
deep peroneal nerve

趾长伸肌
extensor digitorum longus

胫骨前肌
tibialis anterior

足背动脉
dorsal artery of foot

踇长伸肌
extensor hallucis longus

足背外侧皮神经
lateral dorsal cutaneous nerve
of foot

图 437　小腿前区局部解剖 3
Topography of the anterior crural region 3

腓肠肌
gastrocnemius

腓骨长肌
peroneus longus

肌支
muscular branches

腓骨短肌
peroneus brevis

腓总神经
common peroneal nerve

腓深神经
deep peroneal nerve

腓浅神经
superficial peroneal nerve

胫骨前肌
tibialis anterior

趾长伸肌
extensor digitorum longus

踇长伸肌
extensor hallucis longus

足背外侧皮神经
lateral dorsal cutaneous nerve
of foot

足背静脉弓
dorsal venous arch of foot

图 438　小腿前区局部解剖 4
Topography of the anterior crural region 4

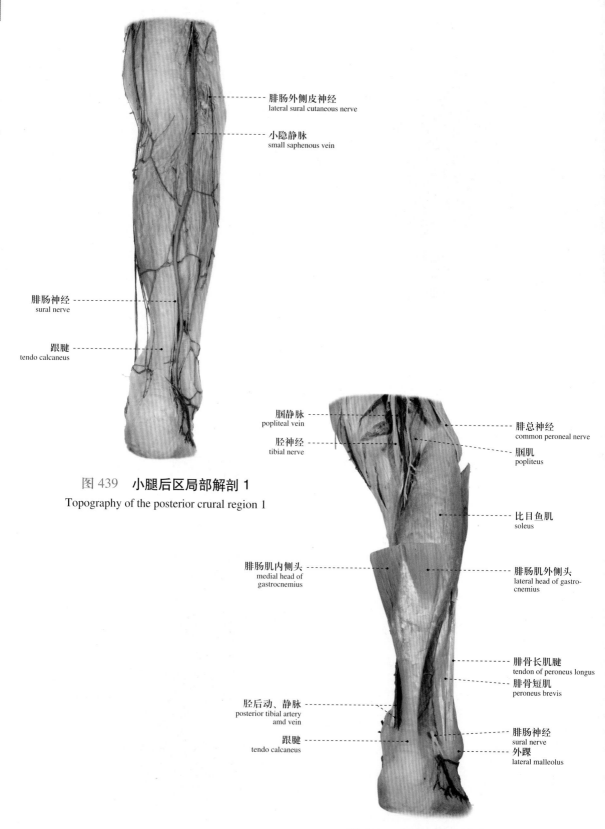

腓肠外侧皮神经
lateral sural cutaneous nerve

小隐静脉
small saphenous vein

腓肠神经
sural nerve

跟腱
tendo calcaneus

图 439　小腿后区局部解剖 1
Topography of the posterior crural region 1

腘静脉
popliteal vein

腓总神经
common peroneal nerve

胫神经
tibial nerve

腘肌
popliteus

比目鱼肌
soleus

腓肠肌内侧头
medial head of
gastrocnemius

腓肠肌外侧头
lateral head of gastro-
cnemius

腓骨长肌腱
tendon of peroneus longus

腓骨短肌
peroneus brevis

胫后动、静脉
posterior tibial artery
amd vein

跟腱
tendo calcaneus

腓肠神经
sural nerve

外踝
lateral malleolus

图 440　小腿后区局部解剖 2
Topography of the posterior crural region 2

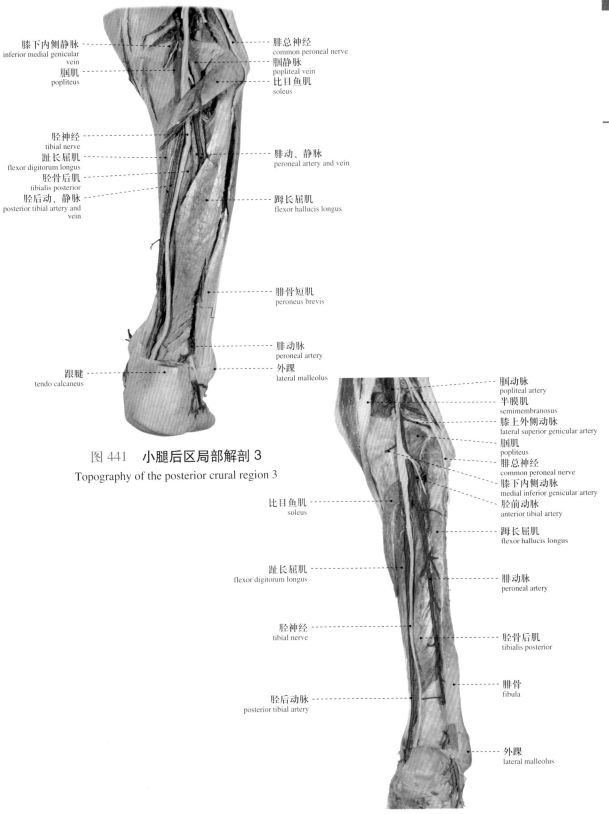

膝下内侧静脉
inferior medial genicular vein

腘肌
popliteus

胫神经
tibial nerve

趾长屈肌
flexor digitorum longus

胫骨后肌
tibialis posterior

胫后动、静脉
posterior tibial artery and vein

跟腱
tendo calcaneus

腓总神经
common peroneal nerve

腘静脉
popliteal vein

比目鱼肌
soleus

腓动、静脉
peroneal artery and vein

姆长屈肌
flexor hallucis longus

腓骨短肌
peroneus brevis

腓动脉
peroneal artery

外踝
lateral malleolus

图 441　小腿后区局部解剖 3
Topography of the posterior crural region 3

比目鱼肌
soleus

趾长屈肌
flexor digitorum longus

胫神经
tibial nerve

胫后动脉
posterior tibial artery

腘动脉
popliteal artery

半膜肌
semimembranosus

膝上外侧动脉
lateral superior genicular artery

腘肌
popliteus

腓总神经
common peroneal nerve

膝下内侧动脉
medial inferior genicular artery

胫前动脉
anterior tibial artery

姆长屈肌
flexor hallucis longus

腓动脉
peroneal artery

胫骨后肌
tibialis posterior

腓骨
fibula

外踝
lateral malleolus

图 442　小腿后区局部解剖 4
Topography of the posterior crural region 4

踝与足部

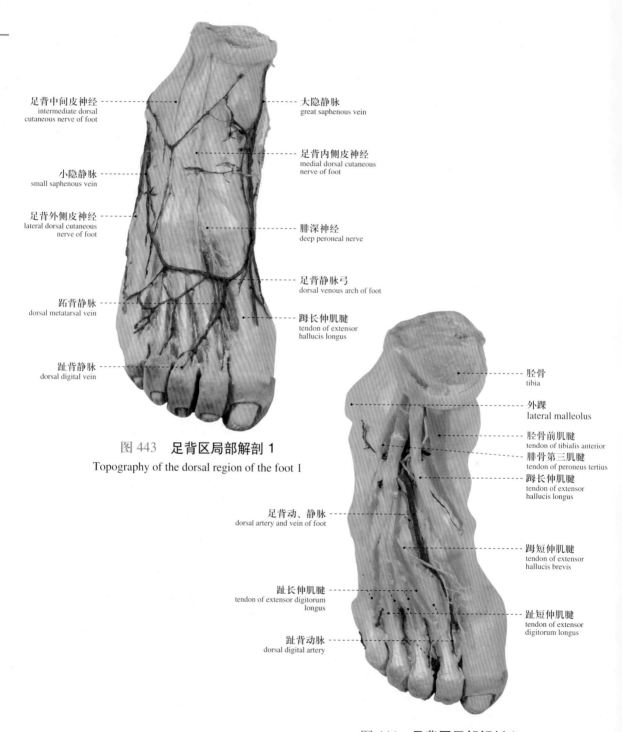

足背中间皮神经
intermediate dorsal
cutaneous nerve of foot

大隐静脉
great saphenous vein

足背内侧皮神经
medial dorsal cutaneous
nerve of foot

小隐静脉
small saphenous vein

足背外侧皮神经
lateral dorsal cutaneous
nerve of foot

腓深神经
deep peroneal nerve

足背静脉弓
dorsal venous arch of foot

跖背静脉
dorsal metatarsal vein

跨长伸肌腱
tendon of extensor
hallucis longus

趾背静脉
dorsal digital vein

图 443　足背区局部解剖 1
Topography of the dorsal region of the foot 1

胫骨
tibia

外踝
lateral malleolus

胫骨前肌腱
tendon of tibialis anterior

腓骨第三肌腱
tendon of peroneus tertius

跨长伸肌腱
tendon of extensor
hallucis longus

足背动、静脉
dorsal artery and vein of foot

跨短伸肌腱
tendon of extensor
hallucis brevis

趾长伸肌腱
tendon of extensor digitorum
longus

趾短伸肌腱
tendon of extensor
digitorum longus

趾背动脉
dorsal digital artery

图 444　足背区局部解剖 2
Topography of the dorsal region of the foot 2

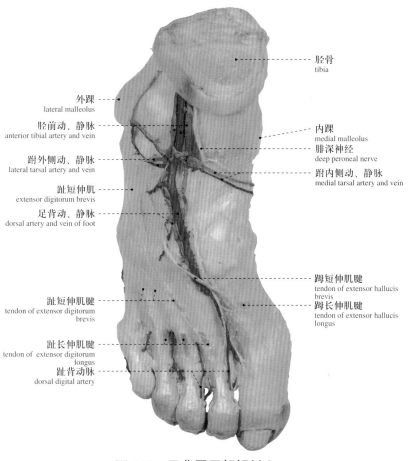

外踝
lateral malleolus

胫前动、静脉
anterior tibial artery and vein

跗外侧动、静脉
lateral tarsal artery and vein

趾短伸肌
extensor digitorum brevis

足背动、静脉
dorsal artery and vein of foot

趾短伸肌腱
tendon of extensor digitorum brevis

趾长伸肌腱
tendon of extensor digitorum longus

趾背动脉
dorsal digital artery

胫骨
tibia

内踝
medial malleolus

腓深神经
deep peroneal nerve

跗内侧动、静脉
medial tarsal artery and vein

跨短伸肌腱
tendon of extensor hallucis brevis

跨长伸肌腱
tendon of extensor hallucis longus

图 445　足背区局部解剖 3
Topography of the dorsal region of the foot 3

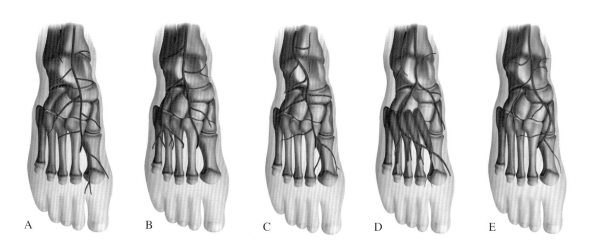

A　　　　B　　　　C　　　　D　　　　E

图 446　足背动脉类型
Types of the dorsalis pedis arteries
A. Ⅰ型；B. Ⅱ型；C. Ⅲ型；D. Ⅳ型；E. Ⅴ型

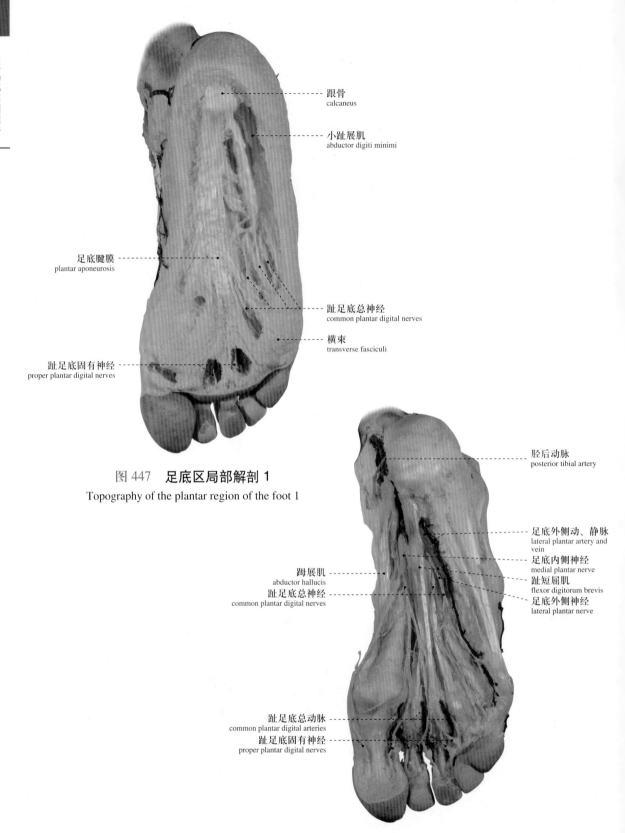

跟骨
calcaneus

小趾展肌
abductor digiti minimi

足底腱膜
plantar aponeurosis

趾足底总神经
common plantar digital nerves

横束
transverse fasciculi

趾足底固有神经
proper plantar digital nerves

图 447　足底区局部解剖 1
Topography of the plantar region of the foot 1

胫后动脉
posterior tibial artery

足底外侧动、静脉
lateral plantar artery and vein

足底内侧神经
medial plantar nerve

趾短屈肌
flexor digitorum brevis

足底外侧神经
lateral plantar nerve

鉧展肌
abductor hallucis

趾足底总神经
common plantar digital nerves

趾足底总动脉
common plantar digital arteries

趾足底固有神经
proper plantar digital nerves

图 448　足底区局部解剖 2
Topography of the plantar region of the foot 2

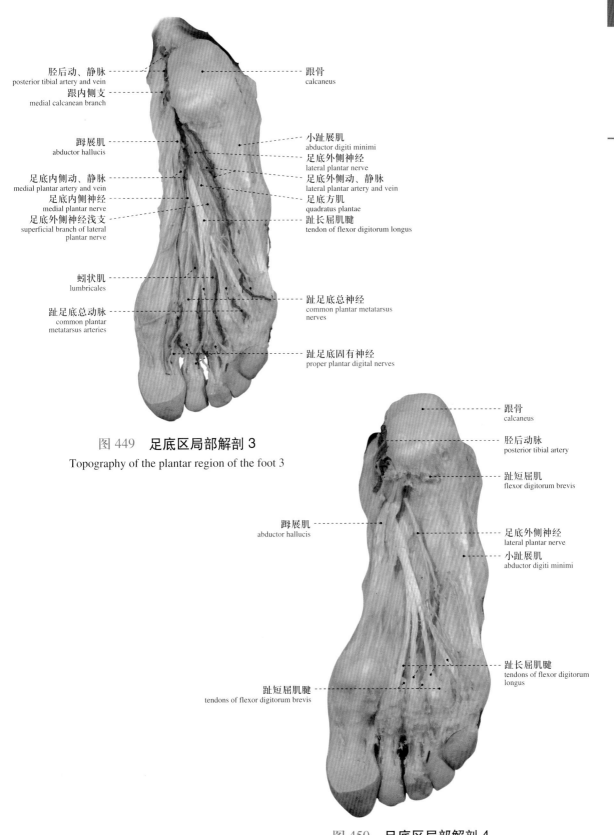

胫后动、静脉
posterior tibial artery and vein

跟内侧支
medial calcanean branch

跟骨
calcaneus

跗展肌
abductor hallucis

小趾展肌
abductor digiti minimi

足底外侧神经
lateral plantar nerve

足底内侧动、静脉
medial plantar artery and vein

足底内侧神经
medial plantar nerve

足底外侧神经浅支
superficial branch of lateral
plantar nerve

足底外侧动、静脉
lateral plantar artery and vein

足底方肌
quadratus plantae

趾长屈肌腱
tendon of flexor digitorum longus

蚓状肌
lumbricales

趾足底总动脉
common plantar
metatarsus arteries

趾足底总神经
common plantar metatarsus
nerves

趾足底固有神经
proper plantar digital nerves

图 449　足底区局部解剖 3
Topography of the plantar region of the foot 3

跗展肌
abductor hallucis

跟骨
calcaneus

胫后动脉
posterior tibial artery

趾短屈肌
flexor digitorum brevis

足底外侧神经
lateral plantar nerve

小趾展肌
abductor digiti minimi

趾长屈肌腱
tendons of flexor digitorum
longus

趾短屈肌腱
tendons of flexor digitorum brevis

图 450　足底区局部解剖 4
Topography of the plantar region of the foot 4

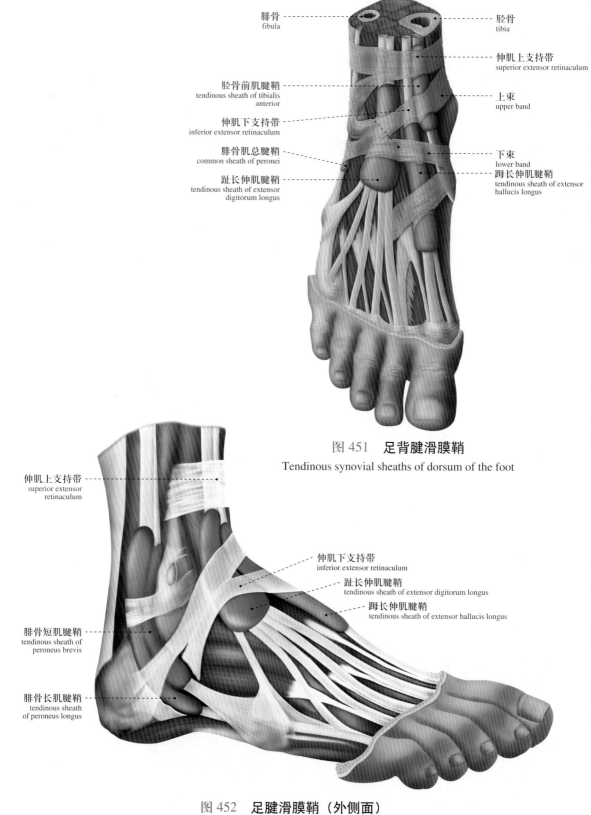

腓骨
fibula

胫骨
tibia

伸肌上支持带
superior extensor retinaculum

胫骨前肌腱鞘
tendinous sheath of tibialis
anterior

上束
upper band

伸肌下支持带
inferior extensor retinaculum

下束
lower band

腓骨肌总腱鞘
common sheath of peronei

踇长伸肌腱鞘
tendinous sheath of extensor
hallucis longus

趾长伸肌腱鞘
tendinous sheath of extensor
digitorum longus

图 451　足背腱滑膜鞘
Tendinous synovial sheaths of dorsum of the foot

伸肌上支持带
superior extensor
retinaculum

伸肌下支持带
inferior extensor retinaculum

趾长伸肌腱鞘
tendinous sheath of extensor digitorum longus

踇长伸肌腱鞘
tendinous sheath of extensor hallucis longus

腓骨短肌腱鞘
tendinous sheath of
peroneus brevis

腓骨长肌腱鞘
tendinous sheath
of peroneus longus

图 452　足腱滑膜鞘（外侧面）
Tendinous synovial sheaths of the foot (lateral aspect)

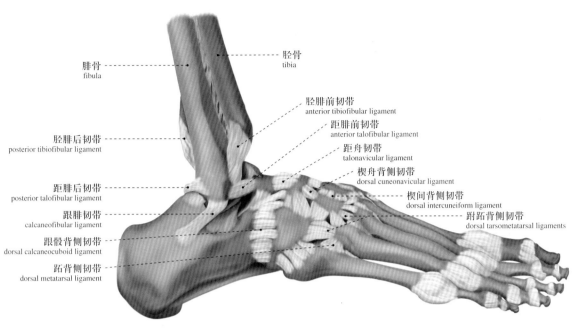

图 453　足的关节和韧带（外侧面）
Joints and ligaments of the foot (lateral aspect)

腓骨
fibula

胫骨
tibia

胫腓前韧带
anterior tibiofibular ligament

距腓前韧带
anterior talofibular ligament

距舟韧带
talonavicular ligament

楔舟背侧韧带
dorsal cuneonavicular ligament

楔间背侧韧带
dorsal intercuneiform ligament

跗跖背侧韧带
dorsal tarsometatarsal ligaments

胫腓后韧带
posterior tibiofibular ligament

距腓后韧带
posterior talofibular ligament

跟腓韧带
calcaneofibular ligament

跟骰背侧韧带
dorsal calcaneocuboid ligament

跖背侧韧带
dorsal metatarsal ligament

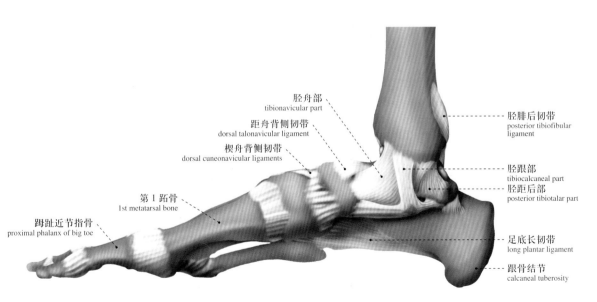

图 454　足的关节和韧带（内侧面）
Joints and ligaments of the foot (medial aspect)

胫舟部
tibionavicular part

距舟背侧韧带
dorsal talonavicular ligament

楔舟背侧韧带
dorsal cuneonavicular ligaments

第 1 跖骨
1st metatarsal bone

踇趾近节指骨
proximal phalanx of big toe

胫腓后韧带
posterior tibiofibular ligament

胫跟部
tibiocalcaneal part

胫距后部
posterior tibiotalar part

足底长韧带
long plantar ligament

跟骨结节
calcaneal tuberosity

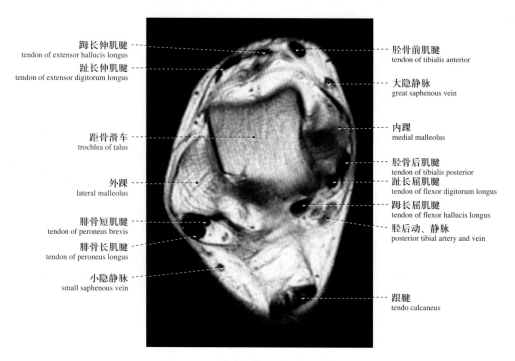

蹞长伸肌腱 tendon of extensor hallucis longus	胫骨前肌腱 tendon of tibialis anterior
趾长伸肌腱 tendon of extensor digitorum longus	大隐静脉 great saphenous vein
距骨滑车 trochlea of talus	内踝 medial malleolus
外踝 lateral malleolus	胫骨后肌腱 tendon of tibialis posterior
	趾长屈肌腱 tendon of flexor digitorum longus
腓骨短肌腱 tendon of peroneus brevis	蹞长屈肌腱 tendon of flexor hallucis longus
腓骨长肌腱 tendon of peroneus longus	胫后动、静脉 posterior tibial artery and vein
小隐静脉 small saphenous vein	跟腱 tendo calcaneus

图 455　踝部磁共振成像（轴位）
MRI of the ankle (axial view)

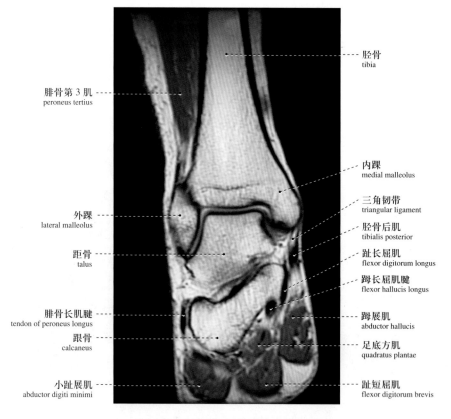

	胫骨 tibia
腓骨第 3 肌 peroneus tertius	
	内踝 medial malleolus
外踝 lateral malleolus	三角韧带 triangular ligament
	胫骨后肌 tibialis posterior
距骨 talus	趾长屈肌 flexor digitorum longus
	蹞长屈肌腱 flexor hallucis longus
腓骨长肌腱 tendon of peroneus longus	蹞展肌 abductor hallucis
跟骨 calcaneus	足底方肌 quadratus plantae
小趾展肌 abductor digiti minimi	趾短屈肌 flexor digitorum brevis

图 456　踝部磁共振成像（冠状位）
MRI of the ankle (coronal view)

参考书目

[1] Schuenke M, Schulte E, Schumacher U. THIEME Atlas of Anatomy, Neck and Internal Organs. Thieme Stuttgart.

[2] Schuenke M, Schulte E, Schumacher U. THIEME Atlas of Anatomy, General Anatomy and Musculoskeletal System. Thieme Stuttgart.

[3] Schuenke M, Schulte E, Schumacher U. THIEME Atlas of Anatomy, Head and Neuroanatomy. Thieme Stuttgart.

[4] Putz R, Sobotta PR. Atlas der Anatomie des Menschen. Band 2, 21st edition. Elsevier, Pte Ltd.

[5] Marieb EN, Hoehn K. Human Anatomy & Physiology. Benjamin Cummings.

[6] Standring S. GRAY'S Anatomy Susan Standring. Churchill Livingstone Elsevier.

[7] Netter FH. Atlas of Human Anatomy. SAUNDERS Elsevier.

[8] Bontrager KL, Lampignano JP. Radiographic Positioning and Related Anatomy. Elsevier, Pte Ltd. Inc.

[9] Moore KL, Persaud TVN. The Developing Human. Saunders Elsevier.

[10] StollerDW. MRI, Arthroscopy,and surgical anatomy of the joints. Lippincott Williams & Wilkins Inc.

[11] Agur AMR. Grant's Atlas of Anatomy. Lippincott Williams & Wilkins Inc.

[12] 王怀经. 局部解剖学. 高等教育出版社.

[13] 李瑞锡, 刘树伟. 局部解剖学. 人民卫生出版社.

[14] 徐国成, 韩秋生, 舒强, 等. 局部解剖学彩色图谱. 辽宁科学技术出版社.

[15] 舒强, 徐国成, 鹿晓理. 局部解剖学. 高等教育出版社.

[16] 郭光文, 王序. 人体解剖彩色图谱. 人民卫生出版社.

[17] 柏树令, 段坤昌, 陈金宝. 人体解剖学彩色图谱. 上海科学技术出版社.

[18] 段坤昌, 王振宇, 李庆生. 颅脑颈部应用解剖学彩色图谱. 辽宁科学技术出版社.

[19] 金连弘. 人体断面解剖学彩色图谱. 人民卫生出版社.

[20] 姜树学, 马述盛. 断面解剖与 MRI、CT、ECT 对照图谱. 辽宁科学技术出版社.

[21] 汪忠镐, 舒畅. 血管外科临床解剖学图谱. 山东科学技术出版社.

[22] 高士濂. 实用解剖图谱, 上肢分册. 上海科学技术出版社.

[23] 高士濂. 实用解剖图谱, 下肢分册. 上海科学技术出版社.

对提供本页书目的作者和出版社，在此一并表示衷心的感谢。